BLOOD INFECTIONS: SCIENTIFIC, CLINICAL AND PUBLIC HEALTH ASPECTS

BLOOD INFECTIONS: SCIENTIFIC, CLINICAL AND PUBLIC HEALTH ASPECTS

VIROJ WIWANITKIT

Nova Science Publishers, Inc.
New York

LIBRARY OF CONGRESS CATALOGING-IN-PUBLICATION DATA

Viroj Wiwanitkit.
Blood infections : scientific, clinical, and public health aspects / Viroj Wiwanitkit.
p. ; cm.
Includes bibliographical references and index.
ISBN-13: 978-1-60021-685-5 (hardcover)
ISBN-10: 1-60021-685-4 (hardcover)
1. Septicemia. 2. Bloodborne infections . 3. Tropical medicine. I. Title.
[DNLM: 1. Hematologic Diseases. 2. Infection. 3. Tropical Medicine--methods. WH 120 V819b 2007]
RC182.S4V57 2007
616.9'44--dc22

2007013512

Published by Nova Science Publishers, Inc. ✦ New York

CONTENTS

Chapter I

What Is "Blood Infection" and How Can It Occur?

The word "blood infection" means a common group of hematological and infectious disorders. Good examples of blood infections are malaria and babesiosis. Most blood infections are endemic in tropical countries and become important public health threaten for the developing countries. However, the blood infections can be seen in non tropical countries as well. There is still limited knowledge on this topic while the wider distribution of the disorder due to the globalization can be expected. Most practitioners should realize and urge to get the information on this topic.

Table 1. Important blood infections and the causative pathogens

Blood infections	Pathogens
1. malaria	*Plasmodium falciparum, Plasmodium vivax*
2. toxoplasmosis	*Toxoplasma gondii*
3. histoplasmosis	*Histoplasma capsulatum*
4. leishmaniasis	*Leishmania donovani*
5. babesiosis	*Babesia microti*

Similar to other types of infection, the blood infection has two important basic compartments: pathogen and host. Early views of pathogenesis and virulence were primarily pathogen centered and were based on the assumption that these characteristics were intrinsic properties of microorganisms, although it was recognized that pathogenesis was neither invariant nor absolute [1]. For host, the host defense mechanism is a basic response to the foreign invader. This defense mechanism can result in having or having not infection. However, new information about the attributes of microbes and their hosts resulted in the understanding that the host-pathogen interaction does not always result in disease [2]. External factors are also important determinants. According to the nature of the interaction various types of interrelations can be distinguished: (a) neutral relations (e.g. epiphytes), (b) mutualistic relations (fertilization, symbiosis), and (c) parasitic relations (incompatibility, the phytopathological host-parasite interactions) [3]. Pathogens can be defined as organisms out of place [3].

Such interrelations occurring on the cellular level include the problems of cell recognition, adherence of the cell surfaces to each other, and intercellular bridging [3]. The recently identified family of Toll-like receptors (TLRs) represents the major group of cellular signaling receptors for pathogens [4]. The discovery of genetic variations of these proteins caused by single nucleotide polymorphisms (SNPs) has led to first studies aimed at elucidating a potential link between genomic variation of the host and susceptibility to infections [4]. Interactions on the individual population and ecosystem levels can be reduced to aspects of the interactions, which involve mutual gene regulation [3]. If such a connection, a peak in a new host population followed by a peak in the pathogen population, is further substantiated for the pathogenic agents in endemic areas of the disease, it may lead to a better understanding of the role of the new host for the pathogen [5].

Mode of Transmission of Blood Infection

In natural, the general mode of transmission of blood infection is usually via vector. Such vectors can be mosquitoes, fly and etc. Malaria is the well-known example of mosquito-borne blood infection, which affects millions of world population annually. Leishmaniasis is a good example of fly-borne blood infection. Some blood infections can be occurred as food borne zoonoses such as toxoplasmosis. In some cases, transplacental transmission causing congenital blood infection such as congenital malaria and congenital toxoplasmosis can be seen. In additional to natural mode of transmission, blood and blood product transfusion becomes another important mode of transmission in the present era corresponding to the increasing number of transfusions.

1. Vector Borne Transmission

Vector borne infectious diseases are emerging or resurging as a result of changes in public health policy, insecticide and drug resistance, shift in emphasis from prevention to emergency response, demographic and societal changes, and genetic changes in pathogens [6]. Vector-borne transmission occurs when a living creature, because of its ecological relationship to others, acquires a pathogen from one living host and transmits it to another. Thus vector-borne transmission is a form of indirect horizontal transmission in which a biological intermediary, often an arthropod, carries a disease agent between animals.

A biological vector is a vector that supports replication of the pathogen. The disease agent and the biological vector are considered to have a long-standing ecological relationship. Biological vectors are usually persistently infected with the disease agent and may even be a required part of that organism's life cycle. The transmission depends upon the attributes and requirements of at least three different living organisms: the pathologic agent, either virus, protozoa, parasite or bacteria; the vector, which are commonly arthropods such as ticks or mosquitoes; and the human host [1 - 2] (figure 1.1). In addition, intermediary hosts such as domesticated and/or wild animals often serve as a reservoir for the pathogen until susceptible human populations are exposed [1 - 2]. Classification of vector borne disease can be based on the types of vectors. Of several vectors, mosquito becomes the most common vectors. Several diseases can be carried by mosquito vector such as dengue infection and malaria. Effective prevention strategies can reverse this trend. Research on vaccines, environmentally safe insecticides, alternative approaches to control, and training programs for health-care workers are needed [6].

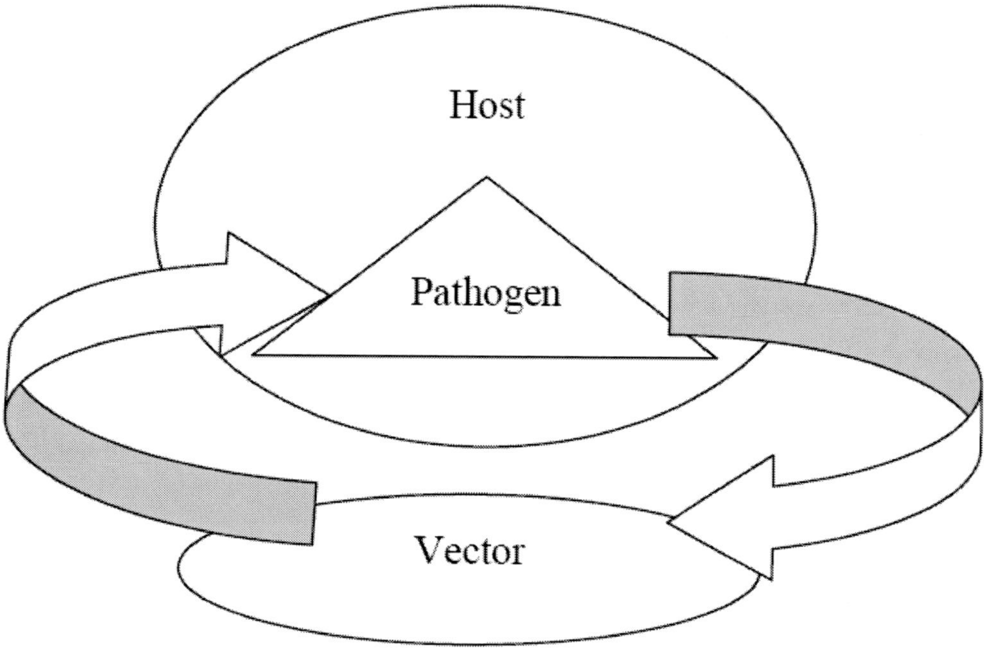

Figure 1.1. The composition of a vector borne transmission.

2. Food and Water Borne Zoonosis

Food and water borne zoonosis is another important mode of transmission of pathogen. Transmission usually starts with the passing of pathogens from the infected animal into the food or water and the human accidentally ingest or drink food or water with contaminants. The contaminated pathogens pass into the intestinal lumen and further cause infection in susceptible host. Transmission of disease can be expected if codes of good practice are not adhered to. However, the food and water borne zoonosis is the common mode of transmission for gastrointestinal infection not blood infection. Nevertheless, some specific food and water borne zoonosis especially for toxoplamosis is considered as important blood infection.

3. Transplacental Transmission

Vertical transmission is the transfer of a pathogen from a parent, usually the mother, to the offspring through reproduction. Basically, the transplacental transmission can be occurred if there is an infection within the mother. Usually, the mothers get infection during the pregnancy, especially in the third trimester adjunctive to the labor period. Infection in early infection rarely results in transplacental transmission and congenital infection since the affected fetus usually dies in utero and abortion is the result. An important considerable fact for the tranplacental transmission is that the pathogen has to pass across the placenta from mother to the fetus. The main determinants for this event are size of pathogen and placenta sieve pore size. The pathogen must have smaller size than the pore size [7]. However, some additional mechanism such as transformation of parasite shape and direct invasion into the tissue of placenta and cross to the fetus can also be seen.

4. Transmission via Blood and Blood Product Transfusion

Since blood transfusion is the insertion of the foreign blood into the patient, there is feasibility for passing of unwanted and undetected blood infection into the recipient. Therefore, blood screening for blood infection is necessary in blood bank. Luckily, over the past decades, the incidence of clinically significant transfusion-transmitted diseases has been dramatically reduced. These reductions have occurred because of a multifocal approach to the collection, processing, and release of blood and blood components [8]. Efforts to make blood transfusion as safe as possible have focused on making the blood in the bag as disease-free as possible [9]. The results have been dramatic, and the costs have been correspondingly high [9]. Although blood services will have to continue to deal with emerging pathogens, efforts to reduce the transfusion of infectious agents presently posing a risk will require high incremental costs and result in only improvements of a small magnitude [9].

5. Transmission via Organ Transplantation

Transplantation medicine is a new branch of medicine. Similar to blood transfusion, transplantation is insertion of new organs, which must contain blood, into the recipient. Therefore, transmission of blood infection can be expected. Malaria is a good example of blood infection with confirmative evidences for the transmission via organ transplantation.

6. Direct Contact and Air Borne Transmission

Neither direct contact nor air borne transmission is the mode of transmission for blood infection in general.

Where Does the Blood Infection Occur?

Generally, blood has two important parts: solid and liquid part. Solid part is the combination of blood cells and platelets while liquid part, known as serum, is the mixture of body fluid and chemicals. Blood infection can be seen in both cells and plasma. However, in terminology, blood infection usually deals with infection of cellular components.

1. Red Blood Cell

Red blood cell is an important target for many pathogens. Malaria is the good examples. Many pathogens invade into blood cell and cause infection. Microscopically, these pathogens can be seen as pathogenic inclusion bodies within red blood cell. Invading of red blood cell and intracellular infection usually end up with the breaking down or lysis of red blood cell, which usually causes severe clinical manifestations.

2. White Blood Cell

White blood cell can be another target for some pathogens. Those pathogens usually involve with the immune system. Both polymorphonuclear cell and mononuclear cell can be the target of pathogen invading. Examining of the buffy coat smear by microscopy can reveals the existence of pathogen within the cytoplasm of white blood cells, however, it is difficult to detect and diagnose.

3. Plasma

Some infections pose their specific clinical presentation as detection of pathogens within the serum of the patients. The examples of these infections are filariasis and relapsing fever. Generally, the microscopic examination can reveal the extracellular organism within the blood film of the patient.

Factor Contributing to Blood Infections

Similar to general disorders in medicine, two main factors contributing to the blood infection are inherited and non-inherited factors.

1. Inherited Factor

Host Susceptibility

Indeed, the inherited factor has been widely studied for its role in response to many blood infections, especially for the response to tropical blood infections. Of those infectious diseases, malaria has been the most widely investigated. Lell *et al* noted that red cell polymorphisms that confer resistance to severe disease are widespread in regions highly endemic for *Plasmodium falciparum* malaria [10]. Lell *et al* proposed that the different presentation of re-infections in severe versus mild cases probably reflected different susceptibility to malaria [10]. Stirnadel *et al* performed a study to investigate the effects of host polymorphisms on malaria morbidity and infection in Tanzania [11]. They found that there were no differences in malariametric indices between infants with the normal TNF alpha promoter gene and those who were heterozygous for this trait and the cases heterozygous for the sickle cell trait had significantly lower parasite densities, but similar prevalence, and MSP-2 infections compared to those with normal hemoglobin [11]. Conclusively, they proposed that the TNF alpha promotor polymorphism appeared not to have any protective effect on malaria in contrast to the sickle cell trait [11].

In hematology, it is widely accepted for the resistance of malaria in the patients with some hemoglobinopathies. The good example is the resistance to malaria in the patients with hemoglobin S or thalassemic disorders. Heterozygous thalassemia and sickle cell disease produce mild hematological symptoms but provide protection against malaria mortality and severe malaria symptoms [12]. Akide-Ndunge *et al* said that two explanations for resistance were considered in the literature - impaired growth of the parasite or enhanced removal by the host immune cells [12]. Haldane's prophetic statement: 'The corpuscles of the anemic heterozygotes are smaller than normal, and more resistant to hypotonic solutions. It is at least conceivable that they are also more resistant to attacks by the sporozoa which cause malaria." is fit for this phenomenon [12].

Susceptibility of Pathogens

In addition to the host susceptibility to the pathogen, the pathogen susceptibility to the anti-pathogen drug is also widely investigated. Le Bras and Durand mentioned that an established and strong drug pressure and a low antiparasitic immunity probably explained the multidrug-resistance encountered in forests of Southeast Asia and South America and frequent genetic recombinations in Plasmodium originate from a high level of malaria transmission, and falciparum chloroquine-resistant prevalence brought to stabilise at an equal level as chloroquine-sensitive malaria in Africa [13]. Finally Le Bras and Durand pointed that in vivo and in vitro tests were insufficient to give an accurate map of resistance and biochemical tools at a low cost were urgently needed for a prospective monitoring of resistance [13]. Filariasis is another infection that is studied for the genetic effect on drug resistance. A P-glycoprotein gene probe, used to analyze restriction fragment length polymorphisms between susceptible isolates and isolates resistant to either benzimidazole; levamisole and benzimidazole; or benzimidazole, ivermectin and closantel, was recently isolated from the human nematode parasite Onchocerca volvulus by Kwa *et al* [14]. In this work, no polymorphism could be correlated with any of the different resistances [14].

2. Non-Inhertied Factor

Sima Zue *et al* proposed that despite enormous progress in medical science, health care coverage in poor underdeveloped tropical countries remains incomplete, uncertain and minimal and the probability of death is high in these countries [15].

In addition, due to difficult field conditions and limited medical facilities in the tropical countries, care is often delayed [15]. As the results, most patients are admitted with advanced, complicated disease to facilities that are often poorly equipped, undersupplied and lacking in qualified personnel, basic medication [15]. These situations also the main problematic concerns for tropical blood infections as well.

Poverty

In the other word, the poverty leads to lack of opportunity to get good health and bring many health disorders especially tropical infections including tropicalblood infections. Recently, Pinikahana mentioned that poverty created preconditions for malaria and ways for its spread, thereby making it difficult to control malaria [16]. Pinikahana also proposed that research need to examine whether cultural beliefs and values or poverty prevent some people from not using bed nets or any other protective device [16].

Therefore, development based on economic growth, to conquer the poverty in the tropical countries in necessary and become the politic strategies for all developing countries. Development stands for an improved quality of life through gains in health, education, living standards, and higher income [17]. However, Brinkmann noted that although all indicators of development: GDP per capita, average life expectancy at birth, and per capita income had been rising in almost all countries, including the "developing" countries over the past decades, economic growth did not lead to the expected disappearance of infectious diseases [17]. Brinkmann also noted that the people who suffered from the adverse effects of economic growth were often different from those who benefit from it [17]. The process of urbanization could be described as one of the major global environmental changes directly affecting human health today and the populations particularly affected are in developing countries where rapid urban growth has been accompanied by massive urban poverty [18]. One of the adverse effects of adverse effects of development, the pollution has also been proposed as an important factor leading to the blood infections at present.

Poor Hygiene

As already mentioned the poor hygiene can become from the poverty. The underprivileged population in the tropics usually poses poor hygienic behaviors. Mata proposed that the physical environment in tropical and the socioeconomic characteristics of the population inhabiting such regions, favor maintenance and transmission of a variety of viruses, bacteria, and parasites that make agricultural progress and social development difficult [19]. Recently, Das *et al* performed epidemiological investigations in six tribal villages in Rajmahal range hill in south Bihar, India and they noted that poor socio-economic condition, lack of sense of hygiene worsened the situation in the presence of asymptomatic carriers [20].

Environmental Temperature and Humidity

Similar to other tropical diseases, the hot environmental temperature in the tropics helps transmit of many tropical infectious diseases. There are many researches on the effect of temperature on important vectors causing vector-borne blood infections. Recently, Bayoh and Lindsay examined how temperature influences the survival of larval stages (larvae and pupae) of *Anopheles gambiae* and subsequent adult production of this most efficient malaria vector. According to this study, larvae developed into adults at temperatures ranging from 16 to 34 degrees C [21]. Within the temperature range at which adults were produced, larval mortality was highest at the upper range 30-32 degrees C, with death (rather than adult emergence) representing over 70% of the terminal events [21]. These data provide fundamental information about *Anopheles gambiae* adult productivity at different temperatures, which may facilitate the construction of process-based models of malaria risk in Africa and the development of early warning systems for epidemics [22].

In addition to the temperature, humidity is another important factor affecting the spreading of the vector-borne infectious diseases. Humidity mainly affects the breeding of mosquitoes. It should be noted that the prevalence of mosquito-borne infectious diseases in the desert area is less common that of rain forest area.

Pollution

Exposures to environmental pollution remain a major source of health risk throughout the world, though risks are generally higher in developing countries, where poverty, lack of investment in modern technology and weak environmental legislation combine to cause high pollution levels [22]. Briggs noted that associations between environmental pollution and health outcome were, however, complex and often poorly characterized [22]. It should be noted that human health may not remain sustainable if damage to the global environment continues [23]. McMichael proposed a simple argument that "Earth is essentially a closed system; humans are proliferating and commandeering more surface area, food and energy; the resultant accumulation of waste gases, depletion of soil and water, and loss of biodiversity is starting to overload Earth's carrying capacity. There are limits in any closed system and our species is now pressing against some of them. These are new problems and we cannot be certain of the consequences for human health. A warmer world will probably have more frequent heatwaves, unstable weather, increased spread of mosquito-borne infectious diseases, and disruptions to agriculture." [23].

Presently, the change in climate is an important consideration point in world health. Epstein noted that Projections from computer models predict that global warming will expand the incidence and distribution of many serious medical disorders [24]. Global warming, aside from indirectly causing death by drowning or starvation, promotes by various means the emergence, resurgence, and spread of infectious diseases [24]. Among the greatest health concerns are diseases transmitted by vectors especially for malaria [24]. Such disorders are projected to become increasingly prevalent because their insect vectors are very sensitive to meteorological conditions [24]. In addition, floods and droughts resulting from global warming can each help trigger outbreaks by creating breeding grounds for insects whose desiccated eggs remain viable and hatch in still water [24].

Some Present Concerns on Blood Infections

1. Emerging Blood Infection in New Settings

The existence of blood infections in many non-tropical countries is considered an important public heath problem at present. These diseases are considered as an important emerging infectious problem in the new settings.

The possible factors contributing to the changing in the epidemiology of tropical blood infection from tropical to non tropical zone include the good transportation system, traveling and tourism, urbanization, mutation of the pathogens and the changing of environmental temperature (as previously mentioned for the "Global Warming").

2. Co-Occurrence of Blood Infections

The co-occurrence of blood infections can be seen and is usually a difficult- to-treat condition in medicine. A good example is a co-occurrence between falciparum and vivax malaria [25 - 26]. Recently Mason and McKenzie performed a mathematical model study and suggested several phenomena that might merit clinical attention, including the potential recrudescence of a long-standing, low-level *Plasmodium falciparum* infection following a *Plasmodium vivax* infection or relapse and the capacity of an existing *Plasmodium vivax* infection to reduce the peak parasitemia of a *Plasmodium falciparum* superinfection [27]. They also simulated the administration of antimalarial drugs, and illustrate some potential complications in treating mixed-species malaria infections and they found that when a mixed-species infection is misdiagnosed as a single-species *Plasmodium vivax* infection, treatment for *Plasmodium vivax* can lead to a surge in *Plasmodium falciparum* parasitemia [27].

3. Co-Manifestation with other Diseases

Sometimes blood infections can be seen accompanied with diseases of other systems. The good example is the occurrence of histoplasmosis in the patient with immunodeficiency system, which other infectious and non-infectious diseases can be detected in the same patients. It should be noted that the occurrence of white blood cell infection usually imply some degrees of impairment of immune system in the patients and the closed evaluation of the patients for other subverted diseases should be done.

REFERENCES

[1] Casadevall A, Pirofski LA. Host-pathogen interactions: redefining the basic concepts of virulence and pathogenicity. *Infect Immun.* 1999;67:3703-13.

[2] Casadevall A, Pirofski LA. Host-pathogen interactions: basic concepts of microbial commensalism, colonization, infection, and disease. *Infect Immun.* 2000;68:6511-8.

[3] Linskens HF. Host-pathogen interaction as a special case of interrelations between organisms. *European Journal of Plant Pathology.* 1968;74:1 – 8.

[4] Schumann RR. Host cell-pathogen interface: molecular mechanisms and genetics. *Vaccine.* 2004;22 Suppl 1:S21-4.

[5] Halpern M, Raats D, Lavion R, Mittler S. Dependent population dynamics between chironomids (nonbiting midges) and Vibrio cholerae. *FEMS Microbiol Ecol.* 2006;55:98-104.

[6] Gluber DJ. Resurgent vector-borne diseases as a global health problem. Available online at www.cdc.gov/ncidod/eid/vol4no3/gubler.htm

[7] Wiwanitkit V. HIV transmission from mother to child: an aspect on the placenta barrier at the nano-level. *Aust. N. Z. J. Obstet. Gynaecol.* 2005;45:539-40.

[8] Luban NL. Transfusion safety: Where are we today? *Ann. N. Y. Acad. Sci.* 2005;1054:325-41.

[9] Brooks JP. Reengineering transfusion and cellular therapy processes hospitalwide: ensuring the safe utilization of blood products. *Transfusion.* 2005;45(4 Suppl):159S-71S.

[10] Lell B, May J, Schmidt-Ott RJ, Lehman LG, Luckner D, Greve B, Matousek P, Schmid D, Herbich K, Mockenhaupt FP, Meyer CG, Bienzle U, Kremsner PG. The role of red blood cell polymorphisms in resistance and susceptibility to malaria. *Clin. Infect. Dis.* 1999; 28:794-9.

[11] Stirnadel HA, Stockle M, Felger I, Smith T, Tanner M, Beck HP. Malaria infection and morbidity in infants in relation to genetic polymorphisms in Tanzania. *Trop. Med. Int. Health.* 1994; 4:187-93.

[12] Akide-Ndunge OB, Ayi K, Arese P. The Haldane malaria hypothesis: facts, artifacts, and a prophecy. *Redox. Rep.* 2003; 8: 311-6.

[13] Le Bras J, Durand R. Molecular aspects of chloroquine and antifols resistance in P. falciparum. *Ann. Pharm. Fr.* 2001; 59: 85-92.

[14] Kwa MS, Okoli MN, Schulz-Key H, Okongkwo PO, Roos MH. Use of P-glycoprotein gene probes to investigate anthelmintic resistance in Haemonchus contortus and comparison with Onchocerca volvulus. *Int. J. Parasitol.* 1998; 28: 1235-40.

[15] Sima Zue A, Chani M, Ngaka Nsafu D, Carpentier JP. Does tropical environment influence morbidity and mortality? *Med. Trop.* (Mars). 2002; 62: 256-9.

[16] Pinikahana J. Socio-cultural factors associated with malaria transmission: a review. *Indian J. Malariol.* 1992;29:121-6.

[17] Brinkmann UK. Economic development and tropical disease. *Ann. N. Y. Acad. Sci.* 1994; 740: 303-11.

[18] Stephens C. The urban environment, poverty and health in developing countries. *Health Policy Plan.* 1995; 10:109-21.

[19] Mata LJ. The environment of the malnourished child. *Basic Life Sci.* 1976; 7: 45-66.

[20] Das NG, Bhuyan M, Das SC. Entomological and epidemiological studies on malaria in Rajmahal range, Bihar. *Indian J. Malariol.* 2000; 37: 88-96.

[21] Bayoh MN, Lindsay SW. Temperature-related duration of aquatic stages of the Afrotropical malaria vector mosquito Anopheles gambiae in the laboratory. *Med. Vet. Entomol.* 2004; 18: 174-9.

[22] Briggs D. Environmental pollution and the global burden of disease. *Br. Med. Bull.* 2003; 68: 1-24.

[23] McMichael AJ. Global environmental change and human health: new challenges to scientist and policy-maker. *J. Public Health Policy.* 1994; 15: 407-19.

[24] Epstein PR. Is global warming harmful to health? *Sci. Am.* 2000; 283: 50-7.

[25] Snounou G, White NJ. The co-existence of Plasmodium: sidelights from falciparum and vivax malaria in Thailand. *Trends Parasitol.* 2004; 20: 333-9.

[26] Mayxay M, Pukrittayakamee S, Newton PN, White NJ. Mixed-species malaria infections in humans. *Trends Parasitol.* 2004; 20: 233-40.

[27] Mason DP, McKenzie FE. Blood-stage dynamics and clinical implications of mixed Plasmodium vivax-Plasmodium falciparum infections. *Am. J. Trop. Med. Hyg.* 1999; 61: 367-74.

Chapter II

MALARIA

INTRODUCTION TO MALARIA

Malaria is a mosquito-borne parasitic infection. It can be said that malaria is a very important tropical mosquito-borne infectious disease. Malaria is caused by protozoan parasites of the genus Plasmodium. Four species of *Plasmodium*, *Plasmodium falciparum*, *Plasmodium vivax*, *Plasmodium ovale* and *Plasmodium malariae* can produce the human disease in its various forms. In addition, there are other species, which infected animal such as *Plasmodium gallinaceum*. In human, malaria is an important is a potentially deadly mosquito-borne disease characterized by cyclical bouts of fever with muscle stiffness, shaking and sweating in the tropical countries [1 – 2]. Despite encouraging trends in dramatically reducing malaria, the rates of disease may be re-emerging in many tropical and non-tropical countries as evidence from an increased annual parasite index. Despite decades of control success and a competent network of countrywide health infrastructure, malaria remains an important health threat in rural communities [3]. Members of 5 anopheline species complexes, *Anopheles dirus*, *Anopheles minimus*, *Anopheles sandicus*, *Anopheles aconitus* and *Anopheles manculatus*, considered to be primary malaria vectors, are also common in many tropical countries.

Although there have been many efforts for decades to produce a vaccine to combat this infection, few have been able to meet the challenges posed by the unusual interplay between this virus and its human host. According to the globalization at present, the malaria becomes an emerging infectious problem not only to the tropical but also to the non-tropical countries. Angell and Cetron said that high-risk illnesses in travelers included childhood vaccine-preventable illnesses, hepatitis A and B, tuberculosis, malaria, and typhoid fever [4]. In addition, the problem of drug resistant malaria is increase at present. Wernsdorfer and Wernsdorfer noted that drug resistance of malaria was the most formidable obstacle in the fight against the disease since it jeopardized the most elementary objective of malaria control, namely the elimination of mortality and the reduction of suffering from malaria [5]. The knowledge on the malaria is, therefore, an interesting topic for general practitioners all over the world.

Worldwide Epidemiology of Malaria

Malarial infections are one of the most important mosquito-borne diseases in the world. With an annual incidence of 300-500 million clinically manifest cases and a death toll of 1.1-2.7 million, malaria is still one of the most important communicable diseases [5]. Wernsdorfer and Wernsdorfer said that about 40% of the world's populations live in areas where malaria is endemic, as against 80% in 1950 [5]. They also noted that although this reflected considerable impact of intensive malaria control, especially between 1950 and 1970, the disease continued to affect large populations in all parts of the tropics and subtropics, and remained most deeply rooted in tropical Africa, the region with 90% of the global malaria incidence [5]. Summaries on some recent reports on the epidemiology of malaria in several regions of the world are hereby presented.

A. Asia

Tropical Asia is the well-known endemic area of malaria. In Southeast Asia, the high prevalence of malaria is mentioned. Hay *et al* noted that stratifying the malaria extent by endemically class and examining regional differences highlighted that nearly 1 billion people are exposed to hypoendemic and mesoendemic malaria in Southeast Asia [6]. In Thailand, noted that rubber tapers in southern region had the highest malaria incidence rate (46.29%) [7]. Similar high prevalence among the hill tribes in the northern region is also noted [8]. Of interest, Wiwanitkit recently reported for the impact of migration of the populations from Myanmar to Thailand on the prevalence of malaria in a Thai-Myanmar border area namely Bangsaparn [9]. Chaveepojnkamjorn and Pichainarong also reported a similar finding in another Thai-Myanmar border area namely [10]. They noted that *Plasmodium falciparum* was the major type of the malaria (60.8%) [10]. A cross-sectional survey of the malaria prevalence among mobile Cambodians in Aranyaprathet, at the Thai-Cambodia border, was conducted in November 2000 [11]. According to this study, the overall prevalence rate was 2.4%, with 93.75% of the infections being due to Plasmodium vivax and 6.25% due to *Plasmodium falciparum* [11]. Kitvatanachai *et al* said that factors associated with malaria infection included being male, being in the 10-59 year age group, having a lower level of education and frequent trans-border crossing [11].

In other Indochina countries, the high prevalence of malaria is noted. Singhasivanon said that there was great diversity in disease patterns in the Indochina countries and at subnational administrative unit area level in each country, so that in the region as a whole there was marked asymmetry in disease distribution, with many areas of high endemicity [12]. Singhasivanon noted that focal expansion of maps in the vicinity of international border areas delineated the differential trans-border malaria distribution that presented a challenge for disease control [12]. Singhasivanon also noted that the malaria pattern was also depicted in environmental context against regional elevation and forest cover profiles, which affected mosquito breeding site distribution and agricultural activity [12]. Concerning Cambodia, Denis and Meek noted that there were around half a million cases of malaria with 5-10,000 deaths per year [13]. They said that malaria control was hampered In Cambodia by multiple drug resistance of *Plasmodium falciparum*, inaccessibility to the major vector, poor security in most malarious areas, and lack of resources [13]. Concerning Laos, Pholsena said that malaria was endemic in all 17 provinces of Laos and transmission was perennial with a "seasonal peak" coinciding with the rainy season [14]. Pholsena noted that the vectors *Anopheles minimus* and *Anopheles balabacensis* in Laos remained susceptible to insecticide and multidrug resistance was not a problem [14]. Concerning Vietnam, malaria is still the most common infectious cause of mortality and morbidity in Vietnam as it is in many developing countries in the tropic [15]. Drug resistance of malaria is an important problem [15].

In Malaysia, malaria is still prevalent. Rahman *et al* noted that malaria was still one of the most important diseases in Malaysia [16]. They said that this was because Malaysia was located within the equatorial zone with high temperatures and humidities, usually important for the transmission of malaria [16]. They mentioned that number of malarial cases was estimated to be around 300,000 before the launching of the Malaria Eradication Program (MEP) [16]. Presently, due to MEP, the prevalence of malaria in Malaysia decreases [16]. Considering Indonesia, Albani noted that malaria was the big infectious problem in the major island group of Java-Bali and the remainder of the archipelago called the Outer Islands [17]. Arbani noted that drug-resistant malaria, forest-related malaria, lack of personnel, supervision and coordination, inadequate resources, and community participation were among the main issues confronting the national malaria control program of Indonesia [17].

In South Asia, malaria endemic countries in the region include Bangladesh, Bhutan, India, Maldives, Nepal and Sri Lanka [7]. In India, malaria is prevalent in the northern region. Dev *et al* said that malaria control itself had amounted to be a challenge, and was detrimental to the all round development of the northeastern region of India [18]. They noted that *Plasmodium falciparum* was the predominant parasite species and was solely responsible for increased morbidity and mortality [18]. They proposed that this region contributed bulk of *Plasmodium falciparum* cases for the rest of India, and its proportions were increasing [18]. In Sri Lanka, malaria is a common infectious disease. Disease surveillance and control are practiced as public health strategies in Sri Lanka [19 – 20]. Considering Bangladesh, Birley said that malaria is historically associated with reduced flooding and embankment construction in the flood plains of Bengal [21]. Birley noted that the reduction in health risk could be attributed to the intensification of land use and human population density [21]. Birley also proposed that although there were many mosquito species, the abundance of the former malaria vector appeared to have declined as environmental change removed its breeding sites [21].

Concerning the Middle East, malaria is not endemic. One of the possible factors might be due to the low humidity in this area. However, the imported cases from the nearby area especially South Asia and Africa are reported. Ismaeel *et al* said that malaria was eradicated in Bahrain for many decades ago, however, because of a large immigrant population, cases of imported malaria continued to be seen [22]. However, Ismaeel *et al* noted that there was a consistent decline in the number of imported malaria cases in Bahrain From 1992 to 2001 and there were no cases of locally acquired malaria during this period [22]. They also noted that low level of vector breeding spots with Anopheles mosquito larvae suggests that the potential for reemergence of local transmission remains low [22]. The similar decrease of malarial prevalence trend was also reported in Oman [23].

In East Asia, there are also the reported cases of malaria in these temperate countries. In China, the high prevalence of malaria is mentioned in the lowest region, namely Yunan [24].

The high prevalence of malarial infection is believed to be due to the transmission form the north of Southeast Asia region. Several programs in the control of malaria in Yunan Province are launched [24 – 25]. In Japan, Malaria has been successfully eradicated since 1961 in Japan and now only imported malaria cases are encountered [26]. However, Kano and Kimura noted that as the number of Japanese people who were going abroad and also the number of foreigners who were visiting Japan increases, so did the chance for Japanese doctors to see imported malaria or transfusion-transmitted malaria cases [26]. Concerning the imported malarial patients in Japan, about 45% of patients are *Plasmodium falciparum* and another 45% *Plasmodium vivax* infections [26]. Kano and Kimura said that the former species was likely to be seen in travelers coming back from African countries and the latter was mainly from Asian countries [26]. They proposed that the important issue was that patients in Japan had not been diagnosed promptly nor treated properly because doctors in Japan are no longer familiar with tropical medicine [26].

B. Africa

Very high prevalence of malaria is documented in Africa. At present, malaria affects 300-500 million people and causes about 1 million deaths, primarily in Africa [27]. Le Mire *et al* said that 80 % of malaria cases occurred in sub-Saharan Africa [28]. Snow *et al* noted that the great burden of malaria in Africa included chronic anemia, low birth weight, and enhancement of the severity of other childhood diseases [29]. Worrall *et al* estimated that in Africa, there were more than 12 million malaria episodes and 155,000-310,000 malaria deaths per year attributable to epidemics if control options were not implemented or well timed, which was equivalent to some 4% of estimated annual malaria cases worldwide and 12-25% of estimated annual worldwide malaria deaths, including up to 50% of the estimated annual worldwide malaria mortality in persons above 15 years of age [30]. In addition, Keiser *et al* recently estimated for an annual incidence of 24.8-103.2 million cases of clinical malaria attacks among urban dwellers in Africa [31]. They also noted that malaria not only remains a leading cause of morbidity and mortality, but it also impeded socioeconomic development, particularly in sub-Saharan Africa [31].

There are many interesting reports on the epidemiology of malaria in Africa. Some are quoted here. In Kenya and Uganda, malaria epidemics have long been known to recur in the African highland [32]. Efforts to develop systems of early warning and detection for epidemics are outlined here with special emphasis on the Highland Malaria Project (HIMAL) [32]. John *et al* recently studied the risk of *Plasmodium falciparum* infection during a malaria epidemic in highland Kenya, 1997 [33]. They concluded that the observed pattern was in contrast with the age-related protection from infection reported in areas of stable, intense transmission, and demonstrated that during malaria epidemics, both children and adults in highland areas of Kenya were at high risk of infection [33]. In Tanzania, Lusingu *et al* said that young children living in the high transmission village carried a very high anemia burden, which could be attributed to malaria [34]. They noted that overall incidence of febrile malaria was also highest in the high transmission village particularly among those under five years of age [34]. Based on these data, Lusingu *et al* suggested that in rolling back malaria, available resources in prevention programs should primarily be focused on young children, particularly those residing in areas of high malaria transmission [34].

C. North America

North America is not considered as an endemic area of malaria; however, malaria became an important imported emerging infection in recent few years. Within the last decade witnessed unprecedented global malarial epidemic activity in the American hemisphere. The globalization and easily accessible air transportation are believed to be the key factors in this finding. DeHart said that vectors for yellow fever, malaria, and dengue had been identified on aircraft and should be considered as an important health issue of air travel [35]. Newman *et al* said that nearly 1500 malaria cases occur each year in the United States; most were among U.S. travelers [36].

D. Latin America and South America

There are many recent reports on the epidemiology of malaria from Latin America and South America. During the last years, malaria had a significant increase in Latin America, emerging again as one critical health problem in the Region of the Americas [37]. Dourado *et al* said that falciparum malaria had become a major problem to health planning in Latin America, particularly because widespread drug-resistant strains of *Plasmodium falciparum* had been observed [38]. Castillo-Salgado said that more than 1.04 million new cases were reported in 1990 and this resurgence of malaria needed a comprehensive strategy for its prevention and control [37]. Concerning French Guiana, Carme noted that malaria was the most prevalent infection [39]. Carme said that the most common species was *Plasmodium falciparum* which was responsible for three quarters of all bouts of malaria while *Plasmodium vivax* was mostly present in endemic areas inhabited by Amerindian communities [39]. In addition, Carme noted that *Plasmodium malariae* was rarer [39]. Concerning Brazil, Singer and de Castro showed that land use patterns, linked to social organization of the community and the structure of the physical environment, played a key role in promoting malaria transmission [40]. In addition, Singer and de Castro also noted that the location of each occupied area was itself an important determinant of the pattern of malaria risk [40]. Based on lessons learned from spatial and temporal characterization of malaria risk, they proposed policies for malaria mitigation in the Brazilian Amazon [40]. Nevertheless, Bastos *et al* noted that new outbreaks of cases of HIV and malaria were likely to occur among Brazilian injecting drug users (IDUs), and might conceivably contribute to the development of treatment-resistant strains of malaria in this population [41]. They proposed that health professionals should be alert to this possibility, which could also eventually occur in IDU networks in developed countries [41].

E. Europe

Similar to North America, malaria has been imported into Europe for few years. Castela *et al* said that imported pediatric malaria is not rare in France and only the improvement of prophylaxis could decrease the incidence of malaria in France [42]. Ladhani *et al* studied the imported malarial cases in UK and found that the majority of children with malaria in this study were UK-born, school age, of Black African ethnicity and were visiting family in

Africa, often with other family members [43]. They said that most children had low level parasitemia and uncomplicated malaria, and the patients responded rapidly to antimalarial treatment [43].

F. Australia

Malaria is considered as an important emerging infection in Australia. Imported cases of malarial infections are reported. Generally, three elements must be present for endemic malaria: infected humans, susceptible mosquitoes and a suitable climate [44]. Walker noted that all these three occur in parts of Australia and yet this country had always been a region of marginal malaria endemicity [44]. Historically, with the exception of a large epidemic in Cairns during the Second World War, most outbreaks have occurred in small, isolated populations of the Northern Territory and the last epidemic was at the Roper River Mission in the Northern Territory in 1962 [44]. The malaria in the north of Australia is believed to be transmitted from the southernmost part of Southeast Asia. Australia was declared to be free of endemic malaria in 1983, only sporadic cases of local transmission have been reported [44]. However, the number of reported malaria cases is increasing each year with several deaths reported recently [45]. Walker noted that it was stressed that climate change in only one component in a complex epidemiological setting, and that other aspects such as human activity were probably more important [44]. In addition, with global warming, malarial infection may become more common and more widespread within Australia [46].

VECTOR AND TRANSMISSION

Malaria is an important tropical protozoa infectious disease. The mosquito vector is *Anopheles* spp. Like all other mosquitoes, the anophelines breed in water, and each species having its preferred breeding grounds, feeding patterns and resting place [47]. Their sensitivity to insecticides is also highly variable [47]. Concerning the life cycle, Plasmodium develops in the gut of the mosquito and is passed on in the saliva of an infected insect each time it takes a new blood meal [47]. The parasites are then carried by the blood in the victim's liver where they invade the cells and multiply [47] (table 1). After 9-16 days they return to the blood and penetrate the red cells, where they multiply again, progressively breaking down the red cells [47].

The bioecological parameters, which were of special importance in the epidemiology of malaria, include three levels: the nature of mosquito-man contacts, the susceptibility of the mosquito to the pathogen and multiplication of the latter, and the transmission. Hurd and Carter suggested that programmed cell death occurred during the early stages of the development of the malaria parasite in its vector [48]. Hurd and Carter noted that malaria infection induced apoptosis in the cells of two mosquito tissues, the midgut and the follicular epithelium [48]. They noted that putative signal molecules that might induce parasite and vector apoptosis included nitric oxide, reactive nitrogen intermediates, oxygen radicals and endocrine balance [48]. Finally, they concluded that programmed cell death might play a critical role in regulation of infection by the parasite and the host, and contributed to the success or not of parasite establishment and host survival.

Table 1. Characteristics of pre-erythrocyte and erythrocyte stages of different malaria species

Type of malaria	pre-erythrocyte stage		Erythrocyte Stage	
	Period (day)	Number of merozoite	Period (day)	Number of merozoite
Vivax	7 – 8	10,000	5 – 6	12
Falciparum	5 – 7	30,000	8 – 16	16
Ovale	8 – 9	15,000	5- 10	8
Malariae	11 – 15	15,000	5 – 23	8

In addition to vector transmission, other modes of transmission for malarial infection are also documented. Some pregnant women may also be susceptible to dengue and if they experience malaria, the vertical transmission of the plasmodium protozoa to their babies can be expected. The intrapartum malaria is an interesting tropical intrapartum infection. There are some previous reports on this infection. In areas of stable endemicity, the main consequences are maternal anemia and intra-uterine growth retardation resulting in low birthweight (LBW) particularly after first pregnancy [49]. In addition, recent studies have demonstrated that frequency and severity of placental malaria are greater in pregnant women with concurrent HIV infection [49]. The intrapartum malaria can bring several intrapartum complications, of which cerebral malaria is the most serious form [49 – 50]. Okoko et al proposed that the significantly higher risk of maternal malaria and consequences in primigravidae compared with multigravidae suggested that there were more to mere immunosuppression in pregnancy [50]. They noted that malaria infection of placenta caused a shift from Th2 to Th1 cytokine profile that might be detrimental to pregnancy [50]. They also proposed that increased susceptibility in the first pregnancy could be explained by the absence of anti-adhesion antibody in the primigravida that was being exposed for the first time to a different strain of malaria parasite sub-population that adhere exclusively to chondroitin sulfate A and hyaluronic acid (HA) in the placenta [50]. Vertical transmission due to intrapartum malaria was mentioned. In congenital anemia, affected children are usually presented with severe anemia and hepatosplenomegaly [51]. Marques *et al* said that despite congenital malaria was being considered a rare event it was a preventable disease and these cases should draw attention to the importance of adequate treatment during pregnancy [51]. Ahmed *et al* noted that the diagnosis of congenital malaria should be considered in infants with suspected congenital infection who were born to mothers with a history of living in or travel to endemic areas [52].

In additional to vertical transmission, malaria due to blood transfusion is also mentioned [53 – 54]. Dodd said that of greatest concern among several parasites known to transmit by blood transfusion are malaria [53]. Dodd noted that malaria might be imported into non-endemic areas as a result of population movements and in some cases, the natural range of the parasite was increasing as a result of environmental change [53].Screening for malaria in donated blood is recommended in the endemic areas of malarial infection [55].

Genetic and Molecular Biology of Malaria

Genetic is one of important intrinsic factors and the mechanisms controlling the ability of vectors to transmit pathogen [56]. In addition to the genetic pattern in vector, the effect of genetic polymorphism in human in susceptibility and resistance of disease is proposed. May and Horstmann said that certain human genetic variants occurred only in areas endemic for malaria [57]. May and Horstmann noted that these variants protected against fatal malaria complications and cause inhibition of growth or development of malaria parasites in vitro [57]. Among these are the hemoglobins (Hb) S and C, alpha-thalassaemias, glucose-6-phosphate dehydrogenase deficiency, as well as a deletion in the erythrocyte band 3 protein [57]. Clegg and Weatherall said that the thalassemia was believed to provide protection against malaria, as a natural selection process selection to sickle cell, and it is thought that, in malarial regions of the world, natural selection had been responsible for elevating and maintaining their gene frequencies [58]. They mentioned that population and molecular genetic analysis of thalassemia variants, and microepidemiological studies of the relationship between alpha-thalassemia and malaria in the southwest Pacific, had provided unequivocal evidence for protection [58]. In addition, some of this protection appeared to derive from enhanced susceptibility in very young thalassemic children to both *Plasmodium falciparum* and, especially, *Plasmodium vivax*, and this early exposure appeared to provide the basis for better protection in later life [58]. Hb S occurs in high frequency in Africa where previously exposed to falciparum malaria [59]. Heterozygosity for the mutant sickle hemoglobin confers protection from severe *Plasmodium falciparum* infection [60]. Hebbel said that that this protection derived from the instability of sickle hemoglobin, which clustered red cell membrane protein band 3 and triggered accelerated removal by phagocytic cells [60]. Evidence for similar protective effects has been obtained for HbD and HbE, glycophorins A and C as well as for a number of immunologically relevant molecules such as human leukocyte antigens, tumor-necrosis-factor a and the inducible nitric oxide synthase [57]. Chotivanich *et al* said that HbAE erythrocytes have an unidentified membrane abnormality that renders the majority of the RBC population relatively resistant to invasion by *Plasmodium falciparum* [61]. Chotivanich *et al* said that this would not protect from uncomplicated malaria infections but would prevent the development of heavy parasite burdens and was consistent with the "Haldane" hypothesis of heterozygote protection against severe malaria for hemoglobin E [61]. Wiwanitkit also noted that the predilection occurrence of this Hb Tak in the northern region of Thailand might reflect to the natural selection process to response to the local biological hazard especially malaria [62]. These protective genetic variants indicate that malaria in endemic areas has caused a substantial selection of the human genome [57].

Presently, there are many studied about the role of the vector genetic in the diffusion of malaria. Conclusively, population genetic studies of vectors are essential for (a) the determination of their taxonomic status and consequently the definition of their vectorial role in the transmission of pathogenic agents; (b) the evaluation of the species genetic variability and the estimation of their capacities of adaptation to selection pressure; (c) an estimation of gene flow among populations in order to evaluate their degree of isolation and gene circulation, especially resistance genes [63].

Pathophysiology and Clinical Manifestation

A. Pathophysiology of Malaria

There are many studies on the pathophysiology of malaria. There is now wide acceptance of the concept that the similarity between many acute infectious diseases be they viral, bacterial, or parasitic in origin, is caused by the overproduction of inflammatory cytokines initiated when the organism interacts with the innate immune system [64]. Many established proinflammatory mediators, such as tumor necrosis factor (TNF), interleukin-1, and lymphotoxin, the roles of nitric oxide and carbon monoxide, which are chiefly inhibitory, are discussed for its role in pathogenesis of malaria [64]. Clark *et al* also proposed for the potential roles of two more recently recognized contributors, overactivity of the enzyme poly(ADP-ribose) polymerase 1 (PARP-1) and the escape of high-mobility-group box 1 (HMGB1) protein from its normal location into the circulation [64]. In severe malarial cases, especially for those with the two major syndromes of cerebral malaria and severe malaria anemia, more complex pathogenesis is mentioned [65]. As previously mentioned, the occurrence of severe malaria is determined by both parasite and human host factors [66]. Maitland and Marsh said that it had become apparent that death from severe malaria might arise from a wider spectrum of pathophysiological disorders with many features in common with the derangements seen in sepsis syndrome [65]. They noted that amongst these derangements acidosis had emerged as a central feature of severe malaria and the major predictor of a fatal outcome [65].

At molecular level, Rasti *et al* said that more than 50% of *Plasmodium* spp genes were transcribed constitutively in all the developmental stages of parasite life cycle and functional disruption of these genes might have implications for parasite growth and development [66]. They noted that available microarray data indicate that *Plasmodium falciparum* preferentially expresses rif and stevor gene families at gametocyte and sporozoite stages while var genes were predominantly expressed at the erythrocytic stage [66]. At cellular level, Lang *et al* noted that infection of erythrocytes by the malaria pathogen *Plasmodium falciparum* led to activation of several distinct anion channels and a non-selective, Ca2+-permeable cation channel, which were presumably activated by the oxidative stress generated by the pathogen [67]. They proposed that activation of the non-selective cation channel allowed entry of Ca2+ and Na+, both of which were required for intracellular growth of the pathogen then the entry of Ca2+ stimulated an intraerythrocytic scramblase that facilitated bi-directional phospholipid migration across the bilayer, resulting in breakdown of the phosphatidylserine asymmetry of the cell membrane [67]. They also noted that the exposure of phosphatidylserine at the outer surface of the cell membrane was presumably followed by binding to phosphatidylserine receptors on macrophages and subsequent phagocytosis of the affected erythrocyte and the lysosomal degradation might eventually eliminate the pathogen [67]. Rasti *et al* noted that sequestration and antigenic variation are two of the evasion mechanisms utilized by *Plasmodium falciparum* in order to escape the human host defenses [66]. Lang *et al* concluded that the channel might play a dual role in pathogen survival and absence of the channels was not compatible with pathogen growth, enhanced channel activity accelerates erythrocyte apoptosis that might represent a host defense mechanism serving to eliminate infected erythrocytes [67].

B. Clinical Manifestation of Malaria

Malaria is a common tropical disease with the mosquito as the vector. It is the most important parasitic disease of people, affecting over 200 million people and causing more than one million deaths each year. Humans are infected when a female anopheles mosquito injects a small, mobile form of the parasite, called a sporozoite, into the blood while having a meal then these sporozoites are carried to the liver, where they reproduce [8, 47]. By this process a single sporozoite eventually produces several thousand of what are called daughter merozoites, which discharge from burst liver cells into the blood and it is at this stage that the symptoms is first noticed [8, 47]. Once they are in the blood stream, the merozoites enter the red blood cells therefore the parasite can then be seen in red blood cells when they are examined under the microscope [8]. Within the red blood cell further reproduction takes place and between six and 24 daughter merozoites are released [8, 47]. Each of these is capable of invading a new red cell, and so the cycle is repeated [68].

Symptoms of malaria generally take around six days to appear after infection [8]. Wide range of malarial symptoms is described [8]. Most symptoms are very vague and non-specific [8]. Generally, malaria can be presented as asymptomatic case or mild symptomatic case, also progress rapidly to coma and death in the nonimmune patient [8]. Some patients complain for a headache, fatigue and muscleache [8]. High fever is common; however, these symptoms are similar to a viral illness and can be mistaken for flu [8]. Some people presented with, chest pain, abdominal pain, joint pains and diarrhea which suggest something other than a viral illness [8]. Murphy and Oldfield said that the classical malarial symptoms in which fever spikes, chills and extreme shakings were the most common clinical manifestation of malaira [69]. According to a recent study of Suyaphan *et al* in Thailand, the most common symptom was fever (96.8 %), following by chill (60.6 %) and headache (28.7 %) [8]. The result from this study confirmed the classical presentation of malaria as fever with chill [8]. Of interest, Suyaphan *et al* said that most of the patient usually presented with more than one symptom and some unusual presentations as petichiae, abnormal menstruation and jaundice were reported in this study [8].

Concerning the laboratory abnormality in malaria, aberration of hematological laboratory parameters is common. Presentation of inclusions as malarial parasite (figure 1) or malarial pigment is the key for diagnosis of malarial infection. Concerning the three series of blood cells, all are affected by malarial infection. Considering red blood cell, anemia, as a resulted from malarial infection, is widely mentioned. Severe and refractory anemia lead to hypoxia and cardiac decompensation in malarial patients [70]. Those fatal malaria are common for falciparum malaria. Several mechanisms have been proposed to play a role in the pathogenesis of malarial anemia, such as erythrocyte lysis and phagocytosis, and sequestration of parasitized red blood cells [70]. Concerning erythrocyte lysis, it is believed to due to several cytokine productions especially TNF [71]. Waitumbi *et al* looked for changes in the red cell surfaces of children with severe malarial anemia that could explain this accelerated destruction and they found that red cells from patients with severe anemia were more susceptible to phagocytosis and also showed increased surface IgG and deficiencies in CR1 and CD55 compared with controls [72]. In addition, red cell surface CD59 was elevated in cases of severe anemia compared with asymptomatic controls but not as compared with symptomatic controls [72]. Waitumbi *et al* concluded that the surface of red cells of children with severe *Plasmodium falciparum* anemia was modified by the deposition of IgG and alterations in the levels of complement regulatory proteins and these changes could contribute to the accelerated destruction of red cells in these patients by mechanisms such as phagocytosis or complement-mediated lysis [72]. Concerning microvascular sequestration of parasitized red blood cells, Weatherall *et al* said that after an acute malarial infection there was a steady fall in the hemoglobin level with an inappropriate reticulocyte response [73]. They proposed that this form of anemia might result from a combination of acute sequestration of iron in the reticuloendothelial system associated with a shortened red cell survival [73]. In addition, Davis *et al* studied the mathematical model of the microvascular sequestration phenomenon and found the mean fall in hematocrit over 84 hours in the patients conformed to a three-term equation [74]. Concerning the autoimmune hemolytic anemia, this phenomenon is very rare in malaria and not proposed as a common mechanism for malarial anemia [70].

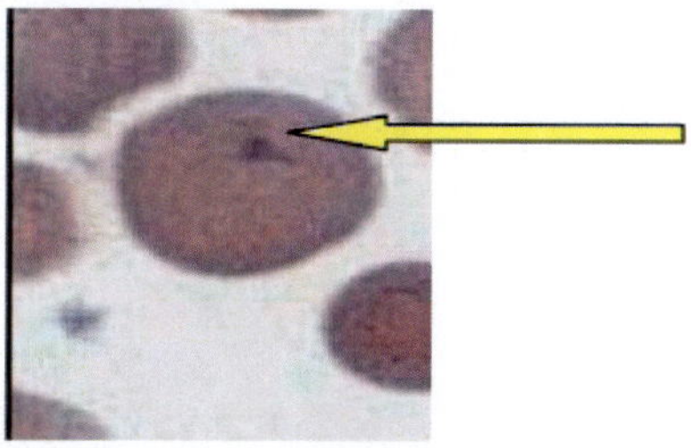

* Wright stain, X 1,000, malarial parasite is indicated by the yellow arrow as a blue inclusion.

Figure 1. Malarial parasite in red blood cell.

Thrombocytopenia and hypofibrinogenemia are the two most common hemostatic defects. Malaria can cause infection-induced thrombocytopenia [75]. Recently, Wiwanitkit and Suyaphan reported a high prevalence of thrombocytopenia among the patients infected with vivax malaria [76]. Mohanty *et al* found an inverse relationship between the platelet count and platelet antibody levels in serum supporting the view that thrombocytopenia in malaria might be partly immune-mediated [77]. They said that platelet aggregation responsed to agonists such as ADP, adrenaline, collagen and ristocetin revealed hyperactivity [77]. Mohanty *et al* also proposed that ultrastructural study of unstimulated platelets from patients revealed several changes such as centralization of dense granules, glycogen depletion, and formation of pseudopods and microaggregates, indicating in vivo activation of the platelets, which may also lead to thrombocytopenia [77]. In addition, Abdalla said that megakaryocytes were found to be increased in number in patients with acute malaria; a proportion of these cells had rounded nuclei, probably indicating accelerated platelet turnover [78].

As previously mentioned, the leukocyte disorder in the patients with malaria is mentioned. Abdalla said that lymphocytosis in the bone marrow and reactive lymphocytes, monocytosis and mild neutrophilia in the peripheral blood could be seen in acute malaria [78]. Abdalla also noted that giant metamyelocytes were also commonly seen in bone marrow of patients but were thought to be part of dysmyelopoiesis and not due to vitamin B12 or folate deficiency [78]. In addition, Abdalla mentioned that phagocytosis of erythrocytes, parasitized cells and nucleated cells was more commonly seen in macrophages in acute malaria, while phagocytosis of small particles such as merozoites was observed in neutrophils [78].

In additional to hematological manifestation, the other uncommon clinical presentations of malaria are also documented. Hepatic manifestation is an interesting uncommon presentation of malaria. The abnormality of liver function test is also reported. Recently, Wiwanitkit proposed that jaundice is not an uncommon presentation in the patients with malarial infection [79]. Yuda and Ishino said that malarial transmission to the human host was established by sporozoite infection of the liver and sporozoites are released from the mosquito salivary glands and carried by the blood flow to the liver sinusoid [80]. They noted that traversal of the sinusoidal cell layer and subsequent hepatocyte infection were the most important events in sporozoite liver invasion, but the molecular basis of both events remained to be elucidated [80]. They also said that this process was homologous to midgut epithelium penetration by the malarial ookinete, because identical or paralogous genes were critically involved in both processes [80]. Recent studies had revealed that NKT cells participate in some types of liver injuries especially for malaria hepatitis [81]. Malarial cirrhosis is an interesting topic of malarial infection. In 1981, Islam *et al* performed a clinical analysis of 293 cases of cirrhosis from two moderate-sized hospitals in Dacca and found that 10.24 % of the patients had the past history of malaria [82]. Until present, it can be confirmed that there is malarial hepatitis but the existence of malarial cirrhosis is controversy [83 – 85]. However, Rothenberg *et al* stated that chronic liver diseases, especially cirrhosis, were not known as ascertained late lesions of malaria [86].

Diagnosis of Malaria

There are many current advances in malarial diagnosis. However, most diagnoses in the endemic area usually based on clinical history and basic screening test especially for blood smear interpretation. There are two major blood smear preparation techniques for malarial investigation, thin film and thick film preparations. Lee *et al* said that thin and thick blood film microscopy is the gold standard for malaria diagnosis [87]. A thin blood smear is a drop of blood that has been spread across a large area of the slide while a thick blood smear is a drop of blood on a glass slide [88]. Thin blood smears are most useful in determining what species of malaria is causing the infection (table 2) while thick blood smears are most useful for detecting the presence of parasites because they allow a larger sample of blood to be examined, often there are few parasites in the blood at the time the test is done [88].

Table 2. Characteristic of different species of malaria in thin film

Species	stripped	Ring stage	trophozoite	schizont	gametocyte
Falciparum	Maurer'clefts	Multiple, marginal	Rare	Rare	Crescent
Vivax*	Schuffner's dot	Single	Round	Round	Round
Malariae	Ziermann's stripping	Single	Banded	Rosette	Round
Ovale	Schuffner' dot	Single	Similar to malariae	Similar to malariae	Round

* red blood cell enlargement is common.

In recent years, there have been important developments in malaria diagnostic tests including fluorescence microscopy of malaria parasites stained with acridine orange, dipstick immunoassays that detect species-specific parasite antigens, and more recently, detection of parasite nucleic acids after amplification by PCR [87]. With some of these methods, sensitivities and specificities approaching and even exceeding those of the thin and thick film can be attained [87]. Concerning fluorescence microscopy, Kawamoto and Billingsley said that it was an efficient method for the detection of malaria parasites using low-cost, paired filters adapted for standard light microscopes and acridine orange staining [89]. Concerning Dipstick test, there are many available test kits at present. Recently, Shah and Deshmukh conducted an interesting study to determine efficacy of a malarial dipstick test, Parasight-F (an HRP-II antigen dipstick method to detect *Plasmodium Falciparum*) in Indian children and found that Parasight-F was an effective tool for diagnosis of *Plasmoduim falciparum* malaria in children [90]. They noted that parasitic index; prior treatment with antimalarials or severity of falciparum malaria had no effect on the sensitivity of Parasight-F test [90]. Concerning PCR-based tests for plasmodium DNA or RNA, Lee *et al* noted that these tests were more sensitive and specific than other tests for malarial parasites and a specific application for PCR diagnosis of malaria could be blood donor screening [87]. They noted that there were many clinical trials of blood donor screening for malarial parasites by PCR, in which pooled donor samples are screened to increase efficiency and reduce costs [87]. Finally, Lee *et al* proposed that the new diagnostic methods might have specific applications in particular settings, depending on the purpose and location of testing, and other factors such as cost, desired sensitivity and specificity, speed and ease of use [87].

Pathology and Complication

A. Pathology

Several malarial pathological findings are documented. The main alteration is on the red blood cell as previously mentioned. The destruction of red blood cell, relating to immunopathology, is proposed. Sherman *et al* noted that the human malaria parasite aged the red blood cell during its intracellular development [91]. They said that during the process of erythrocyte senescence the parasitized cell becomes less dense and deformable, its biconcave disc shape became more spherical and was covered with microscopic protuberances (knobs); the amounts of membrane cholesterol and phospholipids were altered and phosphatidylserine (PS) was externalized [91]. They noted that the malaria-infected cell is osmotically fragile, more permeable to a wide variety of molecules via new permeation pathways (NPP), and there is surface deposition of immunoglobulins and complement and there were declines in sialic acid, reduced glutathione, tocopherol and ATP [91]. They also mentioned that hemichromes were deposited on the inner surface of the red cell membrane and there was clustering of the anion transporter, band 3 protein, as well as exposure of neoantigens, which contributed to antigenic variation and adhesivity of the parasitized erythrocyte [91].

Since red blood cell carrying malarial parasites can wander thorough the bodies, the multisystemic pathological findings due to malaria can be expected. Dondorp *et al* noted that autopsy studies, but also in vivo observations of the microcirculation, demonstrated variable obstruction of the microcirculation in severe malaria [92]. They noted that principal cause of this was cytoadherence to the vascular endothelium of erythrocytes containing the mature forms of the parasite, leading to sequestration and obstruction of small vessels [92]. In addition, they noted that parasitized red cells became rigid; compromising their flow through capillaries whose lumen had been reduced by sequestered erythrocytes [92]. They also mentioned that adhesive forces between infected red cells (auto-agglutination), between infected and uninfected red cells (rosetting) and between uninfected erythrocytes (aggregation) could further slow down microcirculatory flow and a more recent finding was that uninfected erythrocytes also become rigid in severe malaria [92]. They finally proposed that reduction in the overall red cell deformability has a strong predictive value for a fatal outcome [92].

B. Complication

Many complications of malaria are documented in medicine. Rane *et al* said that there was an upward trend in deaths due to malaria and complications accounted for majority of deaths and cerebral malaria topped the list [93]. They noted that other complications observed were adult respiratory distress syndrome (ARDS), acute septicemic malaria, acute renal failure (ARF) and disseminated intravascular coagulation (DIC) [93]. Concerning cerebral malaria, it is accepted as the most serious complication. It is characterized by sequestration of parasitized red blood cells in cerebral capillaries and venules [94]. Mturi *et al* said that cerebral malaria was one of the most common nontraumatic encephalopathies in the world [95]. Wassmer *et al* said that although the exact cause of cerebral malaria remained unclear, evidence had clearly implicated metabolic disturbances and host immune responses [94]. They found that significantly greater accumulation of platelets occurred in capillaries and venules of the patients who died from cerebral malaria than from other diseases [94].

Wassmer *et al* then investigated the role of platelets in IE cytoadhesion in vitro, using CD36-binding IE (IECD36) and CD36-deficient (CD36DEF) brain microvascular endothelial cells and found that platelets could induce strong IECD36 binding to CD36DEF ECs and, conversely, could hide constitutively expressed falciparum receptors such as chondroitin sulfate A [96]. Considering the genetic basis of cerebral malaria, Hirayama noted that the TNF promoter (TNFP)-D allele was significantly associated with cerebral malaria [97]. Aguillon *et al* said that TNF alpha polymorphism was also associated with cerebral malaria [98].

Concerning lung complications in malaria, Taylor and White said that pulmonary edema that resulted from increased pulmonary capillary permeability was the most important pulmonary manifestation of malaria and it was a common feature of severe malaria [99]. Mortality rate is high [99]. The pathophysiologic basis is unclear [99]. Jindil *et al* said that ARDS was common in severe falciparum malaria [100]. TNF is believed to play an important role in development of ARDS in malaria. Similar to cerebral malaria, the direct and indirect effects of TNF on endothelial cells might be the major underlying factor for development of ARDS [101] Lucas *et al* found that lung mcirovascular endothelium from ARDS patients presented a procoagulant profile and a higher production capacity of interleukin-6 (IL-6) and IL-8 when compared with those from controls [101]. Boulos *et al* said that pulmonary involvement occurred in 3 to 10% of the cases of *Plasmodium falciparum* malaria and represented one of the most serious complications of this infection, with a lethality of about 70% [102]. They noted that cell activation by cytokines, produced by lymphocytes and macrophages during the immune response, and express receptors and molecules of adhesion, allowing for sequestration of parasitized erythrocytes and adherence of cells, which would produce locally inflammatory mediators [102]. They propose that the inflammatory reaction and lesion of endothelial cells that ensue, together with the hemodynamic alterations induced by the capillary blockade due to the sequestration of parasitized erythrocytes and leukocytes, caused alterations of the vascular permeability and transfer of liquid to intertitial space and alveoles [102]. Boulos *et al* said that clinical manifestations of pulmonary involvement may start suddenly at any time during the course of malaria, even after disappearance of circulating parasites and hyperparasitemia, renal failure and pregnancy are predisposing factors [102]. They noted that the prognosis depended on how fast the diagnosis is established and convenient treatment initiated [102].

Concerning ARF in malaria, Zinna *et al* said that while the incidence of acute renal failure in malaria is less than 1%, mortality is reported to be as high as 45% in those with renal failure [103]. They noted that falciparum malaria associated with ARF was associated with a high morbidity, but early presentation and intervention with appropriate antimalarial and renal replacement therapy was associated with improved survival and recovery of renal function [103]. Eiam-ong said that ARF was mediated by a complex interaction of mechanical, immunologic, cytokine, humoral, acute phase response, nonspecific factors, and hemodynamic factors [104 - 105]. Acute tubular necrosis (ATN) is the principal pathologic lesion in falciparum malaria-induced ARF [105]. Eiam-ong noted that parasitized erythrocytes played a central role in all aforementioned pathogenic factors of ARF [104 - 105]. Eiam-Ong also mentioned that because of the hypercatabolic state of falciparum malaria-induced ARF, hemodialysis as well as peritoneal dialysis should be immediately performed when there was a rapid increase of creatinine concentration [104 - 105]. Of interest, Eiam-Ong noted that *Plasmodium malariae*, in contradistinction, could cause chronic glomerulopathy that may relentlessly progress to end-stage renal disease [104].

Concerning DIC in malaria, several defects in blood coagulation can be seen. Gorski *et al* said that clinically significant bleeding was relatively uncommon in malaria and occurred in approximately 5% of patients [106]. They noted that severe haemostatic abnormalities are of complex origin and are manifested in thrombocytopenia, decreased activity of coagulation factors and symptoms of vascular diathesis [106]. Thy also said that DIC could be demonstrated, especially the cases with cerebral malaria as co-complication [106].

TREATMENT

The concept of treatment is similar to other infections: getting rid of the pathogen or control of the infection and supportive or symptomatic treatment. In malaria, many antimalarial drugs are available for a long time. The selection of antimalarial drugs depends on the species and the reported resistance pattern in each setting (table 3) [107]. Randomized controlled trials have not revealed any significant benefit of the artemisinin derivatives over quinine in quinine sensitive areas [108]. Also, if quinine is administered in the recommended way, the side effects are no greater than artemisinins [108]. Drug resistant is a very important problem in using of antimalrial drug, Historically, first case of chloroquine resistance was along the Thai-Combodian border in the late 1950s then Southeast Asia has played an important role as a focus for the development of drug resistance in *Plasmodium falciparum* [109]. In addition, the onset of chloroquine resistance marked the beginning of a new chapter in the history of malaria in Southeast Asia and by 1973 chloroquine finally had to be replaced by the combination of sulphadoxine and pyrimethamine (SP) as first line drug for the treatment of uncomplicated malaria in Thailand and more than 10 African countries have also switched their first line drug to other newly developed drug [109]. Farooq and Mahajan said that many molecular markers for antimalarial resistance had been identified, including pfmdr-1 and pfcrt polymorphisms associated with chloroquine resistance and dhfr and dhps polymorphisms associated with SP resistance [109]. They noted that polymorphisms in pfmdr-1 might also be associated with resistance to chloroquine, mefloquine and artemisinin [109]. An important precaution of using antimalarial drug is drug - induced hemolysis in the patients with glucose-6-phosphate dehydrogenase (G-6-PD) deficiency, which is endemic in the same area as malaria. It should be noted that G6PD status is recommended before primaquine or tafenoquine is prescribed in the endemic area [110]. However, the G6PD deficiency, on the other hand, is a protective factor for malaria [110]. Wajcman and Galacteros noted that red blood cells with low G6PD activity offer a hostile environment to parasite growth and thus an advantage to G6PD deficiency carriers [110].

Table 3. Simplified guideline for selection of antimalarial drugs

Species	sensitive	resist
Vivax	chloroquine and primaquine	chloroquine and (increased dose) primaquine
Falciparum	quinine sulfate and doxycycline or mefloquine	quinine dihydrochloride (intravenous)
Ovale	similar to vivax	similar to vivax
malariae	chloroquine	chloroquine

* dosage of each drug is adjusted according to the recommendation of each setting.

In additional to specific treatment, the supportive and symptomatic treatment is also important in taking care of malarial patients. Since several associated systemic complications like hypoglycemia, hypovolemia, hyperpyrexia, renal failure, bleeding disorders, anemia, lactic acidosis and pulmonary edema may contribute in the pathogenesis of coma, and are responsible for high mortality, the meticulous supportive care along with intravenous administration of antimalarial drugs are corner-stone of the treatment [111]. Singhal said that supportive care, early diagnosis and management of complications were as essential as antimalarial therapy [108]. Pamba and Maitland noted that reduction in case fatality could only come through the wider appreciation of the need for and application of supportive therapies to treat the life-threatening complications of malaria [112]. In severe malarial infection, fluid management is very important. Pamba and Maitland said that hypovolaemia had emerged as a common feature of children presenting with severe malaria complicated by acidosis [112]. They noted that early recognition and prompt treatment might lead to improvements in outcome [112]. As soon as the patient is clinically stable and able to swallow, oral treatment should be given and the intravascular volume should be maintained at the lowest level sufficient for adequate systemic perfusion to prevent development of acute respiratory distress syndrome [113]. In addition, renal replacement therapy should be initiated early [113]. Therapeutic red cell-exchange (TREX) has been used with much interest over the years to correct severe anemia [113 - 114]. Singhal said that the role of exchange blood transfusion in the management of severe malaria was still controversial and it might be considered in the presence of high parasites counts, more than10%, with multiorgan dysfunction if adequate quantities of safe blood were available [108].

PREVENTION

The prevention of malaria is the good method to control this parasitic disease. Since this disease is vector-borne transmission, the control of vector is important in primary prevention. Bed nest and pesticide are widely used aiming at primary prevention. Further more details will be presented in the final chapter. Advances in prevention of malaria are the attempts to develop the vaccine and transgenic vector for controlling this disease. Concerning the vaccination for malaria, there are many interesting recent reports on this topic. Tongren *et al* said that it had been repeatedly argued that the discovery and implementation of a safe and effective vaccine against malaria was a major priority in the control of the disease [115]. Concerning transgenic vector for controlling of malaria, engineering mosquitoes with a genetic trait that confers resistance to malaria or causes population suppression is a task [116]. In addition, chemoprophylaxis of malaria is recommended for the traveler entering malarial endemic area [117]. In addition, chemoprophylaxis is also highly effective in reducing mortality and morbidity from malaria in young children and pregnant women living in endemic areas [118]. Greenwood said that intermittent preventive treatment, in which full therapeutic doses of a drug were given at defined intervals, had the potential to provide some of the benefits of sustained chemoprophylaxis in pregnant women and young children without some of its drawbacks and was a promising new approach to malaria control [118]. Hatz said that exposure prophylaxis substantially reduced the risk of infection [119]. Drugs for chemoprophylaxis is indicated. Petersen said that use of malaria chemoprophylaxis was a balance between the risk of infection and death, and the risk of side effects [120]. Three levels of chemoprophylaxis are used: chloroquine in areas with sensitive *Plasmodium falciparum*, chloroquine plus proguanil in areas with low level chloroquine resistance, and atovaquone/proguanil, doxycycline or mefloquine in areas with extensive resistance against chloroquine and proguanil [120]. Hatz also noted that if malaria infection was readily diagnosed, the infection could always be successfully treated [119].

REFERENCES

[1] Chareonviriyaphap T, Bangs MJ, Ratanatham S. Status of malaria in Thailand. *Southeast Asian J. Trop. Med. Public Health.* 2000; 31: 225-37.

[2] Phillips RS. Current status of malaria and potential for control. *Clin. Microbiol.* 2001; 14: 208 – 26.

[3] Thimasarn K, Jatapadma S, Vijaykadga S, Sirichaisinthop J, Wongsrichanalai C. Epidemiology of Malaria in Thailand. *J. Travel Med.* 1995; 2:59-65.

[4] Angell SY, Cetron MS. Health disparities among travelers visiting friends and relatives abroad. *Ann. Intern. Med.* 2005; 142: 67-72.

[5] Wernsdorfer G, Wernsdorfer WH. Malaria at the turn from the 2nd to the 3rd millenium. *Wien. Klin. Wochenschr.* 2003; 115 Suppl 3: 2-9.

[6] Hay SI, Guerra CA, Tatem AJ, Noor AM, Snow RW. The global distribution and population at risk of malaria: past, present, and future. *Lancet Infect Dis.* 2004; 4: 327-36.

[7] Kondrashin AV. Malaria in the WHO Southeast Asia region. *Indian J. Malariol.* 1992; 29: 129-60.

[8] Suyaphun A, Wiwanitkit V, Suwansaksri J, Nithiuthai S, Sritar S, Suksirisampant W, Fongsungnern A. Malaria among hilltribe communities in northern Thailand: a review of clinical manifestations. *Southeast Asian J. Trop. Med. Public Health.* 2002; 33 Suppl. 3: 14-5.

[9] Wiwanitkit V. High prevalence of malaria in Myanmar migrant workers in a rural district near the Thailand-Myanmar border. *Scand. J. Infect. Dis.* 2002; 34: 236-7.

[10] Chaveepojnkamjorn W, Pichainarong N. Malaria infection among the migrant population along the Thai-Myanmar border area. *Southeast Asian. J. Trop. Med. Public Health.* 2004; 35: 48-52.

[11] Kitvatanachai S, Janyapoon K, Rhongbutsri P, Thap LC. A survey on malaria in mobile Cambodians in Aranyaprathet, Sa Kaeo Province, Thailand. *Southeast Asian J. Trop. Med. Public Health.* 2003; 34: 48-53.

[12] Singhasivanon P. Mekong malaria. Malaria, multi-drug resistance and economic development in the greater Mekong subregion of Southeast Asia. *Southeast Asian J. Trop. Med. Public Health.* 1999; 30 Suppl 4: i-iv.

[13] Denis MB, Meek SR. Malaria in Cambodia. *Southeast Asian J. Trop. Med. Public Health.* 1992; 23 Suppl 4: 23-8.

[14] Pholsena K. The malaria situation and antimalaria program in Laos. *Southeast. Asian J. Trop. Med. Public Health.* 1992; 23 Suppl 4: 39-42.

[15] Hien TT, VinhChau NV, Vinh NN, Hung NT, Phung MQ, Toan LM, Mai PP, Dung NT, HoaiTam DT, Arnold K. Management of multiple drug-resistant malaria in Viet Nam. *Ann. Acad. Med. Singapore.* 1997; 26: 659-63.

[16] Rahman WA, Che'Rus A, Ahmad AH. Malaria and Anopheles mosquitos in Malaysia. Southeast. *Asian. J. Trop. Med. Public. Health.* 28, 599-605(1997)

[17] Arbani PR. Malaria control program in Indonesia. *Southeast Asian J. Trop. Med. Public Health.* 1992; 23 Suppl 4, 29-38.

[18] Dev V, Bhattacharyya PC, Talukdar R. Transmission of malaria and its control in the northeastern region of India. *J. Assoc. Physicians India.* 2003; 51: 1073-6.

[19] Samarasinghe L. Malaria control program in Sri Lanka. *Southeast Asian J. Trop. Med. Public Health.* 1992; 23 Suppl 4: 61-5.

[20] Wickremasinghe AR, Gunawardena DM, Mahawithanage ST. Use of routinely collected past surveillance data in identifying and mapping high-risk areas in a malaria

endemic area of Sri Lanka. *Southeast Asian J. Trop. Med. Public Health.* 2002; 33: 678-84.

[21] Birley MH. An historical review of malaria, kala-azar and filariasis in Bangladesh in relation to the Flood Action Plan. *Am. J. Trop. Med. Hyg.* 1993; 87: 319-34.

[22] Ismaeel AY, Senok AC, Jassim Al-Khaja KA, Botta GA. Status of malaria in the Kingdom of Bahrain: a 10-year review. *Am. J. Trop. Med. Hyg.* 2004; 11: 97-101.

[23] Scrimgeour EM, Mehta FR, Suleiman AJ. Infectious and tropical diseases in Oman: a review. *Am. J. Trop. Med. Hyg.* 1999; 61: 920-5.

[24] Qian H, Tand L. Prevention and control of malaria in China, in last 50 years. *Zhonghua Liu Xing Bing Xue Za Zhi.* 2000; 21: 225-7.

[25] Zhao SN. Epdemiological evaluation of a 20-year program in the control of malaria in Mun-hai County Yunan Province. *Zhonghua Liu Xing Bing Xue Za Zhi.* 1985; 6: 150-2.

[26] Kano S, Kimura M. Trends in malaria cases in Japan. *Acta Trop.* 2004; 89: 271-8.

[27] Hartl DL. The origin of malaria: mixed messages from genetic diversity. *Nat. Rev. Microbiol.* 2004; 2: 15-22.

[28] Le Mire J, Arnulf L, Guibert P. Malaria: control strategies, chemoprophylaxis, diagnosis, and treatment. *Clin. Occup. Environ. Med.* 2004; 4: 143-65.

[29] Snow RW, Korenromp EL, Gouws E. Pediatric mortality in Africa: plasmodium falciparum malaria as a cause or risk? *Am. J. Trop. Med. Hyg.* 2004; 71(2 Suppl): 16-24.

[30] Worrall E, Rietveld A, Delacollette C. The burden of malaria epidemics and cost-effectiveness of interventions in epidemic situations in Africa. *Am. J. Trop. Med. Hyg.* 2004; 71(2 Suppl), 136-40.

[31] Keiser J, Utzinger J, Caldas de Castro M, Smith TA, Tanner M, Singer BH. Urbanization in sub-saharan Africa and implication for malaria control. *Am. J. Trop. Med. Hyg.* 2004; 71(2 Suppl): 118-27.

[32] Abeku TA, Hay SI, Ochola S, Langi P, Beard B, de Vlas SJ, Cox J. Malaria epidemic early warning and detection in African highlands. *Trends Parasitol.* 2004; 20: 400-5.

[33] John CC, Koech DK, Sumba PO, Ouma JH. Risk of Plasmodium falciparum infection during a malaria epidemic in highland Kenya, 1997. *Acta Trop.* 2004; 92: 55-61.

[34] Lusingu JP, Vestergaard LS, Mmbando BP, Drakeley CJ, Jones C, Akida J, Savaeli ZX, Kitua AY, Lemnge MM, Theander TG. Malaria morbidity and immunity among residents of villages with different Plasmodium falciparum transmission intensity in North-Eastern Tanzania. *Malar J.* 2004; 3: 26.

[35] DeHart RL. Health issues of air travel. *Annu. Rev. Public Health.* 2003;24:133-51.

[36] Newman RD, Parise ME, Barber AM, Steketee RW. Malaria-related deaths among U.S. travelers, 1963-2001. *Ann. Intern. Med.* 2004; 141: 547-55.

[37] Castillo-Salgado C. Epidemiological risk stratification of malaria in the Americas. *Mem. Inst. Oswaldo Cruz.* 1992; 87 Suppl 3: 115-20.

[38] Dourado HV, Abdon NP, Martins SJ. Falciparum malaria. Epidemiology in Latin America, biologic and clinical considerations, treatment, and prophylaxis. *Infect. Dis. Clin. North Am.* 1994; 8: 207-23.

[39] Carme B. Human parasitoses in French Guiana. *Presse Med.* 2001;.30: 1601-8.

[40] Singer BH, de Castro MC. Agricultural colonization and malaria on the Amazon frontier. *Ann. N. Y. Acad. Sci.* 2001; 954:184-222.

[41] Bastos FI, Barcellos C, Lowndes CM, Friedman SR. Co-infection with malaria and HIV in injecting drug users in Brazil: a new challenge to public health? *Addiction.* 1999; 94: 1165-74.

[42] Castela F, Legros F, Lagardere B. Imported malaria in children in France. *Arch. Pediatr.* 2003; 10: 758-65.

[43] Ladhani S, El Bashir H, Patel VS, Shingadia D. Childhood malaria in East London. *Pediatr. Infect. Dis. J.* 2003; 22, 814-9.

[44] Walker J. Malaria in a changing world: an Australian perspective. *Int. J. Parasitol.* 1998;28:947-53.

[45] Currie B. The diagnosis and treatment of malaria in Australia. *Aust. Fam. Physician.* 1993; 22:1773-6.

[46] Currie BJ, Brewster DR. Childhood infections in the tropical north of Australia. *J. Paediatr. Child. Health.* 2001; 37: 326-30.

[47] Malaria. Available at http://www-micro.msb.le.ac.uk/224/Malaria.html

[48] Hurd H, Carter V. The role of programmed cell death in Plasmodium-mosquito interactions. *Int. J. Parasitol.* 2004; 34: 1459-72.

[49] Cot M, Deloron P. Malaria during pregnancy: consequences and interventional perspectives. *Med. Trop. (Mars).* 2003; 63: 369-80.

[50] Okoko BJ, Enwere G, Ota MO. The epidemiology and consequences of maternal malaria: a review of immunological basis. *Acta Trop.* 2003; 87: 193-205.

[51] Marques HH, Vallada MG, Sakane PT, Boulos M. Congenital Malaria. Case reports and a brief review of literature. *J. Pediatr (Rio. J.).* 1996; 72: 103-5.

[52] Ahmed A, Cerilli LA, Sanchez PJ. Congenital malaria in a preterm neonate: case report and review of the literature. *Am. J. Perinatol.* 1998; 15: 19-22.

[53] Dodd RY. Transmission of parasites by blood transfusion. *Vox Sang.* 1998; 74 Suppl 2, 161-3.

[54] Nurse GT. Transfusion of malarial or other parasites in blood. *S. Afr. Med. J.* 1993; 83: 79-80.

[55] Wiwanitkit V. Screening test in laboratory medicine. *Chula Med. J.* 2001; 42: 1031 – 8.

[56] Failloux AB, Vazeille-Falcoz M, Mousson L, Rodhain F. Genetic control of vectorial competence in Aedes mosquitoes. *Bull. Soc. Pathol. Exot.* 1999; 92: 266-73.

[57] May J, Horstmann R. Influence of human genetic variants on resistance and immunity against malaria. Bundesgesundheitsblatt. *Gesundheitsforschung. Gesundheitsschutz.* 2004; 47: 1000-8.

[58] Clegg JB, Weatherall DJ. Thalassemia and malaria: new insights into an old problem. *Proc. Assoc. Am. Physicians.* 1999; 111: 278-82.

[59] Roberts DJ, Williams TN. Haemoglobinopathies and resistance to malaria. *Redo Rep.* 2003; 8: 304-10.

[60] Hebbel RP. Sickle hemoglobin instability: a mechanism for malarial protection. *Redox Rep.* 2003; 8: 238-40.

[61] Chotivanich K, Udomsangpetch R, Pattanapanyasat K, Chierakul W, Simpson J, Looareesuwan S, White N. Hemoglobin E: a balanced polymorphism protective against high parasitemias and thus severe P falciparum malaria. *Blood.* 2002; 100: 1172-6.

[62] Wiwanitkit V. Haemoglobin Tak, an unstable haemoglobin from Thailand. *Haema.* 2004; 7: 310-312.

[63] Manguin S, Fontenille D, Chandre F, Lochouarn L, Mouchet J, Kengne P, Guillet P. Anopheline population genetics. *Bull. Soc. Pathol. Exot.* 1999; 92: 229-35.

[64] Clark IA, Alleva LM, Mills AC, Cowden WB. Pathogenesis of malaria and clinically similar conditions. *Clin. Microbiol. Rev.*2004; 17: 509-39.

[65] Maitland K, Marsh K. Pathophysiology of severe malaria in children. *Acta Trop.* 2004; 90: 131-40.

[66] Rasti N, Wahlgren M, Chen Q. Molecular aspects of malaria pathogenesis. *FEMS Immunol. Med. Microbiol.* 2004; 41: 9-26.

[67] Lang F, Lang PA, Lang KS, Brand V, Tanneur V, Duranton C, Wieder T, Huber SM. Channel-induced apoptosis of infected host cells-the case of malaria. *Pflugers Arch.* 2004;448:319-24.

[68] Clark IA, Schofield L. Pathogenesis of malaria. *Parasitol. Today.* 2000; 16: 451-4.

[69] Murphy GS, Oldfield EC 3rd. Falciparum malaria. Infect. *Dis. Clin. North Am.* 1996; 10: 747-75.

[70] McDevitt MA, Xie J, Gordeuk V, Bucala R. The anemia of malaria infection: role of inflammatory cytokines. *Curr. Hematol. Rep.* 2004; 3: 97-106.

[71] McGuire W, Knight JC, Hill AV, Allsopp CE, Greenwood BM, Kwiatkowski D. Severe malarial anemia and cerebral malaria are associated with different tumor necrosis factor promoter alleles. *J. Infect. Dis.* 1999; 179: 287-90.

[72] Waitumbi JN, Opollo MO, Muga RO, Misore AO, Stoute JA. Red cell surface changes and erythrophagocytosis in children with severe plasmodium falciparum anemia. *Blood.* 2000; 95: 1481-6.

[73] Weatherall DJ, Abdalla S, Pippard MJ. The anemia of Plasmodium falciparum malaria. *Ciba Found Symp.* 1983; 94: 74-97.

[74] Davis TM, Krishna S, Looareesuwan S, Supanaranond W, Pukrittayakamee S, Attatamsoonthorn K, White NJ. Erythrocyte sequestration and anemia in severe falciparum malaria. Analysis of acute changes in venous hematocrit using a simple mathematical model. *J. Clin. Invest.* 1990; 86: 793-800.

[75] Wilson JJ, Neame PB, Kelton JG. Infection-induced thrombocytopenia. *Semin. Thromb. Hemost.* 1982; 8: 217-33.

[76] Wiwanitkit V, Suyaphan A. Prevalence of thrombocytopenia in vivax malarial patients: an observation. *Platelets.* 2003; 14: 395.

[77] Mohanty D, Marwaha N, Ghosh K, Sharma S, Garewal G, Shah S, Devi S, Das KC. Functional and ultrastructural changes of platelets in malarial infection. *Trans. R. Soc. Trop. Med. Hyg.* 988; 82: 369-75.

[78] Abdalla SH. Hematopoiesis in human malaria. *Blood Cells.* 1990; 16: 401-16.

[79] Wiwanitkit V. Jaundice as co-presentation in Thai malarial patients. *J. Indian Med. Assoc.* 2004; 102: 107.

[80] Yuda M, Ishino T. Liver invasion by malarial parasites--how do malarial parasites break through the host barrier? *Cell Microbiol.* 2004; 6:1119-25.

[81] Tsutsui H, Adachi K, Seki E, Nakanishi K. Cytokine-induced inflammatory liver injuries. *Curr. Mol. Med.* 2003; 3: 545-59.

[82] Islam N, Khan M, Ahmed Z. Cirrhosis of liver. *Bangladesh Med. Res. Counc. Bull.* 1981; 7: 45-51.

[83] Mahi PN, Tandon HD. Malarial hepatitis. *J. Indiana State Med. Assoc.* 1955; 25 ,507-11.

[84] Gyergyay F, Hermann E. Etiopathogenetic factors in liver cirrhosis. *Med. Interna.* (Bucur). 1956; 8: 669-79.

[85] Franken HF, Snoos A. Is there a malaria cirrhosis? *Munch. Med. Wochenschr.* 1996; 108: 879-83.

[86] Rothenberg G, Schubert S. Assessment of late complications of malaria in travelers to the tropics. *Z. Gesamte Inn. Med.* 1983; 38: 46-7.

[87] Lee SH, Kara UA, Koay E, Lee MA, Lam S, Teo D. New strategies for the diagnosis and screening of malaria. *Int. J. Hematol.* 2002; 76 Suppl 1: 291-3.

[88] Thick and thin blood smears for malaria. Available at http://my.webmd.com/hw/health_guide_atoz/hw118744.asp

[89] Kawamoto F, Billingsley PF. Rapid diagnosis of malaria by fluorescence microscopy. *Parasitol Today.* 1992; 8: 69-71.

[90] Shah I, Deshmukh CT. A bedside dipstick method to detect Plasmodium falciparum. *Indian. Pediatr.* 2004; 41: 1148-51.

[91] Sherman IW, Eda S, Winograd E. Erythrocyte aging and malaria. *Cell Mol. Biol.* (Noisy-le-grand). 2004; 50:159-69.

[92] Dondorp AM, Pongponratn E, White NJ. Reduced microcirculatory flow in severe falciparum malaria: pathophysiology and electron-microscopic pathology. *Acta Trop.* 2004;89:309-17.

[93] Rane SR, Bapat VM, Holla W. Malaria still a threat to life--a postmortem study. *Indian J. Pathol. Microbiol.* 2003; 46: 17-9.

[94] Wassmer SC, Coltel N, Combes V, Grau GE. Pathogenesis of cerebral malaria: facts and hypotheses. *Med. Trop.* (Mars). 2003; 63: 254-7.

[95] Mturi N, Musumba CO, Wamola BM, Ogutu BR, Newton CR. Cerebral malaria: optimising management. *CNS. Drugs.* 2003; 17: 153-65.

[96] Wassmer SC, Combes V, Grau GE. Pathophysiology of cerebral malaria: role of host cells in the modulation of cytoadhesion. *Ann. N. Y. Acad. Sci.* 2003; 992: 30-8.

[97] Hirayama K. Genetic factors associated with development of cerebral malaria and fibrotic schistosomiasis. *Korean J. Parasitol.* 2002; 40: 165-72.

[98] Aguillon JC, Cruzat A, Cuenca J, Cuchacovich M. Tumor necrosis factor alpha genetic polymorphism as a risk factor in disease. *Rev. Med. Chil.* 2002; 130: 1043-50.

[99] Taylor WR, White NJ. Malaria and the lung. *Clin. Chest. Med.* 2002; 23: 457-68.

[100] Jindal SK, Aggarwal AN, Gupta D. Adult respiratory distress syndrome in the tropics. *Clin. Chest. Med.* 2002; 23: 445-55.

[101] Lucas R, Lou J, Morel DR, Ricou B, Suter PM, Grau GE. TNF receptors in the microvascular pathology of acute respiratory distress syndrome and cerebral malaria. *J. Leukoc. Biol.* 1997; 61: 551-8.

[102] Boulos M, Costa JM, Tosta CE. Pulmonary involvement in malaria (review). *Rev. Inst. Med. Trop. Sao Paulo.* 1993; 35: 93-102.

[103] Zinna S, Vathsala A, Woo KT. A case series of falciparum malaria-induced acute renal failure. *Ann. Acad. Med. Singapore.* 1999; 28: 578-82.

[104] Eiam-Ong S. Malarial nephropathy. *Semin. Nephrol.* 2003; 23: 21-33.

[105] Eiam-Ong S. Current knowledge in falciparum malaria-induced acute renal failure. *J. Med. Assoc. Thai.* 2002; 85 Suppl 1: S16-24.

[106] Gorski J, Nahorski W, Slonecka A, Birkholz A. Disturbances of hemostasis in malaria. *Wiad Parazytol.* 1993; 39: 339-43.

[107] Farooq U, Mahajan RC. Drug resistance in malaria. *J. Vector Borne Dis.* 2004; 41: 45-53.

[108] Singhal T. Management of severe malaria. *Indian. J. Pediatr.* 2004; 71: 81-8.

[109] Indonesian Society of Medicine. Consensus of Malaria Management 2003 (part 2). *Acta Med. Indones.* 2004; 36: 187-93.

[110] Wajcman H, Galacteros F. Glucose 6-phosphate dehydrogenase deficiency: a protection against malaria and a risk for hemolytic accidents. *C. R. Biol.* 2004; 327: 711-20.

[111] Garg RK. Cerebral malaria. *J. Assoc. Physicians India.* 2000; 48: 1004-13.

[112] Pamba A, Maitland K. Fluid management of severe falciparum malaria in African children. *Trop. Doct.* 2004; 34:67-70.

[113] Trampuz A, Jereb M, Muzlovic I, Prabhu RM. Clinical review: Severe malaria. *Crit. Care.* 2003; 7: 315-23.

[114] Valbonesi M, Bruni R. Clinical application of therapeutic erythrocytapheresis (TEA). *Transfus. Sci.* 2000; 22: 183-94.

[115] Tongren JE, Zavala F, Roos DS, Riley EM. Malaria vaccines: if at first you don't succeed... *Trends Parasitol.* 2004; 20: 604-10

[116] Christophides GK. Transgenic mosquitoes and malaria transmission. *Cell Microbiol.* 2005; 7: 325-33.

[117] Wiwanitkit V. Amazing Thailand Year 1998-1999 Tourist's health concepts. *Chula Med. J.* 1998; 42: 975-984.

[118] Greenwood B. The use of anti-malarial drugs to prevent malaria in the population of malaria-endemic areas. *Am. J. Trop. Med. Hyg.* 2004; 70: 1-7.

[119] Hatz CF. Prophylaxis and therapy of malaria in the practice. *Internist.* (Berl). 2004; 45: 677-83

[120] Petersen E. Malaria chemoprophylaxis: when should we use it and what are the options? *Expert Rev. Anti. Infect. Ther.* 2004; 2: 119-32.

Chapter III

BABESIOSIS

WHAT IS BABESIOSIS?

Human babesiosis is caused predominantly by *Babesia microti* and *Babesia divergens*, a protozooan parasites of red blood cells [1]. Both are transmitted by *Ixodes ricinus* ticks, also the primary vector of Lyme disease [1]. Babesia is a tick-transmitted protozoal parasite that can cause malaria-like symptoms and hemolytic anemia [2]. Clinical manifestation varied widely from asymptomatic infection to a serve rapidly fatal disease [1]. Asplenic, elderly, and immunocompromised patients are at greatest risk for severe disease; however babesiosis can be serious in immunologically normal persons [2].

The emergence of Lyme borreliosis as the most prevalent arthropod disease of humans in the temperate northern hemisphere has resulted in renewed interest in human babesiosis, transmitted by the same tick vectors [3]. The advent of new molecular tools has made possible a reappraisal of the main parasites involved. *Babesia divergens* is probably restricted to European cattle, though there are several nearly identical species [3]. In USA, *Babesia microti* is more common. There is increasing evidence to suggest that human babesiosis in the USA may be caused by babesial parasites that a re antigenically and genotypically distinct from *Babesia microti* [2]. Presently, *Babesia microti* occurs as a world-wide species complex rather than as a single species [3].

EPIDEMIOLOGY OF BABESIOSIS

Babesiosis is a zoonosis that affects several animals. The species of babesia is different for each specific host animals: *Babesia canis* (dogs), *Babesia equi* (horses), *Babesia bovis* (cattle), *Babesia microti* (rodents). However, some *Babesia spp.* are not host specific and can be transmitted to humans. These species are *Babesia microti* and *Babesia divergens*. The epidemiology of babesiosis is different for human and animals.

A. Canine Babesiosis

Canine babesiosis is a worldwide infection [4 – 6]. *Babesia canis* and *Babesia gibsoni* are two organisms commonly known to infect dogs. Both organisms have *Ixodid* tick vectors and are found throughout Asia, Africa, Europe, the Middle East, and North America, with *Babesia canis* being more prevalent [5]. Infection by *B. gibsoni* is increasing in frequency, particularly in North America, although no specific species of ticks in this region have been proven to transmit the disease. However, *Rhipicephalus sanguineus* and *Dermacentor variabilis* are believed to be potential vectors of disease [6]. There also is evidence that some direct animal-to-animal transmission may occur, as when an infected dog with oral abrasions bites a naïve dog. Kennel settings with poor tick surveillance and control are at a higher risk for housed animals to develop babesiosis [6]. Analysis of the DNA from two organisms causing babesiosis in North America and Asia, once believed to be *Babesia gibsoni*, has shown that the two organisms belong to different species [7].

B. Bovine Babesiosis

Babesia divergens is an intraerythrocytic protozoan parasite, transmitted by the tick *Ixodes ricinus*, and is the main agent of bovine babesiosis in Europe. It is not only a cause of significant loss to the cattle industry [8]. In 1981 Purnell wrote "bovine babesiosis caused by *Babesia divergens*, also known as redwater fever, is considered the most important tick-transmitted disease in cattle"[9]. The following years saw a decline in disease outbreaks, probably due in part to the introduction of effective prophylactic treatment and live vaccination in some countries [8]. For USA, both *Babesia bigemina* and *Babesia bovis* are reported as the cause of outbreak of bovine babesiosis [10]. Bovine babesiosis caused by *Babesia divergens* can also be seen in Asia and Africa. Of interest, *Babesia divergens* can also infect immunocompromised humans, causing medical emergencies characterized by rapid fulmination and parasitemias that may exceed 70% [8]. Enzootic stability (herd immunity) in bovine babesiosis occurs when the rate of transmission (inoculation rate) of *Babesia* spp by the tick vector is sufficient to immunize a majority of susceptible calves before the loss of calfhood resistance [11]. More prolonged low winter temperature condition is found to be in a naturally occurring state of enzootic instability [11].

C. Equine Babesisosis

Equine babesiosis or piroplasmosis can be seen worldwide. *Babesia equine*, *Babesia caballi* and *Babesia divergens* are reported in equine babesisosis. For equine babesiosis, significant biases in the distribution of cases of babesiosis are found with regard to season, sex and coat color [12].

D. Human Babesiosis

For human, babesiosis is more common in the Western hemisphere. Human babesiosis can be seen in both Europe and USA [13 – 14]. As previously mentioned, human babesiosis is predominantly caused by *Babesia microti* (rodent-borne piroplasm) and by *Babesia divergens*. The first demonstrated case of human babesiosis in the world was reported in Europe, in 1957 [15]. The vast majority of European cases have been caused by Babesia divergens in splenectomised patients, and although rare, this disease is very dangerous, requiring aggressive treatment [14]. The majority of infections is subclinical or follows a mild chronic course, but dangerous acute infections can occur in immunocompromised patients [14]. Until present, hundreds of cases of human infection with Babesia spp. have been reported in the USA [15]. The spectrum of human babesiosis in the USA is broad, and ranges from an apparently silent infection to a fulminant [13]. In Europe, babesiosis is considerably rarer, but more lethal (42% mortality rate in Europe and 5% in the USA, for clinically apparent infections) and mostly in splenectomized patients [13]. Various determinants are involved in the severity of infection, such as age, immunocompetence and coinfection with other pathogens (*Borrelia burgdorferi*) [13]. Occasionally, in addition to *Babesia microti*, infection in America is caused also by a newly recognized species, so-called WA1 piroplasm [13, 15]. A few other cases of human babesial infection have been described in China, Egypt, Mexico, South Africa and Taiwan [15].

Pathogenic Organism for Babesia

As previously mentioned, the two main pathogenic organisms for human babesiosis are *Babesia microti* and *Babesia divergens*. Generally, the babesia has rounded or pear shape. The size of intraerythrocytic protozoa measure 1-3 microns. The organisms resemble *Plasmodium falciparum*; however, babesia parasites present two distinguishing features. Babesia parasites vary more in shape and in size and they do not produce pigment. Most of organisms can be seen in ameboid or ring form. In cell dividing stage, the parasite can have 2 -4 daughter cells (merozoites).

For animal species, the morphological appearances are usually similar. There is an interesting species namely *Babesia bigemina* which is a large babesia that is pleomorphic but characteristically is seen and identified by the pear-shaped bodies joined at an acute angle within the mature erythrocyte. Large round forms measure 2 μm and the pear-shaped, elongated ones are 4-5 μm [16].

Table 3.1. Morphological appearance of difference *Babesia* species [4]

Species	Morphology	Host
Babesia bigemina	4.5 by 2.5 μm (Large, round and pryiform, acute angle)	Cattle
Babesia bovis	2.4 by 1.5 μm (small, more rounded obtuse angle)	Cattle
Babesia divergens	1.5 by 0.4 μm (small, narrow and obtuse angle)	Cattle
Babesia jakimovi	4.5 by 2.5 μm (Large, round and pryiform, acute angle)	Cattle and wild ruminants
Babesia ovata	4.5 by 2.5 μm (Large, round and pryiform, acute angle)	Cattle
Babesia equi	1.0-2.0 μm (small and rounded, Maltese cross is common)	Horses
Babesia trautmanni	3.5x2.0 μm (large, narrow and long, acute angle)	Swine

LIFE CYCLE OF BABESIA

Babesia is an important tick borne disease. The life cycle of babesia follows the general pattern of vector borne disease. The triads of pathogen, vector and host can be seen. Concerning the pathogen, several species of babesia are identified and becomes important problem for veterinarian medicine all around the world. For human, there are only two important species as previously mentioned. Concerning the vectors, specific vector for specific species of babesia can be seen (table 3.2).

Table 3.2. Morphological appearance of difference *Babesia* species [4]

Species	Vector
Babesia bigemina	*Boophilus annulatus, Boophilus decoratus, Boophilus. microplus*
Babesia bovis	*Boophilus annubtus, Boophilus microplus, Ixodes* spp.
Babesia divergens	*Ixodes ricinus*
Babesia jakimovi	*Ixodes ricinus*
Babesia ovata	*Haemaphysalis longicornis*

For human babesiosis, *Ixodes ricinus* is the specific vector for *Babesia divergens* and *Ixodes dammini* (deer tick) is the specific vector for *Babesia microti* [17].

Concerning the host, *Babesia microti* life cycle involves two hosts, which includes a rodent, primarily the white-footed mouse, *Peromyscus leucopus* [18]. During a blood meal, a *Babesia*-infected tick introduces sporozoites into the mouse host [18]. Sporozoites enter erythrocytes and undergo asexual reproduction (budding) [18]. In the blood, some parasites differentiate into male and female gametes although these cannot be distinguished at the light microscope level. The definitive host is a tick [18]. Once ingested by an appropriate tick, gametes unite and undergo a sporogonic cycle resulting in sporozoites [18]. Transovarial transmission has been documented for "large" *Babesia* spp. but not for the "small" babesiae, such as *Babesia microti* [18]. Human enters the cycle when bitten by infected ticks. During a blood meal, an infected tick introduces sporozoites into the human host [18]. Sporozoites enter erythrocytes and undergo budding and multiplication of the blood stage parasites is responsible for the clinical manifestations of the disease [18]. Human is a dead-end host [18].

For *Babesia divergens*, when the tick bites, sporozoites are injected into the blood stream and penetrate the erythrocytes, multiples by budding then the red cell ruptures and daughter parasites invade new erythrocytes for further asexual multiplication [19]. Some of the sporozoites injected by the tick vector follow a different path of intra-erythrocytic development, growing slowly and "folding" to form accordion-like structures which are destined to undergo further development in the tick vector [19]. Within the intestine of the tick, the accordion-like stage eventually fuses with another, to form a zygote [19]. Further development outside the intestine occurs in a variety of tissues, the salivary glands and ovaries being especially important for transmission [19]. Trans-ovarial transmission of *Babesia divergens* also takes place so that newly hatched tick larvae are already infected [19]. Similar to the case of *Babesia microti* infection, human enters the cycle when bitten by infected ticks and the similar pattern of infected red blood cell changes can be seen [19]. Comparing the life cycle of the babesia to malaria, there is no exoerythrocytic or tissue stage for babesia.

Pathophysiology of Babesia

The main clinical manifestations of human bebesiosis are due to the rupture of infected red blood cells as previously mentioned. According to this situation, the hemoglobinemia, hemoglobinuria, hemolytic jaundice and renal failure can be seen in the infected patients. Concerning the lysis of red blood cells, the increasing number of babesia within the cell is the main cause and lysis of red blood cells is for entering new uninfected red blood cells.

Similar to other infection, when an organism enters into human bodies, host defense will occur. Immunological reaction to babesia can be seen. *Babesia bovis* and its bovine host interact in many ways, resulting in a range of disease and infection phenotypes [20]. Host responses to the parasite elicit or select for a variety of responses on the part of the parasite, the full range of which is not known [20]. One well-established phenomenon, thought to aid parasite survival by evasion of host adaptive immune responses, is the sequential expansion of antigenically variant populations during an infection, a phenomenon referred to as "antigenic variation" [20]. This can also be seen in some human cases infected with *Babesia microti*. For human, immune response to babesia occurs via both cellular and humoral immune response mechanisms. However, the role of cellular immune response is more significant. As is emerging in other fields, study of interleukin-1 alone and synergistically with TNF and IFN-gamma, warrants further exploration in this parasitic disease [21]. Recently et al performed a study to characterized the cytokine response and T-cell requirements of mice infected with the intraerythrocytic parasites *Babesia microti* and WA1 [22]. According to this study, babesia-infected CD4-/- mice experienced a longer duration of parasitemia, indicating that CD4+ T cells participate in parasite elimination [22]. This study demonstrates differences in immune responses during fatal or resolving Babesia infections, and they identify TNF-alpha as an important mediator of the WA1-associated pathogenesis

[22]. Norimine et al found that a novel 78-kDa fatty acyl-CoA synthetase (ACS1) of *Babesia bovis* stimulated memory CD4+ T lymphocyte responses in *Babesia bovis* -immune cattle [23]. These reports can confirm the important of CD4+ T cell for response to babesia infection. In addition to CD4+ T cell, serum levels of tumor necrosis factor-alpha, interferon-gamma, interleukin-2 (IL-2), IL-6, E-selectin, vascular cell adhesion molecule-1, and intercellular adhesion molecule-1 are also highly elevated in the acute phase while normal levels of these mediators are observed one month after treatment [24]. Shaio and Lin suggested that CD8+ T cells and NK cells may be involved in the host defense mechanisms against acute babesiosis [24]. Aguilar-Delfin et al performed another study on the model of acute babesiosis with the WA1 Babesia [25]. Aguilar-Delfin et al suggested that a crucial part of the response that protected from the pathogenic Babesia WA1 was mediated by macrophages and NK cells, probably through early production of IL-12 and IFN-gamma, and induction of macrophage-derived effector molecules like nitric oxide [25].

Several host factors are involved in the response to the infection. Therefore, the clinical manifestations of diseases are different among different host species. For human, the difference of underlying immune status of the patients plays important role in determine of the severity of disease. Since cellular immunity is important protective mechanism for babesiosis, the immune deficiency status can lead to more severe disease [26]. Babesiosis should be considered in the differential diagnosis of HIV-infected patients with fevers and/or anemia in areas where the infection is endemic [27]. HIV-infected patients who are severely immunosuppressed, even those without a history of splenectomy, may present with severe manifestations of babesiosis and develop a chronic infection, which may require therapy to prevent relapse of disease [27]. In addition, spleen is an important organ corresponding to this infection. On animal model, the ability of immune rats to resist challenge with *Babesia divergens* depends upon mechanisms which are largely spleen independent [28]. Histological studies on livers collected from immune rats showed that lymphocytes are accumulated in the Liver and these consisted of B and T cells leukocytes accumulating in the liver might therefore be very important in the development of acquired immunity to *Babesia divergens* in splenectomised rats [28]. There are also some reports in animal that the asymptomatic infected animal can present overt clinical symptoms after splenectomy. For asplenic human host, the patient's lymphocytes usually reveal profound depression in mitogenic responses during acute disease [29]. Rosner et al proposed that Babesiosis must be considered as one of the not uncommon organisms responsible for the postsplenectomy sepsis syndrome and one for which there is no current prophylaxis [30].

Concerning the pathogenic invading property, the babesia can enter the host cell via the receptor method. *Babesia microti* has a tropism for mature erythrocytes [31]. Although reticulocytes are rarely infected, the delayed reticulocytosis in susceptible strains may result from parasite or host activities to limit renewal of the mature erythrocyte pool, thereby preventing an overwhelming parasitemia [31]. Alkhalil et al said that while both babesia and plasmodia increase host erythrocyte permeability to a diverse collection of organic solutes, they utilized fundamentally different mechanisms [32].Alkhalil et al found that plasmodial surface anion channel (PSAC)-like channels nor significant increases in whole-cell anion conductance were seen after *Babesia divergens* infection, which was different from *Plasmodium falciparum* [32]. Gaffar et al said that *Babesia bovis* merozoites invaded human, ovine, equine, porcine and caprine erythrocytes by a sialic acid-dependent mechanism followed by developmental arrest after a single round of cell fission [33]. Such invasion is dependent on the presence of sialic-acid containing membrane receptors on erythrocytes that interact with merozoite ligands that are probably already accessible during pre-incubation prior to invasion [33]. Zintl et al suggest that *Babesia divergens* was not host specific at the level of host cell attachment and invasion [34]. They found that parasite survival appeared to be decided once the organism has gained access into the cell [34]. They also found that treatment of bovine and non-bovine erythrocytes with neuraminidase decreased their susceptibility to invasion by up to 97% implicating sialic acid as an important erythrocyte ligand for babesia, but the addition of either bovine or human N-acetylneuraminyl-lactose to B. divergens cultures in bovine erythrocytes had no inhibitory effect [35].

Clinical Manifestation of Babesiosis

A. Bovine Babesiosis [36]

For cattle, Babesiosis should be suspected in cattle with fever, anemia, jaundice, and hemoglobinuria in endemic areas, particularly if there are signs of erythrocyte hemolysis. The differential diagnosis for bovine babesiosis includes anaplasmosis, trypanosomiasis, theileriosis, bacillary hemoglobinuria, hemobartonellosis, leptospirosis, and eperythrozoonosis. Rabies, other encephalitides, and toxins must also be considered in cattle exhibiting nervous signs.

B. Canine Babesiosis

The mechanisms causing the clinical manifestations in canine babesiosis are similar to other types of babesiosis. According to the study of Mathe et al, hepatopathy, pancreatitis, acute renal failure and disseminated intravascular coagulation were frequent complications, while immune-mediated hemolytic anaemia, acute respiratory distress syndrome and cerebral babesiosis were rarely observed [37]. According to another survey in Africa, cerebral babesiosis, enterorrhagia, 'red' or hemoconcentrated babesiosis, acute renal failure and pulmonary babesiosis or 'shock lung', amongst others, as the most prevalent forms of complicated babesiosis [38].

C. Human Babesiosis

The clinical signs and symptoms of babesiosis are related to the parasitism of red blood cells by *Babesia.* Fever, hemolytic anemia, and hemoglobinuria may result from *Babesia* infection [39]. Most of the infected usually give no exact history of having a tick bite. Generally, the incubation period of this infection varies from 1 to 4 weeks. Physical examination usually reveals fever with slightly hepatosplenomegaly. As with malaria, capillary blockage/microvascular stasis may occur as a result of red blood cell fragments, which explains liver, splenic, renal, and central nervous system (CNS) involvement [39]. With malaria, cells of the reticuloendothelial system in the spleen remove damaged red blood cell fragments from the circulation [39]. Therefore, splenectomy can affect the clinical pattern of human babesiosis. The patient, who had previously undergone splenectomy, usually has a more severe and prolonged illness [40].

DIAGNOSIS FOR BABESIOSIS

Clinical manifestations of babesiosis range from subclinical illness to fulminant disease resulting in death [41]. Prompt and accurate diagnosis is difficult because the signs and symptoms are non-specific [41]. Patients from areas endemic for babesiosis who present with malaria like illness should have a workup for babesiosis with the following direct and indirect tests. A complete blood count is a useful screening test since anemia and thrombocytopenia are commonly observed and parasites may be visualized on blood smear [41]. Conclusive diagnosis of this disease generally depends upon microscopic examination of thin blood smears [41]. The presence of hemolytic anemia with a blood picture of dysmorphic red cell and reticulocytemia can be seen. Howell-Jolly bodies indicative of splenic dysfunction, leukopenia, lymphopenia, thrombocytopenia can be detected. Wright or Giemsa stain on thin blood smears reveals the ring forms of babesisosis. Repeated examinations for many blood films are recommended. Patients with *Babesia* infection, in addition to having intraerythrocytic ring forms, also may demonstrate merozoites arranged in a tetrad configuration that resembles a Maltese cross. Quantitatively stained buffy-coat smears concentrate WBCs and increase the likelihood of demonstrating *Babesia* in the peripheral blood. The ability to identify babesiosis depends on the expertise and experience of the microbiologist or physician and the degree of parasitemia. According to the rat model study of Ike et al, a macrocytic hypochromic anemia with an increase of the reticulocyte count was detected as a rise in the parasitized erythrocyte rate [42]. In addition, white blood cell counts also remarkedly increased with the increases of both neutrophils and active-shaped monocytes, and thus these cells particularly play an important role in eliminating the parasite [42]. Atypical lymphocytes may be present, as they are in malaria, and the number of atypical lymphocytes is not related to the degree of parasitemia or the severity of illness. According to another study on canine babesiosis, there was a statistically significant difference between the thrombocyte counts of dogs with babesiosis when grouped by parasitaemia scores [43]. Concerning other hematological tests, an elevated erythrocyte sedimentation rate is common.

Considering the clinical chemistry test, change in liver function test can be seen. Elevated transaminase levels, an elevated alkaline phosphatase level, hyperbilirubinemia, and a decreased haptoglobin level can be presented. Increased serum transaminase levels usually are mildly and transiently elevated. A decreased haptoglobin level suggests a significant degree of intravascular hemolysis. Indeed, the nature of hemolytic jaundice is corresponding to the pathophysiology of this infection. Erwin and Hutchinson noted that pallor and jaundice were the most consistent observations at necropsy for canine babesiosis [44]. Lactate dehydrogenase (LDH) is another useful test for diagnosis of babesiosis. Increased LDH levels reflect the degree of parasitemia/severity of babesia. In 1995, Shikano et al studied on LDH isoenzyme pattern and reported that at least 5 bands were detected in *Babesia rodhaini*, while only one band in *Babesia microti* [45]. Since each subunit of LDH is known to be coded by different gene [45]. These results suggest that *Babesia microti* and *Babesia microti* are able to be differentiated genetically [45]. It was concluded that the extensive changes to muscle and to creatine kinase (CK) and LDH were caused by anoxia due primarily to shock and stasis of the circulation induced by the parasites [46].

It is noted that total serum protein, albumin, globulin, globulin fractions (alpha, beta and gamma globulins) and an acute-phase protein (alpha1-acid glycoprotein) were evaluated in dogs with naturally occurring babesiosis [47]. Serum protein electrophoresis (SPEP) usually shows polyclonal gammopathy indicative of B-lymphocyte hyperreactivity SPEP (polyclonal gammopathy) in response to T-lymphocyte suppression by *Babesia.*

Urinalysis should be obtained to check for hemoglobinuria. For canine babesiosis, proteinuria, and renal tubular casts and epithelial cells in urine sediment, are commonly observed in both complicated and uncomplicated babesiosis, but do not necessarily reflect or predict renal failure [48]. The degree of hemoglobinuria is related to the intensity of the *Babesia* infection. Serum creatinine measurements should be obtained to assess potential renal insufficiency. However, it must consider other causes of an increased serum creatinine before pointing these changes to *Babesia* infection. De Sally et al concluded that urea and creatinine did not behave in a similar and predictable manner over a range of azotaemia in canine babesiosis and were therefore not ideally suited for the detection of renal disease in this clinical setting [49].

For serology, immunoglobulin M (IgM) or IgG indirect fluorescent-antibody (IFA) tests *B microti* titers may be ordered in patients thought to have babesiosis, which has negative findings on peripheral smears especially for low levels of parasitemia. A single IgM IFA titer of 1:64 or greater is diagnostic of babesiosis. Increased IgG IFA *Babesia* titers indicate past exposure rather than current infection. IFA is effective in real clinical usage especially for seroepidemiology study [50]. However, the cross reaction for IFA was reported for other species of babesia and malaria. In addition to IFA, enzyme-linked immunosorbent assay (ELISA) for detection of *Babesia microti* antigen is also developed. Lao et al found that ELISA was effective in diagnosis for human babesisosi [51]. In additional to basic serology test, animal inoculation is also another alternative for diagnosis of babesiosis. Inoculation into hamster or gerbil can result in parasitemia within 2 - 4 weeks for positive cases. The most modern test for diagnosis of babesiosis is the diagnosis by polymerase chain reaction [52 - 53]. This test may be used to help diagnose recrudescent. PCR amplification with primers to the fragment from a gene encoding the nuclear small-subunit ribosomal RNA (SS-rDNA) may provide a sensitive tool also for the laboratory diagnosis of human babesiosis [54]. Since Babesia frequently are overlooked, however, because parasitemia tends to be sparse, often infecting fewer than 1% of erythrocytes early in the course of the illness, identification of amplifiable babesial DNA by PCR has comparable sensitivity and specificity to microscopic analysis of thin blood smear for detection of babesia in blood [55].

TREATMENT FOR BABESIOSIS

Treatment of human babesiosis can use the general principle for treatment of infectious disease: controlling of infection and getting rid of pathogen. Correctly identifying the infectious agent is important for treatment planning and prognosis [56]. The currently recommended therapy for babesiosis is a 7-10-day course of clindamycin (600 mg every 6 h) and quinine (650 mg every 8 h) [55]. Despite the superficial resemblance of Babesia to malaria, these piroplasms do not respond to chloroquine or other similar drugs [57]. However, the treatment of babesiosis using a clindamycin-quinine combination has been successful [57]. Data in animal models and case-reports in humans have suggested that an atovaquone-azithromycin combination is also effective [57]. Recently, azithromycin (500-600 mg on day 1, and 250-600 mg on subsequent days) and atovaquone (750 mg every 12 h) was found to be equally effective in treating adults experiencing babesiosis [55]. This combination also was associated with fewer adverse reactions than clindamycin and quinine [55]. Exchange transfusion is a potentially life-saving therapy for patients suffering from severe disease with high parasitemia (>5%), significant hemolysis, or renal or pulmonary compromise [55, 58]. Exchange transfusion has been advocated to reduce the level of parasitized red blood cells, to remove cytokines, and to improve the rheologic properties of the blood [59]. Dramatic improvement has been reported, but there are conflicting reports that question the need for exchange transfusion [59].

Prevention of Babesiosis

Prevention of babesiosis can base on the basic principle of prevention of vector borne disease. Potential control methods for hemoparasites that target parasites as they are developing in their respective tick hosts include tick control, vaccines (against ticks and parasites), and drugs (against ticks and parasites). Vector control should be first considered. In all known life cycles, initial infection of tick tissues occurs in midgut epithelial cells and transmission is effected as ticks feed after parasites have developed and multiplied in salivary glands [60]. Many factors reviewed affect development and transmission of hemoparasites by ticks including age of ticks, artificial temperature, climate and/or season, tick stage or sex, hemoparasite variation, concurrent infection of ticks with other pathogens, host cell susceptibility, transovarial transmission, effect of hemoparasites on tick biology, and the effect of infecting parasitemia level in cattle on infection rates in ticks [60]. Corresponding control methods base on the life cycle and ecology of vector should be designed. Control strategies will be dependent upon thorough understanding of parasite developmental cycles, biology of the tick vectors and the immune response of host to ticks and to hemoparasites [60]. The most effective control measures will be those that are targeted against both ticks and the hemoparasites they vector [60]. In contrast to vector control, avoidance of tick bite is another effective preventive method and might be easier. Advising patients about prevention of tick bites, especially in the summer months, may help prevent exposure to dangerous vector-borne diseases [61].

Vaccination against parasitoses of domestic animals is available at present. It has been known for several decades that the soluble parasite antigen (SPA) of several Babesia species can be used as a vaccine against the clinical manifestations of babesiosis [62]. Originally observed in the plasma of infected animals, SPA can also be recovered from the supernatants of in vitro cultures of these parasites [62]. Variable success has been reported for vaccines against the bovine and canine babesia parasites, which seems to be related to antigenic diversity within babesia species [62]. The good example is Pirodog for babesiosis in dogs [63]. It is commercially distributed and has been used in France since May 1988 [64]. Many things remain to be understood concerning individual susceptibility, the immunosuppressive effect of the disease, and the incidence of concomitant infections [64]. For bovine babesiosis, vaccine is also available [65]. Despite considerable research efforts into the development of alternative more consumer friendly vaccines, none is immediately forthcoming and the live attenuated babesiosis vaccines are still used in many countries [66]. Development of successful non-living recombinant vaccines will depend on increased understanding of protective immune mechanisms and availability of parasite genomes [67]. Two antigens from Babesia bovis, 12D3 and 11C5, are two antigens from *Babesia bovis* which is potential for new vaccine development [68]. For human babesiosis, vaccination has never been used. No vaccine is available for human protection [69].

Seromonitoring is another useful tool in prevention of babesiosis. It is a regular rule that the endemic countries must perform seroprevalence survey for the domestic animal hosts as well as epidemiological survey for the vector for the local endemic disease. Considering chemoprophylaxis, the effect of one dose of diminazene at 3 mg/kg bodyweight is sufficient to suppress all the clinical effects of the disease in bovine babesiosis [70]. However, there is no chemoprophylaxis recommendation for human babesisosis.

For prevention of human babesiosis, a focus of the possibility of disease transmission via blood transfusion is necessary. Infectious agents of disease continue to plague transfusion medicine as an increasing number of pathogens are described that pose a potential blood safety risk [71]. Reported cases of transmission, to date, have involved only the transfusion of red blood cells and, more rarely, platelets [72]. Despite the obvious public health issues posed by *Babesia* spp., options for preventing their transmission by blood transfusion remain limited [71]. However, recognition that the *Babesia* spp. are indeed an ongoing and expanding blood safety threat will probably prove instrumental in the development of viable interventions to limit transmission of these agents [71]. Improved strategies to assess and prevent transfusion-associated babesiosis are required [72]. Current measures cannot be relied on to identify infected donors with a high degree of sensitivity or to protect susceptible recipients from this parasite [72]. Photosensitization with pheophorbide derivatives may be a promising approach to inactivation of transfusion-transmissible babesia in blood bank units [73].

REFERENCES

[1] Cichocka A, Skotarczak B. Babesosis--difficulty of diagnosis. *Wiad Parazytol.* 2001;47:527-33.

[2] Babesia research. Available on www.vetmed.ucdavis.edu/VBDP/BABESIA.HTM

[3] Gray JS. Babesia sp.: emerging intracellular parasites in Europe. *Pol. J. Microbiol.* 2004;53 Suppl:55-60.

[4] Cleveland CW. Peterson DS, Latimer KS. An overview of canine babesiosis. Available online at http://www.vet.uga.edu/vpp/clerk/cleveland/index.php

[5] Ano H, Makimura S, Harasawa R. Detection of *Babesia* species from infected dog blood by polymerase chain reaction. *J. Vet. Med. Sci.* 2001; 63:111-113.

[6] Birkenheuer AJ, Levy MG, Savary KC, Gager RB, Breitschwerdt EB. *Babesia gibsoni* infections in dogs from North Carolina. *J. Am. Anim. Hosp. Assoc.* 1999; 35:125-128.

[7] Zahler M, Rinder H, Zweygarth E, Fukata T, Maede Y, Schein E, Gothe R. *Babesia gibsoni* of dogs from North America and Asia belong to different species. *Parasitology*. 2000; 120:365-369.

[8] Zintl A, Mulcahy G, Skerrett HE, Taylor SM, Gray JS. Babesia divergens, a bovine blood parasite of veterinary and zoonotic importance. *Clin. Microbiol. Rev.* 2003 Oct;16(4):622-36.

[9] Purnell RE. Tick-borne diseases of British livestock. Vet Med Rev. 1981; 1:58-69.

[10] Knowles RT, Montrose M, Craig TM, Wagner GG, Long RF. Clinical and serological evidence of bovine babesiosis and anaplasmosis in St. Lucia. *Vet. Parasitol.* 1982;10:307-11.

[11] Smith RD, Evans DE, Martins JR, Cereser VH, Correa BL, Petraccia C, Cardozo H, Solari MA, Nari A. Babesiosis (Babesia bovis) stability in unstable environments. *Ann. N. Y. Acad. Sci.* 2000;916:510-20.

[12] Littlejohn A, Walker EM. Some aspects of the epidemiology of equine babesiosis. *J. S. Afr. Vet. Assoc.* 1979;50:308-10.

[13] Mitrovic S, Kranjcic-Zec I, Arsic-Arsenijevic V, Dzamic A, Radonjic I. Human babesiosis--recent discoveries. *Med. Pregl.* 2004;57:349-53.

[14] Gray J, von Stedingk LV, Granstrom M. Zoonotic babesiosis. *Int. J. Med. Microbiol.* 2002;291 Suppl 33:108-11.

[15] Gorenflot A, Moubri K, Precigout E, Carcy B, Schetters TP. Human babesiosis. *Ann. Trop. Med. Parasitol.* 1998; 92:489-501.

[16] Gonzales EF, Todorovic RA, Adams LG. Ultrastructural de Babesia bigemina. *Rev. Inst. Col. Agropecuario.* 1971; 6: 87-112.

[17] Goethert HK, Lubelcyzk C, LaCombe E, Holman M, Rand P, Smith RP Jr, Telford SR 3rd. Enzootic Babesia microti in Maine. *J. Parasitol.* 2003;89:1069-71.

[18] Babesiosis. Available on http://www.dpd.cdc.gov/DPDX/HTML/Babesiosis.htm

[19] Babesia. Available at http://www.btinternet.com/~ukneqas.parasitologyscheme/Blood_Scheme/Teaching_Information/Babesia_species/babesia_species.html

[20] Allred DR, Al-Khedery B. Antigenic variation as an exploitable weakness of babesial parasites. *Vet. Parasitol.* 2006;138:50-60

[21] Clark IA, Cowden WB. Roles of TNF in malaria and other parasitic infections. *Immunol. Ser.* 1992;56:365-407.

[22] Hemmer RM, Ferrick DA, Conrad PA. Role of T cells and cytokines in fatal and resolving experimental babesiosis: protection in TNFRp55-/- mice infected with the human Babesia WA1 parasite. *J. Parasitol.* 2000;86:736-42.

[23] Norimine J, Ruef BJ, Palmer GH, Knowles DP, Herndon DR, Rice-Ficht AC, Brown WC. A novel 78-kDa fatty acyl-CoA synthetase (ACS1) of Babesia bovis stimulates memory CD4+ T lymphocyte responses in B. bovis-immune cattle. *Mol. Biochem. Parasitol.* 2006;147:20-9.

[24] Shaio MF, Lin PR. A case study of cytokine profiles in acute human babesiosis. *Am. J. Trop. Med. Hyg.* 1998;58:335-7.

[25] Aguilar-Delfin I, Wettstein PJ, Persing DH. Resistance to acute babesiosis is associated with interleukin-12- and gamma interferon-mediated responses and requires macrophages and natural killer cells. *Infect. Immun.* 2003;71:2002-8.

[26] Froberg MK, Dannen D, Bakken JS. Babesiosis and HIV. *Lancet.* 2004;363:704.

[27] Falagas ME, Klempner MS. Babesiosis in patients with AIDS: a chronic infection presenting as fever of unknown origin. *Clin. Infect. Dis.* 1996;22:809-12.

[28] Ben Musa N, Dawoud HA. Immunity of Babesia divergens in the rat. Histology of the infected liver and its possible role in removing PRBC's. *J. Egypt Soc. Parasitol.* 2004;34:791-806.

[29] Brown KS, Tanowitz HB, Rubinstein A, Kunkel M, Wittner M. Babesiosis in asplenic hosts. *Trans. R. Soc. Trop. Med. Hyg.* 1984;78:442-4.

[30] Rosner F, Zarrabi MH, Benach JL, Habicht GS. Babesiosis in splenectomized adults. Review of 22 reported cases. *Am. J. Med.* 1984;76:696-701.

[31] Borggraefe I, Yuan J, Telford SR 3rd, Menon S, Hunter R, Shah S, Spielman A, Gelfand JA, Wortis HH, Vannier E. abesia microti primarily invades mature erythrocytes in mice. *Infect. Immun.* 2006;74:3204-12.

[32] Akhalil A, Hill DA, Desai SA. Babesia and plasmodia increase host erythrocyte permeability through distinct mechanisms. *Cell Microbiol.* 2006 Nov 3;

[33] Gaffar FR, Franssen FF, de Vries E. Babesia bovis merozoites invade human, ovine, equine, porcine and caprine erythrocytes by a sialic acid-dependent mechanism followed by developmental arrest after a single round of cell fission. *Int. J. Parasitol.* 2003;33:1595-603.

[34] Zintl A, Westbrook C, Mulcahy G, Skerrett HE, Gray JS. Invasion, and short- and long-term survival of Babesia divergens (Phylum Apicomplexa) cultures in non-bovine sera and erythrocytes. *Parasitology.* 2002;124:583-8.

[35] Zintl A, Westbrook C, Skerrett HE, Gray JS, Mulcahy G. Chymotrypsin and neuraminidase treatment inhibits host cell invasion by Babesia divergens (Phylum Apicomplexa). *Parasitology.* 2002;125:45-50.

[36] Bovine babesiosis. Available online at http://www.cfsph.iastate.edu/ Factsheets/pdfs/bovine_babesiosis.pdf

[37] Mathe A, Voros K, Papp L, Reiczigel J. Clinical manifestations of canine babesiosis in Hungary (63 cases). *Acta Vet. Hung.* 2006;54:367-85.

[38] Collett MG. Survey of canine babesiosis in South Africa. *J. S. Afr. Vet. Assoc.* 2000;71:180-6.

[39] Cunha B, Barnett B. Babesiosis. Available online at http://www.emedicine.com/ med/topic195.htm

[40] Gombert ME, Goldstein EJ, Benach JL, Tenenbaum MJ, Grunwaldt E, Kaplan MH, Eveland LK. Human babesiosis. Clinical and therapeutic considerations. *JAMA.* 1982;248:3005-7.

[41] Krause PJ. Babesiosis diagnosis and treatment. *Vector Borne Zoonotic Dis.* 2003;3:45-51.

[42] Ike K, Takeuchi K, Uchida Y, Imai S. Hematological findings and antibody responses in Syrian hamster (Mesocricetus auratus) infected with Babesia microti. *J. Vet. Med. Sci.* 2005; 67:457-60.

[43] Kettner F, Reyers F, Miller D. Thrombocytopaenia in canine babesiosis and its clinical usefulness. *J. S. Afr. Vet. Assoc.* 2003;74:63-8.

[44] Erwin PJ, Hutchinson GW. Clinical and pathological findings of Babesia infection in dogs. *Aust. Vet. J.* 1991;68:204-9.

[45] Shikano S, Iwai Y, Shimada T, Ono K, Suzuki N. Isoenzyme patterns of glucose-6-phosphate dehydrogenase, malate dehydrogenase and lactate dehydrogenase in Babesia rodhaini and Babesia microti. *J. Vet. Med. Sci.* 1995;57:129-31.

[46] Wright IG, McKenna RV, Goodger BV. Acute Babesia bovis infections: plasma creatine kinase, lactate dehydrogenase and creatinine levels and associated muscle damage. *Z. Parasitenkd.* 1981;64:297-302.

[47] Lobetti RG, Mohr AJ, Dippenaar T, Myburgh E. A preliminary study on the serum protein response in canine babesiosis. *J. S. Afr. Vet. Assoc.* 2000;71:38-42.

[48] Lobetti RG, Jacobson LS. Renal involvement in dogs with babesiosis. *J. S. Afr. Vet. Assoc.* 2001;72:23-8.

[49] de Scally MP, Lobetti RG, Reyers F, Humphris D. Are urea and creatinine values reliable indicators of azotaemia in canine babesiosis? *J. S. Afr. Vet. Assoc.* 2004;75:121-4.

[50] Hunfeld KP, Lambert A, Kampen H, Albert S, Epe C, Brade V, Tenter AM. Seroprevalence of Babesia infections in humans exposed to ticks in midwestern Germany. *J. Clin. Microbiol.* 2002 Jul;40(7):2431-6

[51] Loa CC, Adelson ME, Mordechai E, Raphaelli I, Tilton RC. Serological diagnosis of human babesiosis by IgG enzyme-linked immunosorbent assay. *Curr. Microbiol.* 2004;49:385-9.

[52] Aguero-Rosenfeld ME. Laboratory aspects of tick-borne diseases: lyme, human granulocytic ehrlichiosis and babesiosis. *Mt. Sinai. J. Med.* 2003;70:197-206.

[53] Weinberg GA. Laboratory diagnosis of ehrlichiosis and babesiosis. *Pediatr. Infect. Dis. J.* 2001;20:435-7.

[54] Skotarczak B, Cichocka A. Isolation and amplification by polymerase chain reaction DNA of Babesia microti and Babesia divergens in ticks in Poland. *Ann. Agric. Environ. Med.* 2001;8:187-9.

[55] Krause PJ. Babesiosis diagnosis and treatment. *Vector Borne Zoonotic Dis.* 2003;3:45-51.

[56] Boozer AL, Macintire DK. Canine babesiosis. *Vet. Clin. North Am. Small Anim. Pract.* 2003;33:885-904, viii.

[57] Weiss LM. Babesiosis in humans: a treatment review. *Expert Opin. Pharmacother.* 2002;3:1109-15.

[58] Krause PJ. Babesiosis. *Med. Clin. North Am.* 2002 Mar;86(2):361-73.

[59] Powell VI, Grima K. Exchange transfusion for malaria and Babesia infection. *Transfus Med. Rev.* 2002;16:239-50.

[60] Kocan CM. Targeting ticks for control of selected hemoparasitic diseases of cattle. *Vet. Parasitol.* 1995;57:121-51.

[61] Bratton RL, Corey R. Tick-borne disease. *Am. Fam. Physician.* 2005;71:2323-30.

[62] Schetters T. Vaccination against canine babesiosis. *Trends Parasitol.* 2005;21:179-84.

[63] Eckert J, Deplazes P. Vaccines against parasitic diseases of domestic animals. *Tierarztl. Prax.* 1996;24:322-9.

[64] Moreau Y, Vidor E, Bissuel G, Dubreuil N. Vaccination against canine babesiosis: an overview of field observations. *Trans. R. Soc. Trop. Med. Hyg.* 1989;83 Suppl:95-6.

[65] Bock R, Jackson L, de Vos A, Jorgensen W. Babesiosis of cattle. *Parasitology.* 2004;129 Suppl:S247-69.

[66] de Waal DT, Combrink MP. Live vaccines against bovine babesiosis. *Vet. Parasitol.* 2006;138:88-96.

[67] Brown WC, Norimine J, Goff WL, Suarez CE, McElwain TF. Prospects for recombinant vaccines against Babesia bovis and related parasites. *Parasite Immunol.* 2006;28:315-27.

[68] Hope M, Riding G, Menzies M, Colditz I, Reverter A, Willadsen P. Potential for recombinant Babesia bovis antigens to protect against a highly virulent isolate. *Parasite Immunol.* 2005;27:439-45.

[69] Brasseur P, Gorenflot A. Human babesial infections in Europe. *Rocz. Akad. Med. Bialymst.* 1996;41:117-22.

[70] Sharma SP, Bansal GC. Chemoprophylaxis with diminazene aceturate in experimental Babesia bigemina infection in cattle. *Res. Vet. Sci.* 1984;37:126-7.

[71] Leiby DA. Babesiosis and blood transfusion: flying under the radar. *Vox. Sang.* 2006;90:157-65.

[72] Pantanowitz L, Telford SR 3rd, Cannon ME. The impact of babesiosis on transfusion medicine. *Transfus. Med. Rev.* 2002;16:131-43.

[73] Grellier P, Santus R, Mouray E, Agmon V, Maziere JC, Rigomier D, Dagan A, Gatt S, Schrevel J. Photosensitized inactivation of Plasmodium falciparum- and Babesia divergens-infected erythrocytes in whole blood by lipophilic pheophorbide derivatives. *Vox Sang.* 1997;72:211-20.

Chapter IV

Mycoplasmosis and Hemobartonellosis

Mycoplasmosis

A. Introduction

Mycoplasmas are prokaryote microorganisms without cellular wall that usually colonize the respiratory and urogenital mucosae [1]. The pathogenic species for mankind are *Mycoplasma pneumoniae*, that produce respiratory infections, among them pneumonia, and *M. genitalium*, *M. hominis* and *Ureaplasma urealyticum*, that produce urinary and genital infections [1]. Mycoplasmas represent a unique and complex group of microorganisms that has been ignored by the majority of diagnostic laboratories, not only because of its fastidious growth, absence of commercial media and of procedures for a rapid diagnosis, but most of all due to a clinical perception established for many years that these microorganisms are of minor importance [2]. Recently, this situation has changed, because there s a better understanding of mycoplasmas clinical importance, they have been recently associated with Human Immunodeficiency Virus (HIV), complications in pregnant women and their neonates and with rheumatological disorders, resulting in a need to cure infected persons [2].

B. Pathogenic Organism

Bacteria of the genus Mycoplasma are the smallest organisms known to be capable of self-replication [3]. They only occur in association with animal host cells on which they are dependant for many pre-formed nutrients since they lack many of the metabolic pathways associated with energy production and the synthesis of cell components found in other species of bacteria [3]. It is generally thought that most species of Mycoplasma are very host specific but there are many reports of mycoplasmas in hosts that are not perceived as their normal habitat [3]. Mycoplasmas are distinguished by their minute size and lack of a cell wall. The total lack of a cell wall explains many of the unique properties of these organisms, including their great sensitivity to detergents and osmotic shock and their resistance to penicillin and other cell-wall antibiotics [4]. The species that can be grown on agar tend to be easy to identify by their unusual fried-egg shaped colonies [4]. There are a number of different genera collectively referred to by the trivial term mycoplasmas, such as *Mycoplasma, Ureaplasma, Spiroplasma, Anaeroplasma, Phytoplasma* and others [4]. Molecular phylogeny places the mycoplasmas among the gram-positive bacteria of low G+C content [4]. It is likely that they were originally gram-positive bacteria and through constant association with a host went through degenerate evolution [4]. There is a notion that strains of mycoplasma species of strict host and tissue specificity exhibit marked genetic homogeneity, suggesting a clonal origin for some species [5]. The regions of the mycoplasma genome carrying the ribosomal RNA (rRNA) genes have been studied using restriction endonucleases, cloning, and hybridization procedures [5]. The mycoplasmal rRNA cistrons cross-hybridized among themselves, and with the seven rRNA cistrons of *Escherichia coli*, demonstrates the marked conservation of structure during evolution of this part of the procaryotic genome [5].

C. Pathogenesis

Mycoplasma can infect many animals including human. Avain mycoplasmosis is a good example of animal mycoplasmosis. The disease is most commonly spread at bird feeders and at roost sites. *M. gallisepticum* does not survive outside the body for any length of time [6]. Transmission usually occurs when large flocks feed or roost closely together and the organism is spread via the eye secretions to neighboring birds [6]. For dogs, the importance of all canine mycoplasmas remains unknown, yet certain species are associated with canine anemia (*M. haemocanis*), respiratory disease (*M. cynos*) and urogenital tract infections (*M. canis*) [7]. For human, mycoplasmosis is usually due to *M. pneumoniae*. Mycoplasma organisms cause infection primarily as extracellular parasites, attaching to the surface of ciliated and nonciliated epithelial cells [8]. The attachment site, or receptor, is a complex carbohydrate structurally akin to antigen I of red blood cells [8]. The antibody response to this receptor results in production of the anti-I antibody or cold agglutinin, which acts as an autoantibody [8].

M. pneumoniae represents one of the common etiological agents causing interstitial pneumonia, but more often a long-lasting tracheobronchitis in children and also in adults [9 - 10]. The incidence of *M. pneumoniae* diseases varies considerably [9 - 10]. *M. pneumoniae* infection occurs worldwide and is the most common cause of community-acquired pneumonia (CAP) in 5- to 20-year-olds [9 - 10]. The pathomechanism of this agent is based on a unique, gliding motility, adhesion to respiratory epithelium cells and the induction of a pathological hyperstimulation of cellular response mechanisms of the host [10]. Antigenic similarities between important functional sites of the adhesin of *M. pneumoniae* and various host molecules might be one of the factors responsible for hindering the host-response mechanism and, moreover, failing to protect the host repeated colonization [10]. Because the airway epithelium is a preferential site for *M. pneumoniae* infection and a major source of the chemokine regulated on activation, normal T cells expressed and secreted (RANTES) and transforming growth factor (TGF)-beta1, Dakhama et al postulated that this microorganism may contribute to the disease by inducing these mediators through direct interaction with airway epithelial cells [11]. Dakhama et al suggested that *M. pneumoniae* infection might contribute to the pathogenesis of chronic asthma at different levels of the airways, by inducing TGF-beta1 in large airways and the chemokine RANTES in small airways [11].

According to an animal model by Hayatsu et al [12], humoral immunity is more important than cell-mediated immunity in resistance of hamsters to *M. pneumoniae* pneumonia, and the antibody secreted in the respiratory tract may be involved in the local defense mechanisms. Attachment of *M. pneumoniae* to host cell by means of a specialized terminus initiates infection [13]. Monoclonal antibodies to a surface protein (Pl) inhibit this process, and react with a region of the tip covered with peplomer-like particles [13]. Since antibodies against the Pl protein are generated by natural and experimental infection and by immunization, the substance may be an important determinant of protective immunity [13].

It has also been suggested that groEL gene of *M. pneumoniae*t might be dispensable in vitro [14]. Bencina et al found that whereas all patients had strong antibody response to the P1 adhesin, only a few had antibodies to GroEL [14].

M. pneumoniae infection exacerbates asthma in children and may play a role in the pathogenesis of chronic asthma [10]. Yano et al found that the effects of mycoplasmal respiratory infections on the airway are multifactorial and involve a complex interplay of airway inflammation and IgE-mediated hypersensitivity [15].

D. Clinical Manifestation

Symptoms of *M pneumoniae* infection are often nonspecific. The onset is usually insidious, with fever, malaise, headache, and cough. Cough is a hallmark of *M pneumoniae* infection [8]. The frequency and severity of cough may increase over the few days after onset and may become debilitating [8]. In patients in whom the infection progresses to lower respiratory tract disease, the original symptoms persist, with a worsening and relatively nonproductive cough [8]. According to a study in Bangkok, The most common clinical manifestations were cough, fever, and headache [16]. According to another study in Saudi Arabia, cough, fever and malaise were the most common symptoms, and crepitations, and wheezes were the most common signs [17]. However, Wadowsky et al said that *M. pneumoniae* was not an important etiologic agent of persistent cough in adolescents and adults [18]. On occasion, white or blood-flecked sputum and parasternal chest pain may be present as a result of muscle strain [8].

As previously mentioned, CAP from the *M. pneumoniae* is common. Pneumonia is the main site of infection with Mycoplasma pneumoniae in paediatric age [19]. Nevertheless it can also give rise to other manifestations, with or without respiratory involvement [19]. Otitis media and sinusitis are uncommon [8]. Encephalitis and meningoencephalitis is the most frequent neurological manifestation, but cases of meningitis, acute transverse myelitis, stroke, and and polyradiculitis, have been reported [19 -20]. The recent introduction in clinical practice of newer molecular diagnostic techniques has helped in establishing a firmer association between *M. pneumoniae* infection and CNS disease especially encephalitis [20]. Clinicians should be aware of the potential association between *M. pneumoniae* infection and several CNS manifestations [20]. Cardiac involvement is potentially severe, including pericarditis and myocarditis [19]. *M. pneumoniae*-associated pericarditis may result in pronounced morbidity unless appropriate therapy is administered [21]. Cold agglutinin haemolytic anemia is the most frequent haematologic manifestation [19]. Hemolytic anemia due to cold agglutinin disease is a known complication of *M. pneumoniae* infection but is rarely observed [22]. Autoantibodies against erythrocyte membrane "I" antigen arise by the interaction of "I" antigen with M. pneumoniae is suspected, since "I" antigen is shown to be a receptor of this agent [22]. Corticosteroid therapy is sometimes necessary for the treatment of marked anemia [22]. Skin, renal, gastro-intestinal, osteoarticular, and other manifestations have also been reported in the literature [19]. Cherry said that the association of exanthem and pneumonia or of hemolytic anemia and pneumonia should suggest the diagnosis of *M. pneumoniae* infection, and an appropriate work-up should be carried out [23]. Postinfectious bronchitis may persist for weeks [8]. *M pneumoniae* infection may complicate asthma, and acute asthma may be the first manifestation of infection [8].

E. Diagnosis of Mycoplasmosis

Diagnosis of *M. pneumoniae* infection is challenging due to the fastidious nature of the pathogen, the considerable seroprevalence, and the possibility of transient asymptomatic carriage [24]. Serology, which is the basic strategy for mycoplasma diagnosis in routine clinical practice, has been improved by the widespread availability of sensitive assays for separate detection of different antibody classes [24]. The most reliable diagnostic test is the enzyme immunoassay, which allows IgG and IgM titration and presents 92% sensitivity and 95% specificity on paired samples [9]. According to a recent seroprevalence report from Malaysia, The male to female ratio was 1:1. The age specific rate was highest amongst patients of the 6-12 years [25] followed by the 13-20 years age groups [25]. For the diagnosis of mycoplasma pneumonia, serology and direct pathogen detection should be combined [24]. Direct antigen detection in sputum specimens is performed using antigen-capture indirect enzyme immunoassay [8]. Relatively high specificity and sensitivity are achieved [8]. Extrapulmonary diseases may be diagnosed by direct pathogen detection alone, but the value of this diagnostic approach is limited by the probably immunologically mediated pathogenesis of some manifestations [24].

Diagnosis carried out by serology and by culture for infections due to genital mycoplasmas are substituted by the new prospects, which may lead to a rapid diagnosis, detection by molecular hybridization [26]. Recently, a complete sequence analysis of the genome of the *M. pneumoniae* was performed by Himmelreich *et al* [27]. After that there are several attempts to develop the diagnostic tools based on molecular microbiology technique [24, 28]. During recent years, various new techniques have been adapted for the diagnosis of *M. pneumoniae* infection, notably in the field of molecular biology [24]. Standard polymerase chain reaction (PCR) is currently the method of choice for direct pathogen detection, but several PCR-related methods provide enhanced sensitivity or more convenient handling procedures, and have been successfully applied for research purposes [24]. Among these techniques are real-time PCR, nested PCR, reverse transcriptase PCR (RT-PCR) and multiplex PCR [24]. Generally, amplification-based methods have replaced hybridization assays and direct antigen detection [24]. Of several primers, the primers namely MP1 and MP2 are widely used for PCR diagnosis of the *M. pneumoniae* [29 - 30]. Here, the author performed a re-evaluation on the PCR test for detection of *M. pneumoniae* using MP1 and MP2 primers. The cross reactions to similar bacterial species were assessed. According to the PCR amplification, the electronic list of bands amplified and a DNA electrophoresis of the bands can be seen. The analysis of the PCR product shows that there are two separated bands, 466 and 469. The sequences of the 466 band and 469 band are shown in table 1. The results from cross – reaction analysis to the other *Mycoplasma spp.* and the other pathogenic member of the class Mollicutes (*Ureaplasma spp*) show no cross reaction. According to the electronic analysis of the product, two bands can be separated. Of interest, the two bands have never been noted before. The limitation in resolution of the PCR tool in the previous study revealed only the 466 band [7]. In addition, there was no report on the sequence of the band. Here, the sequence of the detected bands is also analyzed and presented.

Table 1. Sequences of the bands from amplification for detection of *M. pneumonia*

Band	Sequence
466	GTGAATGGGT TGTTGAATCC GGCGTTGGTG GAAACCTATT TTGGGAACAC GCGAGCGGGT GGTTCGGGGT CCAACACGAC CAGTTCACCC GGTATCGGTT TTAAAATTCC CGAACAAAAT AATGATTCCA AAGCCACCCT GATCACCCCC GGGTTGGCTT GAACGCCCCA GGACGTCGGT AACCTCGTTG TCAGTGGCAC CACGGTGAGC TTCCAGCTCG GCGGGTGGCT GGTCACCTTC ACGGACTTTG TCAAACCCCG CGCGGGTTAC CTCGGTCTCC AGTTAACGGG CTTGGATGCA AGTGATGCGA CGCAGCGCGC CCTCATTTGG GCCCCCCGGC CCTGAGCGGC CTTTCGTGGC AGTTGGGTCA ACCGGTTGGG CCGCGTGGAG AGTGTGTGGG ATTTGAAGGG GGTGTGGGCG GATCAAGCTC AGTCCGACTC GCAAGGATCT ACCACCACCG CAACAA
469	GTGAATGGGC TGTTGAATCC GGCGTTGGTG GAAACCTATT TTGGGACGAC GCGTACGTCT AGCACTGCGA ACCAAAACAG TACAACCGTC CCCGGTATCG GTTTTAAAAT TCCCGAACAA AATAATGATT CAAAGGCTGT GCTGATCACC CCCGGGTTGG CTTGAACGCC CCAGGACGTT GGTAACCTCG TTGTCAGTGG CACCAGCTTC AGCTTCCAGC TCGGCGGGTG GCTGGTCAGC TTCACGGACT TTGTCAAACC CCGCGCGGGT TACCTCGGAC TCCAGTTAAC GGGCTTGGAT GCAAGTGATG CGACGCAGCG CGCCCTCATT TGGGCCCCCC CGGCCCTGAG CGGCCTTTCG TGGCAGTTGG GTCAACCGGT TGGGCCGCGT GGAGAGTGTG TGGGATTTGA AGGGGGTGTG GGCGGATCAA GCTCAGTCCG ACTCGCAAGG ATCTACCACC ACCGCAACA

F. Treatment of Mycoplasmosis

Medical treatment for mycoplasmosis is recommended. Potentially active drugs are tetracyclines, macrolides, ketolides, lincosamides, streptogamines, chloramphenicol, and fluoroquinolones [9]. However, Erythromycin (as others macrolides) is the drug of choice [31]. Antibiotic susceptibility profile and on the development of acquired resistance for this microorganism become a new focus in mycoplasmology. The lack of a cell wall in mycoplasmas makes them intrinsically resistant to beta-lactams and to all antimicrobials which target the cell wall [32]. Intrinsic resistance related to specific mycoplasma species concerns essentially the acrolide-lincosamide-streptogramin-ketolide (MLSK) antibiotic group [32]. *M. pneumoniae* is susceptible to all MLSK antibiotics, except to lincomycin [32]. Among the three antibiotic classes used for the treatment of mycoplasmal infections including tetracyclines, MLSK group, and fluoroquinolones, macrolides and related antibiotics are the drug of choice for respiratory infections caused by *M. pneumoniae* [32]. Both target alterations and efflux mechanisms implicated in acquired antibiotic resistance have been described in mycoplasmas either by genetic mutation or transfer of new genes carried by transposons [32].

HEMOBARTONELLOSIS

A. Introduction

Hemobartonella felis is a gram-negative, non-acid-fast mycoplasma that lives on the surface of the red blood cell [33]. It is a pleomorphic uncultivated wall-less haemotrophic bacterial parasite. Measuring between 0.5 and 1.5 μm in diameter or length, this blood parasite exists as paired cocci, short rods, or small rings on the red blood cell plasma membrane [33]. Hemoplasma infections were associated with male gender, outdoor access, and old age, but not with disease or anemia [34]. In dogs, hemobartonellosis can be caused by H. canis. It should be noted that the clinical symptoms are usually milder than cats. Presently, Haemobartonella and Eperythrozoon species infecting the dog and cat have been reclassified as mycoplasmal parasites and given the names M haemofelis (Ohio or large form of *H. felis*), M haemominutum (California or small form of *H. felis*), and M haemocanis (H. canis) [35]. *H. felis* -OH is apparently more pathogenic than *H. felis*-CA. However, coinfection with both variants can be detected. Messick noted that the prevalence of hemotrophic mycoplasma infections in anemic cats in the USA was about 25% and usually involves *M. haemofelis* [35]. Transmission of the parasite is thought to occur by blood-sucking arthropods such as fleas or by bite wounds [33]. At present, it is beleived that transmission is presumed to be by blood-sucking parasites and possibly bite wounds between cats [36]. *H. felis* can also be vertically transmitted. Prevention requires prudent health management of cats [36].

B. Clinical Manifestation

H. felis is a rickettsial parasite that causes hemolysis and sequestration of feline erythrocytes [36]. It should be considered as a potential primary pathogen or opportunist in any cat presented with signs ranging from episodic malaise to acute anemic collapse [36]. A cat infected with *H. felis* may show mild anemia without clinical signs or may exhibit severe anemia with marked depression or subsequent death [33]. Parasitemic episodes correlate with a decline in the packed cell volume (PCV) [33]. The erythrocyte life span also shortens with each bout of parasitemia [33]. The primary method of red blood cell destruction is immune-mediated, although some direct damage may result from the presence of the parasite [33]. Concerning the hematological manifestations, an acute, severe hemolytic anemia accompanied by markedly increased numbers of nucleated erythrocytes as well as a remarkably elevated leukocyte count can be seen [37]. Presumably, the host makes antibodies against exposed erythrocyte antigens or altered erythrocyte antigens that result from attached organisms [33]. Due to the immune-mediated destruction of the red cell, these cats are Coombs' positive or may occasionally demonstrate autoagglutination [33]. The principal means of sequestration occurred when *H. felis*, located on the erythrocytes was removed by phagocytosis by a cordal macrophage, apparently preceded by the adhesion of extended processes of the macrophage to *H. felis* [38]. The second and least frequent means of removal of *H. felis* was by pitting, a process that did not cause destruction of the host erythrocyte [38]. The *H. felis* was pitted from the parasitized erythrocyte when *H. felis* passed through gaps between reticular cells or when the parasitized erythrocyte passed among the cytoplasmic processes of the reticular cells in the splenic cords [38].

C. Diagnosis of Hemobartonellosis

The best method of diagnosis is observation of *H. felis* infected erythrocytes in the Romanowsky-stained blood film [33]. In addition, organisms may detach from erythrocytes where they can be observed scattered singly or in small aggregates in the background of the smear [33]. The presence of stain precipitate may interfere with the identification of parasitemia, especially if few organisms are present [33]. PCR is a new diagnostic tool to increase the ability in detection of disease. The PCR assay is more accurate than cytologic examination for detection of *H. felis* infection and is an effective clinical tool for the detection and differentiation of both *H. felis* strains known to infect cats [39]. Results of the PCR are usually superior to results of CBC for detecting infection with *H. felis* [40]. According to the study of Berent et al, using PCR analysis, it was possible to detect *H. felis* in blood samples obtained from cats during peak parasitemia, during most of the carrier phase, and after challenge with immunosuppressive drugs [41]. During and immediately after antibiotic treatment, this test may fail to detect the organisms [41].

D. Treatment of Hemobartonellosis

Treatment uses antirickettsial drugs, corticosteroids, and supportive measures.

Clinical recovery requires immune containment of the organism [36]. Treatment does not eliminate the organism from the host [36]. Recently, Dowers et al performed a comparative study to compare treatment with enrofloxacin and doxycycline with no treatment in cats experimentally infected with *H. felis* [42]. Dowers et al concluded that enrofloxacin has anti-*H. felis* effects [42].

References

[1] Roca B. Mycoplasma infections. *Rev. Clin. Esp.* 2006;206:239-42.

[2] Domingues D, Nogueira F, Tavira L, Exposto F. Mycoplasmas: what is the role in human infections? *Acta Med. Port.* 2005;18:377-83.

[3] Pitcher DG, Nicholas RA. Mycoplasma host specificity: fact or fiction? *Vet. J.* 2005;170:300-6.

[4] Mycoplasma. Available at http://www.bact.wisc.edu/Microtextbook

[5] Razin S, Barile MF, Harasawa R, Amikam D, Glaser G. Characterization of the mycoplasma genome. *Yale J. Biol. Med.* 1983;56:357-66.

[6] Mycoplasmosis. Available online at http://www.michigan.gov/dnr/0,1607,7-153-10370_12150_12220-27089--,00.html

[7] Chalker VJ. Canine mycoplasmas. *Res. Vet. Sci.* 2005;79:1-8.

[8] Mycoplasma. Available online at http://www.emedicine.com/ped/topic1524.htm

[9] Blasi F, Tarsia P, Aliberti S, Cosentini R, Allegra L. Chlamydia pneumoniae and Mycoplasma pneumoniae. *Semin. Respir. Crit. Care Med.* 2005;26:617-24.

[10] Jacobs E. Mycoplasma infections of the human respiratory tract. *Wien. Klin. Wochenschr.* 1997;109:574-7.

[11] Dakhama A, Kraft M, Martin RJ, Gelfand EW. Induction of regulated upon activation, normal T cells expressed and secreted (RANTES) and transforming growth factor-beta 1 in airway epithelial cells by Mycoplasma pneumoniae. *Am. J. Respir. Cell Mol. Biol.* 2003;29:344-51.

[12] Hayatsu E, Kawakubo Y, Yayoshi M, Araake M, Wakai M, Yoshida A, Yoshioka M, Nishiyama Y. Immunological responses of hamsters in the acquired immune state to Mycoplasma pneumoniae infection. *Microbiol. Immunol.* 1981;25:1255-63.

[13] Bencina D, Slavec B, Narat M. Antibody response to GroEL varies in patients with acute Mycoplasma pneumoniae infection. *FEMS Immunol. Med. Microbiol.* 2005;43:399-406.

[14] Hu PC, Cole RM, Huang YS, Graham JA, Gardner DE, Collier AM, Clyde WA Jr. Mycoplasma pneumoniae infection: role of a surface protein in the attachment organelle. *Science.* 1982;216:313-5.

[15] Yano T, Ichikawa Y, Komatu S, Arai S, Oizumi K. Association of Mycoplasma pneumoniae antigen with initial onset of bronchial asthma. *Am. J. Respir. Crit. Care Med.* 1994;149:1348-53.

[16] Chaoprasong C, Chanthadisai N, Buasap U, Tirawatnapong S, Wattanathum A. Mycoplasma pneumoniae community-acquired pneumonia at three hospitals in Bangkok. *J. Med. Assoc. Thai.* 2002;85:643-7.

[17] Madani TA, Al-Ghamdi AA. Clinical features of culture-proven Mycoplasma pneumoniae infections at King Abdulaziz University Hospital, Jeddah, Saudi Arabia. *BMC Infect. Dis.* 2001;1:6.

[18] Wadowsky RM, Castilla EA, Laus S, Kozy A, Atchison RW, Kingsley LA, Ward JI, Greenberg DP. Evaluation of Chlamydia pneumoniae and Mycoplasma pneumoniae as etiologic agents of persistent cough in adolescents and adults. *J. Clin. Microbiol.* 2002;40:637-40.

[19] Garnier JM, Noel G, Retornaz K, Blanc P, Minodier P. Extrapulmonary infections due to Mycoplasma pneumoniae. *Arch. Pediatr.* 2005;12 Suppl 1:S2-6.

[20] Tsiodras S, Kelesidis I, Kelesidis T, Stamboulis E, Giamarellou H. Central nervous system manifestations of Mycoplasma pneumoniae infections. *J. Infect.* 2005;51:343-54.

[21] Farraj RS, McCully RB, Oh JK, Smith TF. Mycoplasma-associated pericarditis. *Mayo Clin. Proc.* 1997;;72:33-6.

[22] Nasu K. Mycoplasma infection and hemolytic anemia. *Nippon. Rinsho.* 1996;54:2545-9.

[23] Cherry JD. Anemia and mucocutaneous lesions due to Mycoplasma pneumoniae infections. *Clin. Infect. Dis.* 1993;17 Suppl 1:S47-51.

[24] Daxboeck F, Krause R, Wenisch C. Laboratory diagnosis of Mycoplasma pneumoniae infection. *Clin. Microbiol. Infect.* 2003;9:263-73.

[25] Tay ST, Cheong YM.A review of the serological results obtained in a routine diagnostic laboratory for Mycoplasma pneumoniae infections. *Malays J. Pathol.* 1995;17:35-7.

[26] Bebear C, de Barbeyrac B, Bernet C, Renaudin H. Methods of studying mycoplasma infections. *Ann. Biol. Clin.* (Paris) 1989;47:415-20.

[27] Himmelreich R, Hilbert H, Plagens H, Pirkl E, Li BC, Herrmann R. Complete sequence analysis of the genome of the bacterium *Mycoplasma pneumoniae*. *Nucl. Acids Res.* 1996; 24: 4420-4449.

[28] Loens K, Ursi D, Goossens H, Ieven M. Molecular diagnosis of *Mycoplasma pneumoniae* respiratory tract infections. *J. Clin. Microbiol.* 2003;41:4915-23.

[29] Tumwasorn S, Nilgate S, Udomsantisuk N. Amplification of P1 gene by polymerase chain reaction for detection of Mycoplasma pneumoniae. *J. Med. Assoc. Thai.* 2002;85 Suppl 1:S389-98.

[30] Forsyth MH, Geary SJ. The repetitive element Rep MP 1 of Mycoplasma pneumoniae exists as a core element within a larger, variable repetitive mosaic. *J. Bacteriol.* 1996;178:917-21.

[31] Della Santa L, Crimaldi G, Pellegrini V, Migliaccio P, Pampana A. Pulmonary infections in children. II - Mycoplasma pneumonia. *Minerva Pediatr.* 1994;46147-52.

[32] Bebear CM, Pereyre S Mechanisms of drug resistance in Mycoplasma pneumoniae. *Curr. Drug Targets Infect. Disord.* 2005;5:263-71.

[33] Hemobartonellosis. Available at http://www.vet.uga.edu/vpp/clerk/cowgill/index.php

[34] Willi B, Boretti FS, Baumgartner C, Cattori V, Meli ML, Doherr MG, Reusch CE, Hofmann-Lehmann R. Feline hemoplasmas in Switzerland: identification of a novel species, diagnosis, prevalence, and clinical importance. *Schweiz. Arch. Tierheilkd.* 2006;148:139-40, 142, 144.

[35] Messick JB. New perspectives about Hemotrophic mycoplasma (formerly, Haemobartonella and Eperythrozoon species) infections in dogs and cats. *Vet. Clin. North Am. Small Anim. Pract.* 2003;33:1453-65.

[36] Carney HC, England JJ. Feline hemobartonellosis. *Vet. Clin. North. Am. Small Anim. Pract.* 1993;23:79-90.

[37] VanSteenhouse JL, Taboada J, Dorfman MI. Hemobartonella felis infection with atypical hematological abnormalities. *J. Am. Anim. Hosp. Assoc.* 1995;31:165-9.

[38] Mayde Y. Sequestration and phagocytosis of Haemobartonella felis in the spleen. *Am. J. Vet. Res.* 1979;40:691-5.

[39] Berent LM, Messick JB, Cooper SK. Detection of Haemobartonella felis in cats with experimentally induced acute and chronic infections, using a polymerase chain reaction assay. *Am. J. Vet. Res.* 1998;591215-20.

[40] Westfall DS, Jensen WA, Reagan WJ, Radecki SV, Lappin MR. Inoculation of two genotypes of Hemobartonella felis (California and Ohio variants) to induce infection in cats and the response to treatment with azithromycin. *Am. J. Vet. Res.* 2001;62:687-91.

[41] Jensen WA, Lappin MR, Kamkar S, Reagan WJ. Haemobartonella felis in naturally infected cats. Use of a polymerase chain reaction assay to detect and differentiate two

strains of Haemobartonella felis in naturally infected cats. *Am. J. Vet. Res.* 2001;62:604-8

[42] Dowers KL, Olver C, Radecki SV, Lappin MR. Use of enrofloxacin for treatment of large-form Haemobartonella felis in experimentally infected cats. *J. Am. Vet. Med. Assoc.* 2002;221:250-3.

Chapter V

EHRLICHIOSIS

INTRODUCTION

Ehrlichiosis is a zoonotic disease cause by intracellular bacteria. The disease transmission is via tick bite. Ehrlichiosis is an infectious disease caused by obligate intracellular bacteria in genus Ehrlichia [1]. This disease was first reported in year 1935 in a dog [2]. After that there was a large outbreak of ehrlichiosis within dogs in Vietnam in 1960's [3]. According to this outbreak, there were a number of fatal deaths cases [3]. The corresponding pathogen in this outbreak is *Ehrlichia canis* [3]. This pathogenic organism is classified into family Anaplasmaceae [4]. It is an obligate intracellular bacteria. After entering the body, it will insert into phagocytic cell, macrophage, monocyte or neutrophill depending on the species. The organism will attach with the protein on the cellular surface receptor and enter into the endosome resulting in the inhibition of lysosome fusion process [5]. This pathological process cause an inclusion called "morulae" within the cytoplasm of the infected cell [6]. Each morulae contains the infective agents and those agents will multiply as binary fission, which can result in cell death according to the in vitro experiment [7].

Human infection of Ehrlichia spp was firstly reported in year 1986 as a new disease in UISA [1]. However, the exact cause of disease could not be demonstrated at that time. The patients had fever with unknown origin and blood smear examination reveals white blood cell inclusions. Further serological investigation reveals that the corresponding pathogenic organism is classified within the genus Ehrlichia; hence, this disease is called "human monocytic ehrlichiosis". In addition, there were the reports of Rocky Mountain spotted fever symptoms accompanied with human monocytic ehrlichiosis [8 – 10]. From history taking, most of the infectd cases gave the history of tick bites [9- 12]. The common clinical manifestations among these cases include fever, headache, nausea, vomiting and myalia [10 – 13]. However, these symptoms are usually non specific [10 – 13]. Some cases were asymptomatic. Some cases are mild while fatal illness could be detected sometimes [10 – 13]. Further studies reveal that the identified organism posed similar serological characters to *E. canis* but it posed different DNA sequence [14]. This organism was finally named as *E.chaffeensis* [14]. After the discovery of human monocytic ehrlichiosis, there was a new discovery of human granulocytic ehrlichiosis within neutrophills from patients with febrile illnesses. Further investigation reveals that the corresponding pathogenic organisms for these cases were *Anaplasma phagocytophilla* and *Neorickettsia equi*, which could be seen in the vertebrate animals as well [15].

Epidemiology

Human monocytic ehrlichiosis can be seen in 27 states of USA [6]. The disease can also be seen in Portuguese [16], Mali [17], Venezuela [18]. It usually presents as a nonspecific febrile illness a few days after a tick bite usually between late spring and fall. Considering human granulocytic ehrlichiosis, it can be seen in the upper Midwest and southeastern part of USA [2]. According to a study on 237 cases with human monocytic erhlichiosis during year 1985 to 1990 within 21 states of USA [19], it can be seen that more than 60% of the patients admitted to the hospital are the local people lived in the suburb or rural areas. 7.4% of overall cases lived with in the urban [19]. Most of diseases developed within the period between April and September [19]. Of overall infected cases, it was reported that about 68% had the exact history of tick bite while 15.5% of the cases has no history of tick bite but lived within the area with many ticks [19]. The incubation period of this disease is about 9 days (duration between 0 – 34 days). Generally, human monocytic erhlichiosis occurs within the southeastern part and central of Atlantic states where the local geography is vulnerable for the breeding of tick vectors. The primary tick vectors for this disease, carrying *Erhlichia chaffeensis*, include Lone Star Tick, Amblyomma americanum and dog tick [20 – 22]. Wiscosin et al reported a case series of this infection and said that 8 of 12 patients had a clear history of tick contact before having the fever [23]. The diagnosis of the infection must have a confirmed 4 folds rising of antibodies by immunofluorescence (IFA) or positive polymerase chain reaction (PCR) result.

Clinical Manifestation and Laboratory Diagnosis

Until present, the exact pathophysiology of human erhlichiosis has never been clarified. However, there is a hypothesis that after getting tick bite, the patient will derive the pathogen, erhlichiae, into the lymphatic and blood circulation. Then the pathogenic organic will invade into the monocytes or granulocytes within liver, spleen, veterbral body, lymph nodes and sometimes lungs. In the acute phase, the pathogenic organism will disturb the immune system and can cause the inflammation and infection of cells in circulation system. The resulted granuloma can be seen. Similar to other infections, the severity of infection depends on the immune status of the infected subject and the virulence of the pathogenic organisms [21 – 22].

Clinically, the symptoms of the patients infected with Ehrlichia vary from asymptomatic to severe symptoms. However, the symptoms of this infection are non specific [22]. Although HE and HME are caused by different pathogenic organisms the clinical manifestations of infections are similar and named as human erhlichiosis symptoms. These symptoms included fever, headache, nausea, vomiting, diarrhea, lymphadenopathy, abdominal pain, and etc. During the infection, 36% of the patients might present skin symptoms in monocytic erhlichiosis while fewer patiensts (about 8%) showed skin symptoms in granulocytic erhlichiosis. The estimated illness duration for the patients is generally equal to 23 days (duration 0 – 270 days). Despite the undifferentiated presentation of both ehrlichioses with fever, headache, myalgias, leukopenia, thrombocytopenia, and elevated liver enzyme activities, the diagnostic methods are distinct [24]. Considering the seroloigical technique, immunofluorescence assays (IFA) is widely used [2]. The IFA might have cross reaction with other *Ehrlichia* spp. Therefore, other confirmation tests are necessary. These tests include PCR diagnostic test and determination of morulae in granulocytic cell [2]. Since conventional methods, serological tests, are time-consuming, insensitive, and non-specific, new tools are needed for laboratory diagnostics [25]. Specific diagnostic modalities for acute-phase HGE include buffy coat smear examination and culture [26]. Culture appears to have the greatest sensitivity of the two tests. However, it is very difficult of perform a culture. During recent years, various new techniques have been adapted for the diagnosis of this infection, notably in the field of molecular biology and standard PCR is currently the method of choice for direct pathogen detection [5].Diagnosis carried out by serology was rapidly out of date [25] and is substituted by the new prospects, which may lead to a rapid diagnosis, detection by molecular hybridization [26]. After that there are several attempts to develop the diagnostic tools based on molecular microbiology technique [27]. Several attempts were made to develop Polymerase Chain Reaction (PCR) test for detection of the bacterium using several primers [27]. Of several primers, the primers namely HE1 and HE3 are widely used for PCR diagnosis of the ehrlichisosis [28]. The HE1 and HE3 primers from this diagnostic test are quoted from those used by Standaert *et al* [28]. The details of the mentioned HE1 and HE3 primer are 5'-CAATTGCTTATAACCTTTTGGTTATAAAT-3' and 5'-TATAGGTACCGTCATTATCTTCCCTAT-3', respectively [28]. According to the PCR amplification, the analysis of the PCR product can shows that there is a separated band, 390. The sequence of the 390 band is shown in table 5.1. No cross reaction for this PCR tool was reported. It was concluded that the PCR test for *Ehrlichia* spp detection of using HE1 and HE3 primers has good diagnostic property with no cross reaction to other species.

Table 5.1. The sequences of the 390 band product

TATAGGTACC GTCATTATCT TCCCTATTGA AAGAGTTTTACAACCCGAAG
GCCTTCTTCA CTCACGCGGC ATAGCTGGAT CAGGCTTTCG CCCATTGTCC
AATATTCCCC ACTGCTGCCT CCCGTAGGAG TCTGGACCGTATCTCAGTTC
CAGTGTGGCT GATCGTCCTC TCAGACCAGC TATAGATCATAGCCTTGGTA
AGCCATTACC TTACCAACTA GCTAATCTAACGTAGGCTCATCTAATAGCG
ATAAATCTTT CCCCCGCAGGGATTATACAG TATTACCCAT CATTTCTAAT
GGCTATTCCA TACTACTAGG TAGATTCCTA CGCATTACTC ACCCGTCTGC
CACTAACAATTATTTATAAC CAAAAGGTTA TAAGCAATTG

Concerning the laboratory manifestation of ehrlichiosis, this infection is a disease caused by Ehrlichia spp., which are obligate intracellular, Gram-negative bacteria showing tropism for blood cells (leukocytes and platelets). However, detection of the organism in the blood film requires very high skill in clinical microscopy. The number of infected white blood cells may be less than 0.2%, requiring examination of more than 500 white blood cells. Associated changes prompting careful film review include prominent toxic granulation and atypical large granular lymphocytes [29]. The common hematological findings include neutropenia (50-74%) and decreased platelet count (68-92%). Anemia can be seen in 50 % of the infected cases. Only a few cases demonstrate atypical lymphocytosis. Increased liver enzymes (AST and ALT) can be seen in 86 % -91 %. Generally, the neutropenia and thrombocytopenia accompanied with increased liver enzyme can be seen in the first week of illness while the anemia is usually detected within the second week, corresponding to the prolonged thrombocytopenia [2]. According to a case series reported by Schutze and Jacobs, patients demonstrated thrombocytopenia (92%), elevated liver function tests (91%), lymphopenia (75%), hyponatremia (67%), leukopenia (58%), and anemia (42%) on the initial laboratory examination [30]. Another study by Bakken et al found that most infected cases of HGE had headache, myalgias, chills, and varying combinations of leukopenia, anemia, and thrombocytopenia [31]. In this study, 80 % of the patients tested demonstrated morulae in the cytoplasm of peripheral blood neutrophils [31].

Complication

The complications of ehrlichiosis can result in high fatality. For human monocytic erhlichiosis, the death rate is about 2 – 5% [19, 22]. While the death rate for human granulocyte erhlichiosis is about 7 – 10% [19, 22]. Several complications of ehrlichiosis are reported in the literatures. With increasing disease identification has come recognition that the infections can be severe, with approximately about 50 % of patients requiring hospitalization for complications including respiratory distress, myocarditis, neurological complications, hepatitis, a septic or toxic shock-like disease and opportunistic infections. For kidney complication, mild elevation of creatinine and urinary protein can be seen [32]. Nephrotic syndrome from minimal change glomerulonephritis can also be seen a complication of ehrlichiosis [32]. For canine ehrlichiosis, chronic ehrlichiosis is suspected to be the cause of the dog's renal amyloidosis [33]. For neurological complications, focal neurologic complication of human ehrlichiosis is reported [34]. In addition, seizure and cerebrospinal fluid pleocytosis can be seen in the patients with ehrlichiosis [35 - 36].

There are also other interesting complications of ehrlichisosis. There is a report on the toxic shock syndrome of 6 patients with human ehrlichiosis [37]. These 6 patients have high fever, high blood pressure and multiple organs dysfunction [37]. There are also reported on the cardiac involvement in the patients with human ehrlichiosis. The patients usually present with cardiac failure [38]. Ischemic heart disease corresponding to the human ehrlichiosis is also reported [39]. It is recommended that additional chest radiography should be performed in the patients with human ehrlichiosis. For the death HME cases, bone marrow and hepatic granulomas and multiorgan perivascular lymphohistiocytic infiltrates are usually observed [40]. In HGE, opportunistic fungal and viral infections are important findings [40].

Ehrlichiosis in Immunodeficiency Virus Infection

Ehrlichiosis is a new emerging zoonosis. It may be a life-threatening illness in HIV-infected persons, and the influence of multiple factors, including recent changes in the epidemiology and medical management of HIV infection [41]. As is widely recognized, HIV infection is usually followed by the acquired immunodeficiency syndrome (AIDS) after a variable period during which the individual can develop different types of opportunistic infections whose severity depends on his/her immune status. Talbot et al said that infection in HIV-positive persons typically causes symptomatic disease [42]. According to a recent study of et al, the clinical course and laboratory evaluation of 21 patients coinfected with HIV and *Ehrlichia* spp were reviewed and summarized [41]. In this work, severe manifestations occurred more frequently among patients infected with *E. chaffeensis* than they did among patients infected with *E. ewingii*, and all deaths were caused by *E. chaffeensis* [41]. Paddock et al concluded that ehrlichiosis might be a life-threatening illness in HIV-infected persons, and the influence of multiple factors, including recent changes in the epidemiology and medical management of HIV infection, might increase the frequency with which ehrlichioses occur in this study [41]. del Tami et al said that the presence of *Ehrlichia* spp. in the platelets of HIV-positive patients suggested that ehrlichiosis should be among the differential diagnoses of opportunistic infection in this group of patients [43].

The present knowledge on the incidence of ehrlichiosis among HIV-infected patients is limited. Here, the author reports the experience on the seroepidemiology of ehrlichiosis in Thai hospital population. In this work, ehrlichiosis occurrence was determined in HIV+ patient assisted in a Thai sexually transmitted diseases clinic, King Chulalongkorn Memorial Hospital in period from January/2002 to December/2002. All works were ethically approved and performed under informed consent principles. In order to research, 200 patients were appraised. The blood samples were collected and sent for further examination for by an ELISA for Ehrlichia canis antibodies at Parasitology Laboratory, Department of Clinical Microscopy, Chulalongkorn University. The results verified only 1 positive sample (0.5 %). In this study, the cases with ehrlichiosis are from the group of naïve case without previous history of antiretroviral drug therapy (n = 64) while those who are in the antiretroviral therapy program (n = 136) had no infection. The rate of microsporidiosis is statistical significant higher among the group without antiretroviral drug therapy (3.1 % VS 0 %).

Considering the complication of ehrlichiosis among the HIV infected cases, similar complications, such as cardiopathy [44], to immunocompetent patients can be seen. Recently, Springer and Altice described a HIV-infected patient with a history of lipodystrophy who presented with hepatic insult associated with documented HGE [45]. In this case, despite a normal serum lactate level before the onset of acute coinfection, the patient developed symptomatic hyperlactatemia while receiving appropriate treatment for HGE [45]. Most data now suggest that alterations in host neutrophil function and protection from innate and adaptive immunity also contribute to disease manifestations [46]. It is reasonable to operate from the hypothesis that these host cell functional changes ultimately benefit bacterial survival while inadvertently eliciting clinical disease in poorly adapted hosts [46].

TREATMENT

Effective pharmacotherapy exists to treat each of these diseases, assuming diagnosis is made quickly [47 -49]. Doxycycline and rifampin were found to exert rapidly bactericidal effects, with MBCs in the extracellular culture medium of less than 0.5 and 0.125

microgram/ml, respectively [50]. *E. chaffeensis* was resistant to chloramphenicol, ciprofloxacin, erythromycin, co-trimoxazole, penicillin, and gentamicin, which had MICs greater than 16, 4, 8, 4, 40, and 32 micrograms/ml, respectively [50]. These observations are consistent with the finding that human ehrlichiosis appears to respond to tetracycline therapy, which has been the therapy of first choice [50]. The tetracyclines, but not the beta-lactams, are effective for human ehrlichioses [47 - 49]. Therapy usually starts with doxycycline, but chloramphenicol can also be used. Supportive and symptomatic therapies are also required. However, persistant infection despite therapy with tetracycline and chloramphenicol is also reported [51 - 52]. In these non responsive cases, serious illness with generalized edema, pulmonary infiltrates, acute respiratory distress syndrome, and noncardiogenic pulmonary edema, while receiving replacement intravenous fluids are usually observed [51 – 52]. High fatality can be detected for these cases [51 – 52].

This principle can also be applied for animal ehrlichisosis. Following a positive serological diagnosis of equine ehrlichiosis, treatment with oxytetracycline can be initiated [53]. It is also important to restore the fluid and electrolyte balance by infusion [53]. For canine ehrlichiosis, rapid restoration or improvement of appetite in treated dogs can be observed after treatment with piroxicam and oxytetracycline [54]. Both oxytetracycline and piroxicam are found to be suitable for use in dogs [54]. An increase in the platelet count may be an important indicator for dogs that recover from subclinical ehrlichiosis [55].

For recent advance in human ehrlichiosis, measurement of p44 expression may be a more rapid and simple assay to determine antibiotic susceptibility of the HGE agent in cell culture [56]. Furthermore, it may be used to indicate the presence of infection before morulae are apparent [56]. Since there are new additional evidence on the perinatal transmission of human ehrlichisosis, treatment of HGE during pregnancy becomes a new topic in obstetrics [57]. Since both tetracycline and chloramphenicol are contraindicated in pregnancy, the drug of choice for pregnant with human ehrlichiosis is rifampicin [58]. There are also potential difficulties in diagnosing HGE after plasma exchange, blood transfusion and immunosuppressive therapy [59]. Ehrlichiosis, a potentially curable disease, should be considered in the differential diagnosis of thrombotic microangiopathic disorders [59].

PREVENTION

Similar to other tickborne disease, the best way to prevent this infection is prevention from tick bite. Wearing of bright color dressing is recommended. Informing physicians and occupationally exposed people should reinforce current prevention measures against tick bites [60]. However, prophylactic antibiotic usage is not recommended [20 – 21]. Similar to other vector borne diseases, control of disease in the animal hosts is an effective way for disease control. Chemoprevention of canine monocytic ehrlichiosis with doxycycline is recommended [61]. Disease surveillance is also recommended similar to other infectious disease control. Yabsley et al said that integration of a deer surveillance system with geospatial analyses was useful in developing HME risk maps that will be useful for identifying high-risk areas for public health interventions such as prevention and control efforts [62]. Epidemiologic and environmental surveillance for ehrlichiosis in an endemic area should be done [63]. Vector control is another alternative for prevention of ehrlichiosis.

However, control of tick is basically more difficult than control of animal host or human self prevention. Blagbarn et al said that a combination of imidacloprid and permethrin could prevent transmission of *A. phagocytophilum* to dogs if administered before exposure to infected ticks [64].

It should also concern for prevention of human ehrlichiosis via other transmission methods. The HGE agent in infected blood specimens remained viable during refrigeration at 4 degrees C for up to 18 days [65]. These findings suggest that blood specimens submitted for culture may withstand transportation to a remote laboratory [65]. Kalantapour et al said that HGE should be added to the list of infections potentially transmitted by blood transfusion [65]. For control of the possible transmission via blood transfusion, several concerns on blood bank practice must be set. Leiby et al said that the exposure of blood donors to tick-borne pathogens did suggest a need to better understand the transfusion transmission potential of the pathogenic agents [66]. Although the screening for ehrlichiosis is not included a general practice in blood bank screening for human, it is included in a list for animal [67].

In addition, ehrlichiosis becomes a problematic infection for the patients receiving organ transplantation. Awareness and early diagnosis of the infection is paramount because appropriate therapy leads to rapid defervescence and cure [68]. In additional to new infection, reinfection of human ehrlichiosis is also noted for the transplant cases [69]. If left untreated, particularly in immunosuppressed patients, ehrlichioses may result in multi-system organ failure and death [68]. The affected patients usually present with fever and headache, had negative cultures, and despite broad-spectrum antimicrobial coverage appeared progressively septic [68]. After eliciting a history of tick exposure the patient should be empirically with doxycycline [68]. Human ehrlichiosis should be considered in the differential diagnosis of patients with solid organ transplants, who present with fever and thrombocytopenia [70]. Tan et al noted that although epidemiological exposure was responsible for infection, immunosuppression made patients more likely to succumb to disease [68]. They also proposed that a high index of suspicion and early treatment resulted in a favorable outcome [68].

References

[1] Maeda K, Markowitz N, Hawley RC, Ristic M, Cox D, McDade JE. Human infection with Ehrlichia canis, a leukocytic rickettsia. *N. Engl. J. Med.* 1987;316:853-6.

[2] Bakken JS, Dumler JS, Chen S-M, Eckman MR, Van Etta LL, Walker DH. Human granulocytic ehrlichiosis in upper Midwest United States. *JAMA.* 1994;272:212-8.

[3] Keefe TJ, Holland TJ, Salyer PE, Ristic M. Distribution of Ehrlichia canis among military working dogs in the world and selected civilian dogs in the United States. *J. Am. Vet. Med. Assoc.* 1982 ;181:236-8

[4] Dumler, J. S., A. F. Barbet, C. P. J. Bekker, G.A. Dasch, G. H. Palmer, S. C. Ray, Y. Rikihisa, and F.R. Rurangirwa. Reorganization of Genera in the Families Rickettsiaceae and Anaplasmataceae in the order Rickettsiales; Unification of some species of Ehrlichia with Anaplasma, Cowdria with Ehrlichia, and Ehrlichia with Neorickettsia; Description of six New Species Combinaions; and Designation of Ehrlichia equi and

"HGE agent" as Subjective Synonyms of Ehrlichia phagocytophila. *Int. J. Syst. Evol. Microbiol.2001.* 51: 2145-2165.

[5] Wells M, Rikihisa Y. Lack of lysosomal fusion with phagosome containing Ehrlichia risticii in P388D1 cells: abrogation of inhibition with oxytetracyclin. *Infect. Immune.* 1988;56:3209-15

[6] Dawson JE, Anderson BE, Fishbein DB, Sanchez JL, Goldsmith CS, Wilson KH, et al. Isolation and characterization of an *Ehrlichia* sp. from a patient diagnosed with human ehrlichiosis. *J. Clin. Microbiol.* 1991;29:2741-5.

[7] Dumler JS, Dawson JE, Walker DH. Human ehrlichiosis hematophatology and immunohistologic detection of Ehrlichia Chaffeensis. *Hum. Pathol.* 1993;24:391-6

[8] Fishbein DB, Sawyer LA, Holland CJ, Hayes EB, Okoroanyanwu W, Williams D, et al. Unexplained febrile illnesses after exposure to ticks. Infection with an *Ehrlichia*? *JAMA.* 1987;257:3100-4.

[9] Eng TR, Harkess JR, Fishbein DB, Dawson JE, Greene CN, Redus MA, et al. Epidemiologic, clinical, and laboratory findings of human ehrlichiosis in the United States, 1988. *JAMA.* 1990;264:2251-8.

[10] Rohrbach BW, Harkess JR, Ewing SA, Kudlac J, McKee GL, Istre GR. Epidemiologic and clinical characteristics of persons with serologic evidence of *E. canis* infection. *Am. J. Public Health.* 1990; 80:442-5.

[11] Harkess JR, Ewing SA, Crutcher JM, Kudlac J, McKee G, Istre GR. Human ehrlichiosis in Oklahoma. *J. Infect. Dis.* 1989;159:576-9.

[12] Fishbein DB, Kemp A, Dawson JE, Greene NR, Redus MA, Fields DH. Human ehrlichiosis: prospective active surveillance in febrile hospitalized patients. *J. Infect. Dis.* 1989;160:803-9.

[13] Taylor JP, Betz TG, Fishbein DB, Roberts MA, Dawson J, Ristic M. Serological evidence of possible human infection with *Ehrlichia* in Texas. *J. Infect. Dis.* 1988;158:217-20.

[14] Anderson BE, Dawson JE, Jones DC, Wilson KH. *Ehrlichia chaffeensis*, a new species associated with human ehrlichiosis. *J. Clin. Microbiol.* 1991;29:2838-42.

[15] Chen S, Dumler JS, Bakken JS, Walker DH. Identification of a granulocytotropic *Ehrlichia* species as the etiologic agent of human disease. *J. Clin. Microbiol.* 1994;32:589-95.

[16] Moralis J, Dawson JE, Greence CR, Filipe AR, Galhardas LC, Bacellar F. First europian case of ehrlichiosis. *Lancet.* 1991;338:633-4

[17] Uhaa IJ, Maclean JD, Greence CR, Fishbein DB. A case of human ehrlichiosis acquired in Mali: clinical and laboratory finding. *Am. J. Trop. Mad. Hyg.* 1992;46:161-4

[18] Arraga-Alvarado C, Montero-Ojeda M, Bernardoni A, Anderson BE, Parra O. Human ehrlichiosis: report of the 1st case in Venezuela. *Invest. Clin.* 1996 Mar;37(1):35-49

[19] Fishbein DB, Dawson JE, Robinson LE. Human Ehrlichiosis in the United States, 1985 to 1990. *Ann. Intern. Med.* 1994;120:736-743.

[20] Schaffner W, Standaert SM. Ehrlichiosis -- In Pursuit of an Emerging Infection. [Editorials] *N. Engl. J. Med.* 1996;334(4):262-263.

[21] Glushko GM. Human Ehrlichiosis. *Postgrad. Med.* 1997;101(6):225-230.

[22] Dumler JS, Bakken JS. Ehrlichial Diseases of Humans: Emerging Tick-Borne Infections. *Clin. Infect. Dis.* 1995;20:1102-1110

[23] Wormser G, McKenna D, Aguero-Rosenfeld M, et al. Human Granulocytic Ehrlichiosis- New York, 1995. *MMWR.* 1995;44(32);593-595.

[24] Dumler JS, Bakken JS. Human ehrlichioses: newly recognized infections transmitted by ticks. *Annu. Rev. Med.* 1998;49:201-13.

[25] Aguero-Rosenfeld ME. Laboratory aspects of tick-borne diseases: lyme, human granulocytic ehrlichiosis and babesiosis. *Mt. Sinai. J. Med.* 2003;70:197-206.

[26] Aguero-Rosenfeld ME. Laboratory aspects of tick-borne diseases: lyme, human granulocytic ehrlichiosis and babesiosis. *Mt. Sinai. J. Med.* 2003;70:197-206.

[27] Dumler JS, Brouqui P. Molecular diagnosis of human granulocytic anaplasmosis. *Expert. Rev. Mol. Diagn.* 2004;4:559-69.

[28] Standaert SM, Dawson JE, Schaffner W, Childs JE, Biggie KL, Singleton J Jr, Gerhardt RR, Knight ML, Hutcheson RH. Ehrlichiosis in a golf-oriented retirement community. *N. Engl. J. Med.* 1995;333:420-5.

[29] Hamilton KS, Standaert SM, Kinney MC. Characteristic peripheral blood findings in human ehrlichiosis. *Mod. Pathol.* 2004;17:512-7.

[30] Schutze GE, Jacobs RF. Human monocytic ehrlichiosis in children. *Pediatrics.* 1997;100:E10.

[31] Bakken JS, Krueth J, Wilson-Nordskog C, Tilden RL, Asanovich K, Dumler JS. Clinical and laboratory characteristics of human granulocytic ehrlichiosis. *JAMA.* 1996;275:199-205.

[32] Scaglia F, Vogler LB, Hymes LC, Maki A Jr. Minimal change nephrotic syndrome: a possible complication of ehrlichiosis. *Pediatr. Nephrol.* 1999;13:600-1.

[33] Luckschander N, Kleiter M, Willmann M. Renal amyloidosis caused by Ehrlichia canis. *Schweiz. Arch. Tierheilkd.* 2003;145:482-5.

[34] Carter N, Miller NR. Fourt h nerve palsy caused by Ehrlichia chaffeensis. *J. Neuroophthalmol.* 1997;17:47-50.

[35] Everett ED, Evans KA, Henry RB, et al. Human ehrlichiosis in adults after tick exposure diagnosis using polymerase chain reaction. *Ann. Intern. Med.* 1994;120:730-735.

[36] Dimmitt DC, Fishbein DB, Dawson JE. Human Ehrlichiosis Associated with Cerebrospinal Fluid Pleocytosis: A case report. *Am. J. Med.* 1989;87:677-678.

[37] Fichtenbaum CJ, Peterson LR, Weil GJ. Ehrlichiosis Presenting as a life-threatening illness with features of the Toxic Shock Syndrome. *Am. J. Med.* 1993;95:351-357.

[38] Williams JD, Snow RM, Arciniegas JG. Myocardial involvement in a Patient with Human Ehrlichiosis. *Am. J. Med.* 1995;98:414-415.

[39] Shea W, Calio AJ, Klein NC, et al. Rhabdomyolysis Associated with Ehrlichia chaffeensis Infection. [Report] *Clin. Infect. Dis.* 1995;21:1056-1057.

[40] Walker DH, Dumler JS. Human monocytic and granulocytic ehrlichioses. Discovery and diagnosis of emerging tick-borne infections and the critical role of the pathologist. *Arch. Pathol. Lab. Med.* 1997;121:785-91.

[41] Paddock CD, Folk SM, Shore GM, Machado LJ, Huycke MM, Slater LN, Liddell AM, Buller RS, Storch GA, Monson TP, Rimland D, Sumner JW, Singleton J, Bloch KC, Tang YW, Standaert SM, Childs JE. Infections with Ehrlichia chaffeensis and Ehrlichia ewingii in persons coinfected with human immunodeficiency virus. *Clin. Infect. Dis.* 2001;33:1586-94.

[42] Talbot TR, Comer JA, Bloch KC. Ehrlichia chaffeensis infections among HIV-infected patients in a human monocytic ehrlichiosis-endemic area. *Emerg. Infect. Dis.* 2003;9:1123-7.
[43] de Tami Idel C, Tami-Maury IM. Morphologic identification of Ehrlichia sp. in the platelets of patients infected with the human immunodeficiency virus in Venezuela . *Rev. Panam. Salud. Publica.* 2004;16:345-9
[44] Whitt SP, Everett ED, Roland W, Dolan S. Ehrlichia chaffeensis--associated cardiomyopathy in a patient with AIDS. *Clin. Infect. Dis.* 1999;28:140.
[45] Springer SA, Altice FL. Human immunodeficiency virus infection with human granulocytic ehrlichiosis complicated by symptomatic lactic acidosis. *Clin. Infect. Dis.* 2003;36:e162-4.
[46] Dumler JS. Anaplasma and Ehrlichia infection. Ann N Y Acad Sci. 2005;1063:361-73.
[47] Donovan BJ, Weber DJ, Rublein JC, Raasch RH. Treatment of tick-borne diseases. *Ann. Pharmacother.* 2002;36:1590-7.
[48] Klein NC, Cunha BA. New uses of older antibiotics. *Med. Clin. North Am.* 2001;85:125-32.
[49] Ungvatcharaprakarn V, Yaemsuwan T, Wiwanitkti V. Ehrlichiosis, review literature on human infec. *Songkhanagarind. Med. J.* 2004; 21:301-5.
[50] Brouqui P, Raoult D. In vitro antibiotic susceptibility of the newly recognized agent of ehrlichiosis in humans, Ehrlichia chaffeensis. *Antimicrob. Agents Chemother.* 1992;36:2799-803.
[51] Dumler JS, Sutker WL, Walker DH. Persistent infection with Ehrlichia chaffeensis. *Clin. Infect. Dis.* 1993;17:903-5.
[52] Weaver RA, Virella G, Weaver A. Ehrlichiosis with severe pulmonary manifestations despite early treatment. *South Med. J.* 1999;92:336-9.
[53] van der Kolk JH, de Groot J. Equine monocytic ehrlichiosis (EME), a review. *Tijdschr Diergeneeskd.* 1991;116:721-7.
[54] Adawa DA, Hassan AZ, Abdullah SU, Ogunkoya AB, Adeyanju JB, Okoro JE. Clinical trial of long-acting oxytetracycline and piroxicam in the treatment of canine ehrlichiosis. *Vet. Q.* 1992;14:118-20.
[55] Harrus S, Waner T, Aizenberg I, Bark H. Therapeutic effect of doxycycline in experimental subclinical canine monocytic ehrlichiosis: evaluation of a 6-week course. *J. Clin. Microbiol.* 1998;36:2140-2.
[56] Hsieh T, DiPietrantonio AM, Horowitz HW, Dumler JS, Aguero-Rosenfeld ME, Wormser GP, Wu JM. Changes in expression of the 44-kilodalton outer surface membrane antigen (p44 kD) for monitoring progression of infection and antimicrobial susceptibility of the human granulocytic ehrlichiosis (HGE) agent in HL-60 cells. *Biochem. Biophys. Res. Commun.* 1999;257:351-5.
[57] Casau NC, Hewins ME, Zaleznik DF. Treatment of human granulocytic ehrlichiosis during pregnancy and risk of perinatal transmission. *Scand. J. Infect. Dis.* 2002;34:853-5.
[58] Buitrago MI, Ijdo JW, Rinaudo P, Simon H, Copel J, Gadbaw J, Heimer R, Fikrig E, Bia FJ. Human granulocytic ehrlichiosis during pregnancy treated successfully with rifampin. *Clin. Infect. Dis.* 1998;27:213-5

[59] Modi KS, Dahl DC, Berkseth RO, Schut R, Greeno E. Human granulocytic ehrlichiosis presenting with acute renal failure and mimicking thrombotic thrombocytopenic purpura. A case report and review. *Am. J. Nephrol.* 1999;19:677-81.

[60] Amiel C, Abadia G, Choudat D. Human granulocytic ehrlichiosis in Europe. *Med. Mal. Infect.* 2004;34:111-22.

[61] Davoust B, Keundjian A, Rous V, Maurizi L, Parzy D. Validation of chemoprevention of canine monocytic ehrlichiosis with doxycycline. *Vet. Microbiol.* 2005;107:279-83.

[62] Yabsley MJ, Wimberly MC, Stallknecht DE, Little SE, Davidson WR. Spatial analysis of the distribution of Ehrlichia chaffeensis, causative agent of human monocytotropic ehrlichiosis, across a multi-state region. *Am. J. Trop. Med. Hyg.* 2005;72:840-50.

[63] Fritz CL, Bronson LR, Smith CR, Crawford-Miksza L, Yeh E, Schnurr D. Clinical, epidemiologic, and environmental surveillance for ehrlichiosis and anaplasmosis in an endemic area of northern California. *J. Vector Ecol.* 2005;30:4-10.

[64] Blagburn BL, Spencer JA, Billeter SA, Drazenovich NL, Butler JM, Land TM, Dykstra CC, Stafford KC, Pough MB, Levy SA, Bledsoe DL. Use of imidacloprid-permethrin to prevent transmission of Anaplasma phagocytophilum from naturally infected Ixodes scapularis ticks to dogs. *Vet. Ther.* 2004;5:212-7.

[65] Kalantarpour F, Chowdhury I, Wormser GP, Aguero-Rosenfeld ME. Survival of the human granulocytic ehrlichiosis agent under refrigeration conditions. *J. Clin. Microbiol.* 2000;38:2398-9.

[66] Leiby DA, Chung AP, Cable RG, Trouern-Trend J, McCullough J, Homer MJ, Reynolds LD, Houghton RL, Lodes MJ, Persing DH. Relationship between tick bites and the seroprevalence of Babesia microti and Anaplasma phagocytophila (previously Ehrlichia sp.) in blood donors. *Transfusion.* 2002;42:1585-91.

[67] Reine NJ. Infection and blood transfusion: a guide to donor screening. *Clin. Tech. Small Anim. Pract.* 2004;19:68-74.

[68] Tan HP, Stephen Dumler J, Maley WR, Klein AS, Burdick JF, Fred Poordad F, Thuluvath PJ, Markowitz JS. Human monocytic ehrlichiosis: an emerging pathogen in transplantation. *Transplantation.* 2001;71:1678-80.

[69] Liddell AM, Sumner JW, Paddock CD, Rikihisa Y, Unver A, Buller RS, Storch GA. Reinfection with Ehrlichia chaffeensis in a liver transplant recipient. *Clin. Infect. Dis.* 2002;34:1644-7.

[70] Vannorsdall MD, Thomas S, Smith RP, Zimmerman R, Christman R, Vella JP. Human granulocytic ehrlichiosis in a renal allograft recipient: review of the clinical spectrum of disease in solid organ transplant patients. *Transpl. Infect. Dis.* 2002;4:97-101.

Chapter VI

LEISHMANIASIS

INTRODUCTION

Leishmaniasis is an important tropical vector-borne disease. There are two common forms of leishmaniasis, cutaneous and visceral forms. Leishmanioses are a group of parasitic diseases that affect man and other mammals. They are caused by different species of trypanosomatids of the genus Leishmania [1 – 2]. Leishmaniasis represents a complex of diseases with a clinical and epidemiological diversity [3]. Leishmaniasis remains a severe public health problem and its burden is increasing [3]. The disease is caused by a parasite belonging to the genus Leishmania [3]. Approximately 350 billion people in 88 different countries are thought to be infected with Leishmania spp [3]. The distribution of this re-emerging disease, which is found throughout the world (except in Antarctica), is influenced by various factors linked to both human activity and climatic change [2]. The heteroecious life cycle of the Leishmania includes an invertebrate host (sandflies of the Phlebotomidae family) [2 - 4]. The dog is the main reservoir for many of the

Governed by parasite and host factors and immunoinflammatory responses, the clinical spectrum of leishmaniasis encompasses subclinical (inapparent), localised (skin lesions), and disseminated infection (cutaneous, mucosal, or visceral) [5]. Symptomatic disease is subacute or chronic and diverse in presentation and outcome [5]. Cutaneous leishmaniasis and VL are the two forms of leishmaniasis as previously described. Leishmania species, simultaneously present both cutaneous and visceral clinical signs [2 - 4]. Visceral leishmaniases (VL), with spreading epidemics in India and Sudan, and sporadic cases in mediterranean basin, show clinical, therapeutical and public health aspects varying according to the geographic context [6]. VL is considered an important fatal tropical blood infection.

VL is of higher priority than cutaneous leishmaniasis as it is a fatal disease in the absence of treatment [7]. Anthroponotic VL foci are of special concern as they are at the origin of frequent and deathly epidemics [7]. Leishmaniasis burden remains important: 350 million people at risk, 500,000 new cases of VL per year, 1-1.5 million for cutaneous leishmaniasis: 2.4 millions [7]. Most of the burden is concentrated on few countries which allow clear geographic priorities [7]. Leishmaniasis is still an important public health problem due to not only environmental risk factors such as massive migrations, urbanisation, deforestation, new irrigation schemes, but also to individual risk factors: HIV, malnutrition, genetic, etc [7]. The extent and presentation of the disease depend on several factors, including the humoral and cell-mediated immune response of the host, the virulence of the infecting species, and the parasite burden [8]. Children are at greater risk than adults in endemic areas. Malnutrition contributes to the development of disease, and incomplete therapy of initial disease is a risk factor for recurrence of leishmaniasis [8]. Molecular methods appear to offer the promise of accurate non-invasive tools for the diagnosis of Leishmaniasis [8]. World-wide, with the notable exception of India, pentavalent antimonial compounds remain the most effective and the most affordable therapy for this disease [8]. Lipid formulations of amphotericin B were assessed as short duration treatment and were proved to be effective; however, their cost precludes their wide use in developing countries [8].

Pathogenic Organism

Leishmania is a parasite. Leishmaniasis is primarily a zoonotic disease in which wild and domestic animals including the fox, jackal, rodents and wolves serve as reservoir hosts. Other animals can become infected and these are referred to as secondary or incidental hosts. Of all the potential animal hosts, domestic dogs play important role in transmitting the disease to humans. Leishmaniae spend part of their life cycle in the gut of the sandfly, but their life cycle is completed in a vertebrate host [9]. Leishmania parasites need phlebotomine sand flies to complete their life cycle and to propagate [10]. Within the sandfly gut, the protozoa are carried as extracellular promastigotes [9]. Over the course of 4-25 days, these parasites multiply in the gut and migrate toward the pharynx. As the leishmaniae replicate, they create a blockage in the fly's esophagus [9]. Concerning leishmania-sand fly interactions, the parasites develop from amastigotes to infectious metacyclics, highlighting recent findings concerning the evolutionary adaptations that ensure survival of the parasites [10]. Such adaptations include secretion of phosphoglycans, which protect the parasite from digestive enzymes; production of chitinases that degrade the stomodeal valve of the sand fly; secretion of a neuropeptide that arrests midgut and hindgut peristalsis; and attaching to the midgut to avoid expulsion [10]. Leishmania infections in the vector sandfly are limited to the gut, where contact with tissues, secretions and the medium of sandfly food influence their cycle of development [11]. Leishmania have a digenetic life cycle, involving a motile, extracellular stage (promastigote) which parasitises the alimentary tract of a sandfly vector [12]. Almost immediately the amastigotes transform in to the motile, elongated (10-20 micrometers), flagellate promastigote form [13]. Leishmania can adapt to survive in several hostile environments such as the vector insect midgut, blood and the mammalian macrophage phagolysosome [14]. Several Leishmania glycoconjugates have been implicated as key molecules for these remarkable capabilities [14]. The surface coat of the protozoan parasite Leishmania affords remarkable protection in the harsh environments encountered within the insect vectors and vertebrate hosts [15]. It also provides specificity for the interaction of these parasites with the cells in the sandfly gut and with the human macrophage [15]. Surprisingly few molecules have been identified on the Leishmania surface [15]. The major surface molecules of both promastigotes and amastigotes are the glycoconjugates lipophosphoglycan and a glycoprotein of approximately 63 kDa [15]. These major surface molecules vary structurally between Leishmania species and throughout the life-cycle of the parasite [15].

Bloodfeeding activity by an infected sandfly can result in transmission of infective (metacyclic) promastigotes to mammalian hosts, including humans [12]. When the sandlfy next feeds on a mammalian host, it's proboscis pierces the skin and saliva containing anti-coagulant is injected into the wound to prevent the blood from clotting, the leishmania promastigotes are transferred to the host along with the saliva [13]. Once in the host the promastigotes are taken up by the macrophages where they rapidly revert to the amastigote form [13]. Leishmania promastigotes are rapidly phagocytosed but may survive and transform into non-motile amastigote forms which can persist as intracellular parasites [12, 16]. The leishmania are able to resist the microbiocidal action of the acid hydrolases release form the lysozymes and so survive and multiply inside the macrophages, eventually leading to the lysis of the macrophages [13]. The released amastigotes are taken up by additional macrophages and so the cycle continues [13]. Leishmania amastigotes multiply in an acidic intracellular compartment, the parasitophorous vacuole [12, 16]. pH plays a central role in the developmental switch between promastigote and amastigote stages, and amastigotes are metabolically most active when their environment is acidic, although the cytoplasm of the amastigote is regulated at near-neutral pH by an active process of proton extrusion [12].

The vector of the leishmania is the blood-sucking female of the genus *Phlebotomus* in the old world and *Lutzomyia* in the new world. The insects are 2-3 mm long and are found through-out the tropical and temperate parts of the world [13]. The sandfly larvae require organic matter, heat and humidity for development and so are commonly found in house-hold rubbish, bark of old trees, burrows of old trees and in cracks in house walls [13, 17]. Cross et al said that the greatest sand fly activity and thus the highest risk of sandfly fever and leishmania infections occurred during the spring/summer months [18]. El Sayed et al said that seasonal density changes were correlated with temperature, relative humidity and rainfall prevailing in the area [19]. The sandflies usually feed at night while the host is asleep [20]. However, a phenomenon that could significantly influence the transmission rate: later host-seeking sand flies being more likely to find sleeping, nondefensive, human hosts [20]. Only 30 or so of the over 500 species of Phlebotomine sandflies are known to transmit leishmania parasites, these include *P.argentipes* on the Indian sub-continent, *P.martini* and *P.orientalis* in Africa and the Mediterranean basin, *P.chinensis* and *P.alexandri* in china [13]. In the new world *Lutzomyia logipalpis* is the only one vector [13].

PATHOGENESIS

Parasitic protozoa of the genus Leishmania infect mammalian mononuclear phagocytic cells causing a potentially fatal disease with a broad spectrum of clinical manifestations [21]. In order to invade the host cell Leishmania are able to recruit different surface receptors which may assist engaging the microbicidal responses [21]. Hespanhol et al performed an interesting study to analyze the expression of mannose receptors in primary cultures of skin fibroblasts further characterizing their role during the invasion of promastigotes of Leishmania [22]. After longer periods of Leishmania: fibroblasts contact, the modulation noted in the host mannose receptors was reverted concomitantly to the infection control, suggesting that the parasites were required for the alteration maintenance and providing evidences that the skin fibroblast may display microbicidal mechanisms to control the

Leishmania infection [22]. Extracellular matrix (ECM)-binding proteins on the surface of Leishmania are thought to play a crucial role in the onset of leishmaniasis, as these parasites invade mononuclear phagocytes in various organs after migrating through the ECM [23]. Both the promastigote and amastigote forms of Leishmania bind the basement membrane glycoprotein laminin with high affinity (Kd = 3.56 x 10(-9) M and 3.98 x 10(-9) M respectively) with approximately 9000 and approximately 800 sites per cell [24]. Ghosh et al proposed that propose that the 67 kDa protein is an adhesin involved in the attachment of Leishmania to host tissues [23]. Bandyopadhyay et al suggested a role for the 67 kDa protein in the interaction of the parasite with extracellular matrix elements, which might constitute a basis for the homing of the parasite to its physiological address [25]. In addition, Wilson and Hardin suggested that the major Con A-binding surface glycoprotein from leishmania promastigotes was important in attachment to human macrophages, and might be a factor in parasite virulence for a mammalian host [26].

In the intracellular phase, the pathogenic organism can deactivate and/or subvert the phagocyte signal transduction machinery rendering these cells permissive to infection [21]. Basically, MAP Kinase and JAK/STAT cascades are repressed, and intracellular Ca2+ and the activities of protein tyrosine phosphatases, in particular SHP-1, are elevated [27]. Activation of the JAK2/STAT1alpha signaling pathway is repressed in Leishmania-infected macrophages [28]. This represents an important mechanism by which this parasite subverts the microbicidal functions of the cell to promote its own survival and propagation [28]. Perturbation of macrophage surface with pathogens leads to activate general signal transduction pathways of macrophages, including activation of NADPH oxidase, nitric oxide synthase, and so on [29]. However, the results of macrophage interactions only with Leishmania parasites, which harbor the host macrophages, are discussed [29]. It appears that interference in transduction of regulatory signals during leishmanial invasion lead to an inadequate leishmanicidal response [29]. Reduced basal and IFN-gamma-induced activity of the NOS2 transcriptional unit accompanies the inability of the host to control an intracellular pathogen [30]. The parasitic protozoan Leishmania specifically manipulates the expression of host macrophage genes during initial interactions, as revealed by mRNA differential display reverse transcription-PCR and cDNA microarray analyses [31]. Misra et al conclude that Leishmania down-regulates 7SL RNA in macrophages to manipulate the targeting of many proteins that use the vesicular transport pathway and thus favors its successful establishment of infection in macrophages [31].

Being the most important determinant not only cellular immunity plays the essential role in the control of leishmaniasis, but the virulence, tropism and pathogenicity that is modulated by environmental and genetic factors of their mammalian hosts and sandfly vectors, are the key interactions [3]. These eukaryotic pathogens have evolved with the vertebrate immune system and typically produce long lasting chronic infections [3]. The obligate intracellular leishmania must survive the antimicrobial activities of its host cell, the macrophage, and prevent activation of an effective immune response [32]. In order to do this, it has developed numerous highly successful strategies for manipulating activities, including antigen presentation, nitric oxide and oxygen radical generation, and cytokine production [32]. A critical step in their host interaction is the evasion of innate immune defenses [3]. After transmission of Leishmania parasites by sandflies, disease manifestation of the infection requires mechanisms which allow the parasites to replicate in the mammalian host and to resist, at least initially, its innate and acquired antileishmanial defence [33]. Likewise, lifelong persistence of Leishmania parasites, as it occurs even in cases of clinical healing of the infection, points to the existence of strategies which enable the parasite to partially circumvent the protective adaptive immune response of the host [33]. The quoted defense mechanisms include the passive protection of the parasite against antileishmanial products and the retreat into "safe target cells", the active suppression of the synthesis of reactive oxygen or nitrogen intermediates, the modulation of the host cytokine response, the inhibition of antigen-presentation and T cell-stimulation, and the induction and expansion of counterprotective T helper cells [33].

In mice, IFN-gamma, produced by natural killer (NK) cells (AsGM1+, CD4-, CD8-, CD3), regulates CD4+ T cell subset development and early resistance to leishmania [34]. Rapid Th1 cell development and resistance to infection occur in mice that develop an NK cell response early after infection [34].

The ability to avoid attack by humoral effector mechanisms, such as complement lysis, and to resist killing by lysosomal enzymes and toxic metabolytes is also of particular importance [3].

By remodelling the phagosomal compartments in which they reside and by interfering with signalling pathways that lead to cellular activation, escaping of parasite can be expected [3]. Transforming growth factor-beta (TGF-beta) is a multipotential cytokine with diverse effects on cells of the immune system, including down-regulation of certain macrophage functions. Leishmanial infection induced the production of active TGF-beta, both in vitro and in vivo [35]. TGF-beta is important for determining in vivo susceptibility to experimental leishmanial infection and relates to escape mechanism [35]. In addition, leishmania can also modify the antigen presenting and immunoregulatory functions of dendritic cells, a process that fascilitates their evasion of both innate and adaptive immunity [3]. For cutaneous leishmaniasis, the polarization of Th2/Th1 cells is responsible for the progression of the disease which than leads to the chronic-persistant state [3]. However, the Th2/Th1 paradigm does not apply for VL [3]. Immunosupression rather than polarization is responsible for the systemic and progressive outcome of the disease in VL [3].

Clinical Manifestations

As previously mentioned, there are two main groups of leishmaniasis, cutaneous leishmaniasis and VL. VL is more severe and can be fatal. In some endemic areas, natives have recognized that immunity occurs as a natural course of the disease [9]. Some cultures deliberately inoculate their children on a part of the body that is not usually exposed to avoid later development of a disfiguring scar on an exposed part of the body [9].

A. Visceral Leishmaniasis

VL is a well-known tropical infection. Kala azar or black disease is the Indian name for visceral leishmaniasis. Darkening of the skin can be seen in the infected patients. VL can take different forms ranging from asymptomatic or self-resolving disease to fulminant disease. In addition, its onset can be insidious or sudden. In endemic areas, kala azar may be suspected in a patient with persistent, irregular, or remittent fever; leukopenia; and splenomegaly [36]. Other symptoms include lymphadenopathy and weight loss [36]. Considering VL, the typical symptomatic triad, anemia-fever-enlarged spleen, may be incomplete. The diagnosis of visceral form is conventionally made by the demonstration of amastigotes of the parasite in the aspirated fluid from the bone marrow, the spleen, and rarely from the lymph nodes, or the liver [36]. Doctors should bear in mind that especially immunosuppressed patients can present with atypical and abortive symptoms and that in this group of patients immune diagnosis is unreliable [37]. A diagnosis of a lymphoma related only to the spleen should not be made and splenectomy must not be carried out before reliable exclusion of kala azar, using modern diagnostic tools like PCR [37]. This disease is endemic to several tropical and subtropical countries, but also to the Mediterranean region [38]. As previously mentioned, this infection is transmitted by the sand fly (Phlebotomus, Lutzomyia). Occasional nonvector transmissions also have been reported through blood transfusions, sexual intercourse, organ transplants, excrements of dogs, and sporadically outside endemic areas [38]. Of interest, vertical transmission of VL is also reported [38].

VL is caused by at least 3 species of Leishmania protozoa: *L. donovani*, *L. infantum* and *L. chagasi* [39]. The incidence of the disease is estimated at 500,000 new cases annually. *Leishmania* spp. have a predilection to the reticulo-histiocytary system cells, leading to their proliferation and disruption, and after spreading to the circulation they invade spleen, liver and bone marrow [39]. The hepatic infection is usually self-limiting due to production of multiple cytokine responses including moderate level of TNF while in spleen excess TNF mediates destructive pathology [40]. CD8+ T cells appear to play multiple roles comprising both cytotoxic activity and secretion of cytokines and chemokines [40]. Capacity to produce ThI cytokines is associated with asymptomatic or subclinical self-healing infection. However, in symptomatic patients, Th I cytokine production is not depressed but there appears to be unresponsiveness to the stimuli of these cytokines [40]. Both teenagers and young children may be affected by this disease, whose clinical manifestations may be misleading [41]. The typical symptomatic triad, anemia-fever-enlarged spleen, may be incomplete, especially as a result of the intermittent character of the fever [41]. Patients may remain afebrile for long periods [41]. Concerning anemia, leishmaniasis anemia is an important tropical anemia [42 – 43]. Enhanced formation of oxidative metabolic products can be observed in the erythrocytes of the patients with VL [44]. Decreased activities of the protective enzymes suggest impairment of the defense mechanism against peroxidative threat [44]. These may contribute to some extent to the shortened lifespan of red cells in VL [44]. Major factors contributing to the anemia in VL are haemolysis occurring in both the massively enlarged spleen and liver and hemodilution resulting from expansion of the plasma volume [45]. There is no evidence of significant ineffective erythropoiesis, but a reduced plasma iron in the presence of greatly increased iron stores suggested that reticuloendothelial hyperplasia was accompanied by abnormal iron retention by macrophages typical of the anemia of chronic disorders [45]. According to the study of Karger and Rees, low serum iron and transferrin concentration, low total iron binding capacity and normal to high serum ferritin levels, consistent with anemia of chronic inflammation, was found [46]. Normo- to hypercellular bone marrow with increased erythropoietic activity can be observed [46]. In addition, low haemosiderin content of the bone marrow but normalization of hemoglobin without iron supplementation could argue against a major role of iron deficiency [46]. In addition, coagulation studies did not indicate diffuse intravascular coagulation [46].

Bone marrow leishmaniasis is a specific subtype of VL. Berentsen et al said that the identification of the parasites in bone marrow biopsy, should be performed in pancytopenic patients in the patients of unknown origin who had the history of visiting to the Mediteranian, the endemic area of VL [47]. Here, the author performed a literature review of the reports of bone marrow leishmaniasis in Thailand in order to summarize the characteristics of bone marrow leishmaniasis among Thai patients. According to the search, there have been at least 4 reports [48 - 51] in the literature of 5 cases of bone marrow leishmaniasis in the Thai population, of which no case was lethal. All cases are not immunocompromised. Concerning the clinical manifestations, all except had prolonged fever with unknown origin. From physical examination, all had hepatosplenomegaly. At the time of diagnosis, peripheral blood smear could not demonstrate the parasites. But pancytopenia could be seen in all cases. The bone marrow study was performed and revealed increased bone marrow cellularity, adequate production of magakaryocytes, erythroid and myeloid precursors. The striking findings were active hemophagocytosis with increased proliferation of lymphoidplasma cell line in the bone marrow and amastigotes of *Leishmania donovani* was demonstrated. Considering the treatment, pantavalent antimony compound was used and the excellent improvement and complete recovery of the clinical and hematologic abnormalities were obtained promptly after the administration. According to this study, it can be seen that all bone marrow leishmaniasis cases had the history of visiting to the Middle East. All had the classical triads but smear revealed no organisms. Indeed, in Thailand, other tropical infectious diseases such as malaria can give the picture of triad as well. However, the bone marrow aspiration to find the cause of unexplained pancytopenia can bring the final diagnoses in all cases. In this series, the bone marrow appearance show classical findings according to the bone marrow leishmaniasis. Detection of amastigote is the hallmark of diagnosis. However, some other rare appearances such as myelofibrosis are also reported [52]. Concerning the treatment, the pantavalent antimony is effective. Complete cure can be derived in all cases in this series. For treating VL, pentavalent antimonial compounds are still the first-line agents [53]. However, due to increasing resistance to this agent, many patients at present require other drugs including amphotericin B and pentamidine [53]. Toxic effects of these second-line agents have led to development of drug delivery systems like liposomal amphotericin B, which has shown uniform efficacy in clinical trials [53].

B. Cutaneous Leishmaniasis

Cutaneous leishmaniasis is usually not fatal. Cutaneous leishmaniasis can be caused by several *Leishmania* spp. [54]. For the new world cutaneous leishmaniasis, the pathogenic organisms include *L. tropica mexicana, L. braziliensis,* and *L. amazonensis.* For the old world cutaneous leishmaniasis, the pathogenic organisms include *L. tropica, L. major, L infantum,* and *L. ethiopica.* The disease occurs in varying presentations, from the self-limited and even self-healing cutaneous forms to fatal systemic disease [55]. The clinical manifestations range from simple cutaneous leishmaniasis to a more destructive mucosal inflammation (mucocutaneous leishmaniasis), the latter usually being a complication of infection with *L. braziliensis* or *L. ethiopica.* Lesions of cutaneous leishmaniasis may occur anywhere on the body but the most likely sites are the exposed parts. The initial papule rapidly gives rise to an ulcer [55]. Initially, the lesion is a small, red papule up to 2 cm in diameter [9]. Over several weeks, the papule becomes darker and will crust in the center, eventually ulcerating to present a typical appearance of an ulcer with raised edges and surrounding dusky red skin [9]. The ulcers can be moist or open with seropurulent exudate or dry with a crusted scab [9]. After about 3-6 months, the ulcers heal; leaving a raised border [9].Untreated sores can leave depigmented retracted scars [9]._Diagnosis of cutaneous leishmaniasis is difficult because of the varied symptoms and because making cultures of this parasite is complicated [54]. When faced with a possible leishmanial skin lesion, a skin scraping with microscopic analysis is the best test [56]. Punch biopsies with tissue-impression smears also can be diagnostic [56]. Needle aspiration of tissue fluid from the margin of a lesion can yield fluid for culture to isolate the organism and identify the species [56]. There are also different therapeutic, medical and surgical options, none of which is fully satisfactory [54]. The treatment mainstay is pentavalent antimony [56]. Not all patients require treatment; many lesions heal spontaneously [56]. Antimonials have a high incidence of reversible adverse effects. Other medications used for treatment include amphotericin B, pentamidine isethionate, paromomycin, and antifungals [56].

Mucocutaneous leishmaniasis is a destructive subtype of leishmaniasis [57]. Cutaneous lesions can be single or multiple [9]. Secondary mucosal lesions often develop after the primary lesion has healed [9].Mucosal lesions can progress to involve the entire nasal mucosa and the hard and soft palates [9]. Epidemiological data suggest that a detectable mucosal metastasis occurs in fewer than 5% of patients infected with *L. braziliensis* [58]. The determinants of this complication are still largely obscure [58]. The granuloma usually commences on the nasal septum [58]. In about two-thirds of our patients the lesions remain restricted to the nose [58]. In the rest the pharynx, palate, larynx and lips are involved, in this order [58]. Without treatment, the entire nasal mucosa and palates become deformed with ulceration and erosion of the nasal septum, lips, and palate [9].

Diagnosis of Leishmaniasis

As previously mentioned, diagnosis of VL rests on demonstration of the parasite in bone marrow specimens (several biopsies are often required) or in the spleen [41]. The diagnosis of VL is rarely from the lymph nodes, or the liver [59]. Bacteriologic studies using a special medium are helpful [41]. Serologic tests are sensitive and specific but often become positive only late in the disease [41]. Cultures are grown on NNN medium (media available from the CDC), a biphasic medium, or liquid media with fetal calf serum (eg, Schneider *Drosophila* medium) [9]. The parasite demonstration and isolation rates are rather poor from cutaneous and mucocutaneous lesions due to low parasite load and high rate of culture contamination [59]. Serologic testing is useful with the indirect fluorescent antibody test (IFAT), [9]. However, IFAT may cross-react in patients who have leprosy, tuberculosis, malaria, schistosomiasis, Chagas disease, and African trypanosomiasis [9]. ELISA methods are also available. Recently several recombinant proteins have been developed to accomplish accurate diagnosis. Recombinant kinesin protein of 39 kDa called rK 39 is the most promising of these molecules. The antigen used in various test formats has been proved highly sensitive and specific for visceral leishmaniasis [59]. It is useful in the diagnosis of HIV-Leishmania coinfection and as a prognostic marker [59]. With the recent advances in molecular biology, PCR methods were also developed for diagnosis of VL [60].

For diagnosis of cutaneous leishmaniasis, direct microscopic examination is helpful. Patients usually have a single ulcer that may heal spontaneously, requiring only topical, or no treatment at all [61]. Traditional diagnostic investigations for individual cases include the search of suggestive history and clinical features, the identification of amastigotes by histology or direct microscopy, and the growth of promastigotes in culture [62]. Diagnosis by the PCR seems to be approaching a gold standard status as novel techniques offer considerable advantages in the collection and transport of specimens and DNA extraction procedures that are more efficient in individual and field-based protocols [62]. Several authors have reported consistent 100% specificity with increasing sensitivity that overall is between 92 and 98% [62].

Treatment of Leishmaniasis

For VL, pentavalent antimonials (Sbv) have been successfully used for treatment of kala-azar for decades [63 - 64]. Pentavalent antimonials are the first-line treatment options worldwide except for in Europe and Sbv-unresponsive regions of India [65]. The therapeutic armamentarium for VL is currently plagued with several limitations as the available drugs are toxic, majority are effective only parenterally and need to be administered for extended periods [64]. Recently, miltefosine (hexadecylphosphocholine), a compound originally developed as an antitumour agent has been shown to be an orally effective drugs against kala-azar [66]. The first orally effective drug, miltefosine has been approved for treating VL [66]. In antimony refractory zones, pentavalent antimony has been largely replaced by amphotericin B deoxycholate, but prolonged hospitalization, toxic effects, and requirement for monitoring greatly hamper its widespread application in endemic regions [64]. Lipid formulations of amphotericin B, a remarkable advance in amphotericin B therapy, have greatly reduced toxicity enabling large doses to be delivered over a short period [64]. Amphotericin B deoxycholate is the drug of choice in India, as are its lipid formulations in Europe [65]. However, liposomal amphotericin B is the best antileishmanial formulation, but its prohibitive cost limits its use in endemic countries [65]. Combination of two most potent leishmanicidal drugs amphotericin B and miltefosine which are not dependent on host immune system, may shorten the course of therapy besides encountering unresponsiveness [63]. A combination therapy should be preferred when treating kala-azar associated with HIV/AIDS. Immunotherapy with exogenous Th1 stimulating cytokines or use of antileishmanial vaccine in combination with a potent chemotherapeutic agent is a future option [63]. The important problem in treatment for VL is drug resistance. Historically, Sb(v) has been highly effective in the treatment of VL at a low dose (10 mg/kg) for short durations (6-10 days) [67]. But in the early 1980s reports of its ineffectiveness emerged, and the dose of Sb (v) was eventually raised to 20 mg/kg for 30-40 days [67]. This regimen cures most patients with VL except in India, where the proportion of patients unresponsive to Sib (v) has steadily increased [67]. Notwithstanding the growing incidence of resistance, pentavalent antimony complex has been the mainstay for the treatment of VL during the last several decades [68]. The second line drugs such as amphotericin B, lipid formulations of amphotericin B, paromomycin and recently developed miltefosine are the other alternatives [68]. In spite of significant development in various areas of Leishmania research, there is a pressing need for the technological advancement in the understanding of immune response, drug resistance and the pathogenesis of leishmaniasis that could be translated into field applicable and affordable methods for diagnosis, treatment, and control of the disease [68]. With the introduction of new therapies, including miltefosine in 2002 and paromomycin in 2005-2006, it is essential that there be a strategy to prevent the emergence of resistance to new drugs; combination therapy, monitoring of therapy, and improved diagnostics could play an essential role in this strategy [69].

For cutaneous leishmaniasis, local treatment modalities including topical paromomycin, cryotherapy, localized controlled heat, carbon dioxide laser therapy, or intralesional meglumine antimoniate can be effective against *L. major* or *L. tropica* [70]. Oral fluconazole may be a second-line treatment. Parenteral antimonials are useful for persistent or recurrent Old World leishmaniasis [70]. For New World leishmaniasis, parenteral antimonials represent the first-line treatment in all forms except those caused by Leishmania guyanensis in which pentamidine is preferable [70]. Lesions caused by *L. braziliensis* may evolve into the mucocutaneous form, 'espundia', and should be treated with systemic antimony [61]. Sodium stibogluconate 20mg/kg/day i.v. for 20 days is the appropriate first line treatment in these cases [61]. Although it may cause transient bone marrow suppression, liver damage, a chemical pancreatitis, and disturbances in the electrocardiogram, it appears safe [61]. The success of treatment should be assessed 6 weeks after it has been completed and patients should be followed up for 6 months [61].

Prevention of Leishmaniasis

Vector control principle can be useful for prevention of leishmaniasis since it is a vector-borne disease [71 – 72]. Interruption of the cycle by vector control may offer a cheaper, more practical solution to treatment and improved knowledge of the alternatives available could lead to preventative measures being undertaken in more leishmaniasis foci [72]. Different measures to control phlebotomine sandflies, including residual spraying of dwellings and animal shelters, insecticide treated nets, application of repellents/insecticides to skin or to fabrics and impregnated dog collars are discussed [72]. Indoor residual spraying is a simple and cost effective method of controlling endophilic vectors and DDT remains the insecticide of choice for the control of leishmaniasis [71]. However resistance to insecticide is likely to become more widespread in the population especially in those areas in which insecticide has been used for years [71]. In this context use of slow release emulsified suspension (SRES) may be the best substitute. In this review spraying frequencies of DDT and new schedule of spray have been discussed [71]. It is also noted that DDT resistant *P. argentipes*, particularly in endemic zone is growing [73]. Although effective in urban areas with high concentrations of sandflies, residual spraying of insecticides is no often longer tenable in most situations. In rural areas where dwellings are more dispersed and surrounded by large, untargeted "reservoir" populations of sandflies, residual spraying of houses may be both impractical for logistic reasons and ineffective [72]. Role of biological control and environment management in the control of leishmaniasis has been emphasized [71]. Allethrin (coil) 0.1 and 1.6 per cent prallethrin (liquid) have been found to be effective repellents against *P. argentipes*, the vector of Indian kalaazar [71]. Insecticide impregnated bednets is another area which requires further research on priority basis for the control of leishmaniasis [71]. Vaccine for leishmaniasis is the new hope for prevention. Searching for the leishmaniasis vaccine is the ongoing research at present [74]. Candidates, including live or killed parasites, Leishmania purified fractions, defined recombinant parasite antigens, live recombinant bacteria expressing Leishmania antigens and antigen-encoding DNA plasmids, are on trials [75]. the first vaccine against canine visceral leishmaniosis was recently licensed in Brazil [76]. In the light of recent research, the Leishmune vaccine might be seen as the newest tool for prevention and control of canine visceral leishmaniosis [76]. Therefore, human leishamianiasis vaccine is the light at the end of the tunnel at present.

REFERENCES

[1] Murray HW, Berman JD, Davies CR, Saravia NG. Advances in leishmaniasis. *Lancet.* 2005;366:1561-77

[2] Gallego M. Emerging parasitic zoonoses: leishmaniosis, *Rev. Sci. Tech.* 2004;23:661-76.

[3] Yurdakul P. Immunopathogenesis of Leishmania infections. *Mikrobiyol. Bul.* 2005;39:363-81.

[4] Piscopo TV, Mallia AC. Leishmaniasis. *Postgrad. Med. J.* 2006;82:649-57

[5] Murray HW, Berman JD, Davies CR, Saravia NG. Advances in leishmaniasis. *Lancet.* 2005;366:1561-77

[6] Rosenthal E, Marty P. Visceral leishmaniases. *Rev. Prat.* 2004;54:2211-6

[7] Desjeux P. Leishmaniasis: current situation and new perspectives. *Comp. Immunol. Microbiol. Infect. Dis.* 2004;27:305-18.

[8] Kafetzis DA. An overview of paediatric leishmaniasis. *J. Postgrad. Med.* 2003;49:31-8.

[9] Leishmaniasis. Available online at http://www.emedicine.com/emerg/topic296.htm

[10] Kamhawi S. Phlebotomine sand flies and Leishmania parasites: friends or foes? *Trends Parasitol.* 2006;22:439-45.

[11] Schlein Y. Leishmania and Sandflies: interactions in the life cycle and transmission. *Parasitol. Today.* 1993;9:255-8.

[12] Burchmore RJ, Barrett MP. Life in vacuoles--nutrient acquisition by Leishmania amastigotes. *Int. J. Parasitol.* 2001;31:1311-20.

[13] Transmission of visceral leishmaniasis. Available online at http://homepages.uel.ac.uk/d.p.humber/akhter/trans.htm

[14] Ilg T. Lipophosphoglycan of the protozoan parasite Leishmania: stage- and species-specific importance for colonization of the sandfly vector, transmission and virulence to mammals. *Med. Microbiol. Immunol.* (Berl). 2001;190:13-7.

[15] Moody SF. Molecular variation in Leishmania. *Acta Trop.* 1993;53:185-204.

[16] Killick-Kendrick R. The life-cycle of Leishmania in the sandfly with special reference to the form infective to the vertebrate host. *Ann. Parasitol. Hum. Comp.* 1990;65 Suppl 1:37-42.

[17] Guernaoui S, Boussaa S, Pesson B, Boumezzough A. Nocturnal activity of phlebotomine sandflies (Diptera: Psychodidae) in a cutaneous leishmaniasis focus in Chichaoua, Morocco. *Parasitol. Res.* 2006; 98: 184-8.

[18] Cross ER, Newcomb WW, Tucker CJ. Use of weather data and remote sensing to predict the geographic and seasonal distribution of Phlebotomus papatasi in southwest Asia. *Am. J. Trop. Med. Hyg.* 1996;54:530-6.

[19] el Sayed SM, el Raaba FM, Abd el Nur O. Daily and seasonal activities of some sandflies from Surrugia village, Khartoum, Sudan. *Parassitologia.* 1991;33 Suppl:205-15.

[20] Villaseca P, Llanos-Cuentas A, Perez E, Davies CR. A comparative field study of the relative importance of Lutzomyia peruensis and Lutzomyia verrucarum as vectors of cutaneous leishmaniasis in the Peruvian Andes. *Am. J. Trop. Med. Hyg.* 1993;49:260-9.

[21] Vannier-Santos MA, Martiny A, de Souza W. Cell biology of Leishmania spp.: invading and evading. *Curr. Pharm. Des.* 2002;8:297-318.

[22] Hespanhol RC, de Nazare C Soeiro M, Meuser MB, de Nazareth S L Meirelles M, Corte-Real S. The expression of mannose receptors in skin fibroblast and their involvement in Leishmania (L.) amazonensis invasion. *J. Histochem. Cytochem.* 2005; 53:35-44.

[23] Ghosh A, Bandyopadhyay K, Kole L, Das PK. Isolation of a laminin-binding protein from the protozoan parasite Leishmania donovani that may mediate cell adhesion. *Biochem. J.* 1999;337:551-8.

[24] Ghosh A, Kole L, Bandyopadhyay K, Sarkar K, Das PK. Evidence of a laminin binding protein on the surface of Leishmania donovani. *Biochem. Biophys. Res. Commun.* 1996;226:101-6.

[25] Bandyopadhyay K, Karmakar S, Ghosh A, Das PK. Role of 67 kDa cell surface laminin binding protein of Leishmania donovani in pathogenesis. *J. Biochem.* (Tokyo). 2001;130:141-8.

[26] Wilson ME, Hardin KK. The major concanavalin A-binding surface glycoprotein of Leishmania donovani chagasi promastigotes is involved in attachment to human macrophages. *J. Immunol.* 1988;141:265-72.

[27] Gregory DJ, Olivier M. Subversion of host cell signalling by the protozoan parasite Leishmania. *Parasitology.* 2005;130 Suppl:S27-35.

[28] Forget G, Gregory DJ, Olivier M. Proteasome-mediated degradation of STAT1alpha following infection of macrophages with Leishmania donovani. *J. Biol. Chem.* 2005;280:30542-9

[29] Basu MK, Ray M. Macrophage and Leishmania: an unacceptable coexistence. *Crit. Rev. Microbiol.* 2005;31:145-54.

[30] Perez LE, Chandrasekar B, Saldarriaga OA, Zhao W, Arteaga LT, Travi BL, Melby PC. Reduced nitric oxide synthase 2 (NOS2) promoter activity in the Syrian hamster renders the animal functionally deficient in NOS2 activity and unable to control an intracellular pathogen. *J. Immunol.* 2006;176:5519-28.

[31] Misra S, Tripathi MK, Chaudhuri G. Down-regulation of 7SL RNA expression and impairment of vesicular protein transport pathways by Leishmania infection of macrophages. *J. Biol. Chem.* 2005;280:29364-73.

[32] Olivier M, Gregory DJ, Forget G. Subversion mechanisms by which Leishmania parasites can escape the host immune response: a signaling point of view. *Clin. Microbiol. Rev.* 2005;18:293-305.
[33] Bogdan C, Rollinghoff M. The immune response to Leishmania: mechanisms of parasite control and evasion. *Int. J. Parasitol.* 1998;28:121-34.
[34] Scharton-Kersten T, Scott P. The role of the innate immune response in Th1 cell development following Leishmania major infection. *J. Leukoc. Biol.* 1995;57:515-22.
[35] Lang T, Hellio R, Kaye PM, Antoine JC. Transforming growth factor-beta in leishmanial infection: a parasite escape mechanism. *Science.* 1992;257:545-8.
[36] Singh S, Sivakumar R. Recent advances in the diagnosis of leishmaniasis. *J. Postgrad. Med.* 2003;49:55-60.
[37] Sudeck H. Kala azar. Rare import and significant differential diagnosis. *Internist.* (Berl). 2006;47:825-8, 830-3.
[38] Meinecke CK, Schottelius J, Oskam L, Fleischer B. Congenital transmission of visceral leishmaniasis (Kala Azar) from an asymptomatic mother to her child. *Pediatrics.* 1999;104:e65.
[39] Stefaniak J, Paul M, Kacprzak E, Skoryna-Karcz B. Visceral leishmaniasis. *Przegl. Epidemiol.* 2003;57:341-8.
[40] Malla N, Mahajan RC. Pathophysiology of visceral leishmaniasis - some recent concepts. *Indian J. Med. Res.* 2006;123:267-74.
[41] Lagardere B, Chevallier B, Cheriet R. Kala-azar. *Ann. Pediatr.* (Paris). 1992;39:159-64.
[42] Woodruff AW.Recent work concerning anemia in the tropics. *Semin. Hematol.* 1982;19:141-7.
[43] La Placa G, Muschiato M, Arlati S, Urbano M, Verdura C. Anemia and hepatosplenomegaly: search for the protozoon? *Pediatr. Med. Chir.* 1994;16:475-7.
[44] Biswas T, Ghosh DK, Mukherjee N, Ghosal J. Lipid peroxidation of erythrocytes in visceral leishmaniasis. *J. Parasitol.* 1997;83:151-2.
[45] Pippard MJ, Moir D, Weatherall DJ, Lenicker HM. Mechanism of anaemia in resistant visceral leishmaniasis. *Ann. Trop. Med. Parasitol.* 1986 ;80:317-23.
[46] Kager PA, Rees PH. Haematological investigations in visceral leishmaniasis. *Trop. Geogr. Med.* 1986;38:371-9.
[47] Berentsen S, Langholm R, Reitan O. Visceral leishmaniasis (kala-azar). *Tidsskr. Nor. Laegeforen.* 1990;110:3491-3.
[48] Chutaputti A, Siripool P, Chitchang S, Radomyos P. Visceral leishmaniasis (Kala-azar) : with hypersplenism successfully treated with pentavalent antimony : report of 2 cases. *Intern. Med.* 1986; 2: 262 – 5
[49] Chutaputhi A, Siripool P, Chitchang S, Radomyos P. Visceral leishmaniasis (Kala-azar): a case report. *R. Thai. Army. Med. J.* 1986; 39: 98 – 5
[50] Seksarn P, Chumdermpadetsuk S, Dharmkrong-At A, Likitnukul S, Mitrakul C, Poshyachinda M. Visceral leishmaniasis: a case report. *Chula. Med. J.* 1984; 28: 1161-1170
[51] Tantaterdtham S, Susaengrat W. Visceral leishmaniasis : a case report (from Khon Kaen Regional Hospital). *J. Infect. Dis. Antimicrob. Agents.* 1991; 8 : 161-163
[52] Suvajdzic N, Pavlovic M, Misic S, Cemerikic V, Atkinson HD, Colovic M. Secondary myelofibrosis in visceral leishmaniasis--case report. *Haematologia. (Budap).* 2001;31:167-71.

[53] Aggarwal P, Handa R, Singh S, Wali JP. Kala-azar--new developments in diagnosis and treatment. *Indian J. Pediatr*. 1999;66:63-71.
[54] Garcia-Almagro D. Cutaneous leishmaniasis. *Actas Dermosifiliogr*. 2005;96:1-24.
[55] Khan SJ, Muneeb S. Cutaneous leishmaniasis in Pakistan. *Dermatol. Online J.* 2005;11:4.
[56] Markle WH, Makhoul K. Cutaneous leishmaniasis: recognition and treatment. *Am. Fam. Physician*. 2004;69:1455-60.
[57] Schwartz E, Hatz C, Blum J. New world cutaneous leishmaniasis in travellers. *Lancet. Infect. Dis.* 2006;6:342-9.
[58] Marsden PD. Mucosal leishmaniasis ("espundia" Escomel, 1911). *Trans. R. Soc. Trop. Med. Hyg.* 1986;80:859-76.
[59] Singh S, Sivakumar R. Recent advances in the diagnosis of leishmaniasis. *J. Postgrad. Med.* 2003;49:55-60.
[60] Mortarino M, Franceschi A, Mancianti F, Bazzocchi C, Genchi C, Bandi C. Quantitative PCR in the diagnosis of Leishmania] *Parassitologia*. 2004;46:163-7.
[61] Hepbum NC. Cutaneous leishmaniasis: an overview. *J. Postgrad. Med.* 2003;49:50-4.
[62] Vega-Lopez F. Diagnosis of cutaneous leishmaniasis. *Curr. Opin. Infect. Dis.* 2003;16:97-101.
[63] Jha TK. Drug unresponsiveness and combination therapy for kala-azar. *Indian J. Med. Res.* 2006;123:389-98.
[64] Sundar S, Chatterjee M. Visceral leishmaniasis - current therapeutic modalities. *Indian J. Med. Res.* 2006;123:345-52.
[65] Sundar S, Rai M. Treatment of visceral leishmaniasis. *Expert Opin. Pharmacother.* 2005;6:2821-9.
[66] Sangraula H, Sharma KK, Rijal S, Dwivedi S, Koirala S. Orally effective drugs for kala-azar (visceral leishmaniasis): focus on miltefosine and sitamaquine. *J. Assoc. Physicians India*. 2003;51:686-90.
[67] Sundar S. Drug resistance in Indian visceral leishmaniasis. *Trop. Med. Int. Health.* 2001;6:849-54.
[68] Singh RK, Pandey HP, Sundar S. Visceral leishmaniasis (kala-azar): challenges ahead. *Indian J. Med. Res.* 2006;123:331-44.
[69] Croft SL, Sundar S, Fairlamb AH. Drug resistance in leishmaniasis. *Clin. Microbiol. Rev.* 2006;19:111-26.
[70] Minodier P, Noel G, Blanc P, Uters M, Retornaz K, Garnier JM. Management of cutaneous leishmaniasis in adults and children. *Med. Trop.* (Mars). 2005;65:487-95.
[71] Kishore K, Kumar V, Kesari S, Dinesh DS, Kumar AJ, Das P, Bhattacharya SK. Vector control in leishmaniasis. *Indian J. Med. Res.* 2006;123:467-72.
[72] Maroli M, Khoury C. Prevention and control of leishmaniasis vectors: current approaches. *Parassitologia*. 2004;46:211-5.
[73] Kishore K, Kumar V, Kesari S, Bhattacharya SK, Das P. Susceptibility of Phlebotomus argentipes against DDT in endemic Districts of North Bihar, India. *J. Commun. Dis.* 2004;36:41-4.
[74] Poot J. Search for a vaccine against leishmaniasis] *Tijdschr Diergeneeskd.* 2006;131:694-5.
[75] Gradoni L. An update on antileishmanial vaccine candidates and prospects for a canine Leishmania vaccine. *Vet. Parasitol.* 2001;100:87-103.

[76] Dantas-Torres F. Leishmune vaccine: the newest tool for prevention and control of canine visceral leishmaniosis and its potential as a transmission-blocking vaccine. *Vet. Parasitol.* 2006;141:1-8.

Chapter VII

TRYPANOSOMIASIS

INTRODUCTION

Trypanosomiasis is an important vector borne blood infection. The pathogenic organisms causing trypanosomiasis is the parasite in the genus Trypanosoma. In the peripheral blood smear, it is usually characterized by an undulating membrane. There are three main medically important species: *Trypanosoam brucei gambiense*, *T. brucei rhodesiense* and *T. cruzi*. There are three main types of trypanosomiasis: African sleeping sickness caused by *Trypanosoam gambiense*, East African sleeping sickness caused by *T. rhodesiense* and Chagas disease caused by *T. cruzi*. Africa is the main endemic area for trypanosomiasis. Research on the disease suggests that the development of a vaccine is still far away; even existing drugs are becoming ineffective on account of the emergence of drug-resistant trypanosomes [1]. All this contributes to heavy economic losses and a sociopolitical crisis in the continent, thus underscoring the pressure to intensify research for inexpensive, less toxic and affordable trypanocides [1].

PATHOGENIC ORGANISMS

Trypanosoma spp. is a flagellate of the Kinetoplastida Order, Family Trypanosomatidae, characterized by the presence of one flagellum and a single mitochondrion in which is situated the Kinetoplast, a specialized DNA-containing organelle. Trypanosomes are parasites with a 2-host life cycle: mammalian and arthropod [2]. *T. brucei gambiense* and *T. brucei rhodesiense* are morphologically similar. For *T. brucei gambiense*, the main vertebrate host is human. This parasite is transmitted by vector, tsetse flies, most of which belong to the species *Glossina palpalis*. The life cycle starts when the trypanosomes are ingested during a blood meal by the tsetse fly from a human reservoir while an animal reservoir (zoonotic) is described in the East African form [2]. For African sleeping sickness, the life cycle in tsetse fly of *T. brucei gambiense* is very complex and required at least 3 weeks. For *T. cruzi*, the identification of this parasite by morphological and biological features does not offer difficulties and differential is only required for *T. rangeli*, a non-pathogenic flagellate which infects humans in some areas of Central and South America and is transmitted by some of the same vectors that transmit *T. cruzi* [3]. *T. cruzi* is not a homogeneous population and is composed rather by a pool of strains which circulate in both the domestic and sylvatic cycles involving humans, vectors and animal reservoirs of the parasite [3]. Isolation and study of *T. cruzi* populations from different origins demonstrated the presence of a large range of strains with distinct characteristics [3].

African Sleeping Sickness

African sleeping sickness or mid-African sleeping sickness is caused by *T. brucei gambiense.* There is a dramatic resurgence of human African trypanosomiasis in sub-Saharan Africa. The infection is spreading epidemically in large areas of Central Africa, especially the Southern Sudan, Congo-Zaire, Angola, Uganda and the Central African Republic [4]. It is estimated that some 55 million people are exposed to the risk of infection, of whom only 3.5 million are under surveillance throughout the endemic zone [5]. Available data indicate an average observed prevalence of 0.6% (approximately 20,000 annually reported cases among the people surveyed), which represents only 7% of the total population at risk [5]. The causes of the re-emergence of sleeping sickness as a public health problem include widespread civil disturbance and war, declining economies, reduced health financing and the dismantling of disease control programs [4].

A. Pathogenesis

The major epidemiology factor in African trypanosomiasis is the human-tsetse fly contact [2]. This interaction is influenced by an increasing tsetse fly density, changing feeding habits, expanding human development into tsetse fly–infested areas, and an increasing number of immunologically naïve persons in previously endemic areas [2]. Concerning the vector, tsetse fly generally implies any of several two-winged bloodsucking African flies of the genus Glossina, often carrying and transmitting pathogenic trypanosomes. More than 20 types of tsetse flies are described in Africa. Tsetse fly belongs to the sub-order Cyclorrhapha, and form, along with the families Hippoboscidae, Streblidae and Nycteribiidae, the superfamily Hippoboscoidea [6]. They are now placed within their own family the Glossinidae, with a single genus the Glossina, circumscribed by Wiedemann 1830 [6]. Tsetse flies are yellowish to brown, the abdomen may be uniformly coloured or transversed by stripes according to species [6]. Two visually distinctive characters that are apparent to the eye are the forward projecting proboscis and the unusual hatchet shaped cell formed by the wing venation [6]. A closer examination also reveals that the arista arising from the third antennal segment (a characteristic of Cylorrhapha) has branched setae which is not seen on any other flies [6]. Because the viability of the host often depends on these obligate symbionts, and because these organisms often live in close proximity to disease-causing pathogens, they have been of interest to applied biologists as a potential means to genetically manipulate populations of pest species [7]. Tsetse is mentioned as a heaven for *T. brucei gambiense* [7]. Concerning the confined epidemiology of disease, the particular ecological conditions of parasites and vectors are such that the disease is only found in the intertropical regions of Africa, therefore, this disease is limited to Africa [8].

As previously mentioned, disease transmission to human occurs after biting and inoculating by tsetse flies. Immediately after penetration into the human organism, the trypanosome multiplies at the point of inoculation, producing a local inflammatory reaction [8]. It then invades the whole organism, and the central nervous system (CNS) [8]. The involvement of the CNS leads to an irreversible demyelinating process ending by death without treatment. Apart from the initial stages, it is not easy to determine the phase of the disease that the patient is presenting [8]. The parasite can escape the host immune response by varying the surface glycoprotein coat [8]. Variable surface glycoproteins (VSG) are strongly antigenic and lead to great antibody response with immune lysis [8]. It is accepted that African trypanosome has a precarious existence as an extracellular parasite of the mammalian bloodstream, where it is faced with continuous immune attack [9]. As previously mentioned, a main key to survival is a dense VSG coat, which is repeatedly switched during the course of a chronic infection [9]. During infection, large amounts of VSG molecules are released into the circulation [10]. Their interaction with various cells of the immune system underlies the severe infection-associated pathology [10]. In 1994, Ortiz-Ordonezet al tried to elucidate the role played by the VSG coat and trypanosome surface-related processes in the mechanism of HS lysis of HS-sensitive (HSS) and HS-resistant (HSR) trypanosomes [11]. Ortiz-Ordonezet al said that procyclic forms of *T. brucei gambiense* transformed from either HSS or HSR bloodstream stages were found to be HSR and these procyclic forms were shown to have lost their VSG coat [11]. However, the addition of excess soluble VSG from HSS trypanosomes did not block lysis of HSS trypanosomes [11]. The results in this report, taken together, strengthen the hypothesis that the lytic factor interacts with and moves along the trypanosome surface to be internalized eventually [11]. Diffley said that virulence is related to relative sensitivity of the trypanosomes to immunological assault [12]. Diffley also noted that 400 times more *T. brucei gambiense* became noninfective than and *T. brucei rhodesiense* [12].

But, some heterologous antigenic variants can survive to repopulate blood and other tissues [8]. This mechanism of antigenic variation is under parasite genetic control [8]. Basically, antigenic variation of African trypanosomes results from the controlled expression of a single VSG gene from a repertoire of about 1,000 genes [13]. The transcription of the VSG genes occurs uniquely at telomeres, where the expressed VSG gene is part of a large polycistronic transcription unit that appears to be transcribed by a specialized RNA polymerase [13]. The trypanosome can release numerous pathogenic substances which cause alterations in cytokine/prostaglandin network [8].

B. Clinical Manifestation

Generally, African sleelping sickness can be divided into two main stages. For stage 1 (early, or hemolymphatic, stage), the patients usually develop painless skin chancre that appears about 5-15 days after the bite [2]. The chancre appearance is usually a fluctuant, indurated, tsetse-fly bite site. Taiwo et al said that chancre formation would thus appear to be vital for the induction of comprehensive immune recognition of the metacyclic variable antigen repertoire deposited in the skin by infected tsetse, and hence development of protective immunity [14]. Other skin findings included fleeting, erythematous, macular eruptions [15]. The diagnosis was confirmed by the presence of the organism in peripheral blood smears [15]. In 1984, Barry and Emergy cannulated the afferent and efferent lymphatics of the draining lymph node in goats and examined the onset of a cellular reaction, the emigration of the parasite from the chancre and the development of both antigenic variation and the specific immune response [16]. They found that the chancre first became detectable by day 3 post-infection, peaked by day 6 and then subsided [16]. Lymphocyte output increased 6- to 8-fold by day 10 and the number of lymphoblasts increased 50-fold in this period [16]. Intermittent fever, general malaise, myalgia, and headache can be usually seen 3 weeks after bite [2]. Weight loss is common. Generalized lymphadenopathy can also be observed [2]. Pruritus, urticaria, and facial edema can be seen in some cases [2].

For stage 2 (late, or CNS, stage), the patients usually develop persistent headaches. The classical symptoms, daytime somnolence followed by nighttime insomnia, can be seen. Seizure in children is common. It can be said that the nature of disease evolves from the hemolymphatic Stage I to the meningo-encephalitic Stage II. The latter is generally treated with melarsoprol, an arseniate provoking often a deadly encephalopathy [17]. A precise determination of the evolution stage is therefore very important. Generally, the patients in stage II show: (i) a deregulation of the 24-h distribution of the sleep-wake alternation; (ii) an alteration of the sleep structure, with frequent sleep onset rapid eye movement (REM) periods (SOREMPs) [17]. Buguet et al said that polysomnography might represent a diagnostic tool to distinguish the two stages of African trypanosomiasis [17]. Especially, SOREMPs appear shortly after the central nervous system invasion by trypanosomes [17]. The reversibility of the sleep-wake cycle and sleep structure alterations after appropriate treatment constitutes the basis of an evaluation of the healing process [17]. During stage 2, a broad spectrum of neurological signs appears, which finally lead to a demyelinating and fatal stage if untreated [18]. Treatment of stage 2 is usually toxic and difficult to administer when the CNS is invaded [18].

Courtioux et al found that cytokine/chemokine levels in sera were poorly related to disease stage [18]. They observed a relationship between the presence of trypanosomes or trypanosome-related compounds in CSF and levels of IL-1beta, CXCL-8, CCL-2 and CCL-3 [18]. Thy mentioned that these cytokines and chemokines might be triggered by the parasite and hence were potential markers of CNS invasion [18]. According to a large cohort by Blum et al, headache, sleeping disorder and lymphadenopathy are the most frequent symptoms and signs and they are similar for all stages of the disease [19]. Lymphadenopathy tends to be highest in the advanced second stage [19]. The neurological and psychiatric symptoms increase significantly with the number of WBC in the CSF indicating the stage of progression of the disease [19]. Pruritus is observed in all stages and increases with the number of white blood cell in CSF from 30 to 55% [19]. In children younger than 7 years, lymphadenopathy is less frequently reported [19] than in older children or adults [19].

C. Diagnosis

In African trypanosomiasis, the most significant abnormalities are anemia, hypergammaglobulinemia, elevated erythrocyte sedimentation rate (ESR), thrombocytopenia, and hypoalbuminemia, but not eosinophilia or abnormal liver function [2]. Anemia due to African trypanosomiasis becomes an important tropical anemia. Co-infections with other tropical infections causing anemia should be investigated in suspected cases. The transfer of VSG from trypanosomes to erythrocytes could lead to anemia [20]. According to an animal model study, migration of trypanosome VSG from live trypanosomes to target cells could be shown by preincubating erythrocytes with trypanosomes and subsequently testing the washed erythrocytes for insertion of VSG by their susceptibility to lysis by complement in the presence of an anti-VSG antibody [20].

For definite diagnosis of disease, detection of organism within the peripheral blood smear is the most simple and effective tool. Considering the laboratory protocol, the peripheral blood smear examination should be performed at febrile stage. Wright or Giema stains are required. Lymph node aspirate smear examination is also useful in cases with generalized lymphadenopathy. Lymph node aspirate is commonly used as a rapid test for trypanosomes at a high dry magnification (X 400). It requires immediate search for parasites because they are mobile for only 15-20 minutes [2]. During the sleeping stage, the examination of CSF smear can be useful. The organism appears as an elongated flagellate, containing a nucleus and a kinetoplast, and a flagellum bordering an undulating membrane and extending free anteriorly. A standard assay, card agglutination test for trypanosomiasis (CATT) is useful to diagnose African trypanosomiasis [2]. Inojosa et al said that human African trypanosomiasis but, given the toxicity of the drugs, serology using the card agglutination test should be not used alone to guide treatment after active case finding [21]. Recently, Lutumba et al performed a study to make a decision analysis compared the efficiency of three alternative detection strategies: screening by lymph node palpation (LN) only, CATT only and their combination (LN and CATT) [22]. According to this work, the CATT strategy was the most efficient [22]. This moderate efficacy is due to the low sensitivity of the confirmatory (diagnostic) tests [22]. Substantial efficiency gains can be obtained by adopting a CATT only strategy and resources can be better allocated to more sensitive confirmatory tests or to increasing the coverage of populations at risk [22]. A second confirmatory test is needed [21]. With advancement of molecular biology, PCR diagnostic tool for African trypanosomiasis is available. Several recent studies have described the use of the PCR technique with primers specific for *T. brucei* s.1 to improve the sensitivity and specificity of conventional test methods [23]. Within the framework of active screening, PCR carried out on blood samples prior to serological tests could be helpful in identifying suspected infection [23]. Although the one-time initial investment is high, expenditures on expendables is lower for PCR than conventional techniques while achieving higher sensitivity. For application on cerebrospinal fluid samples, PCR also achieves better sensitivity than conventional techniques and thus can contribute to staging of the disease [23].

D. Treatment and Prevention

Pentamidine, suramin, melarsoprol and the new compound DFMO are available for treatment of African trypanosomiasis [24 - 25]. The administration of pentamidine at the beginning of the nervous stage, when the number of cells in the cerebrospinal fluid does not exceed 20/mn3 is a new approach for treatment [24]. At this time of the disease, patients generally are healthy and the pentamidine therapy avoids the use of the toxic melarsoprol (Arsobal) [24]. An alternative protocol for Arsobal therapy (2, 16 mg/kg/d for 10 consecutive days) has been described from pharmacokinetics data to decrease the rate of relapses and the duration of hospital care [24]. Studies of drug combinations are recommended to determine possible combined or synergistic effects and find ways to reduce toxicity [26]. It should be noted there is no vaccine for this disease. The prevention of vector is the best method. Wearing protective as well as vector control can be a good way in controlling of African trypanosomiasis.

East African Sleeping Sickness

East African sleeping sickness is caused by *T. brucei rhodesiense.* The pattern of this disease is very similar to African sleeping sickness.

A. Pathogenesis

The major epidemiology factor in East African trypanosomiasis is the human-tsetse fly contact [2]. Similar process of transmission to African trypanosomiasis is described [27]. The history of human sleeping sickness in East Africa is characterized by the appearance of disease epidemics interspersed by long periods of endemicity [28]. Despite the presence of the tsetse fly in large areas of East Africa, these epidemics tend to occur multiply in specific regions or foci rather than spreading over vast areas. Many theories have been proposed to explain this phenomenon, but recent molecular approaches and detailed analyses of epidemics have highlighted the stability of human-infective trypanosome strains within these foci [28]. Tsuda et al observed that bloodstream form of *T. brucei rhodesiense* did not show any Programmed cell death (PCD) but had up-regulated expression of TAO [29]. Tsuda et al proposed that inhibition of trypanosome alternative oxidase (TAO) by the addition of ascofranone caused the development of PCD in bloodstream *T. brucei rhodesiense* under low-temperature stress, implying that expression of TAO may contribute to the inhibition of PCD [29]. The trypanosome lytic factor (TLF), a primate specific innate defense mechanism that restricts the host range of African trypanosomes, was also studied in *T. brucei rhodesiense* [30]. Milner et al said that suggest that the trypanosome lytic factor (TLF) resistance in human sleeping sickness trypanosomes is a consequence of the selective, high level expression of a cell surface molecule [30].

B. Clinical Manifestation

There are two stages for East African sleeping sickness, similar to African sleeping sickness. A bite by the tsetse fly is often painful and can develop into a red sore, also called a chancre [31]. Fever, severe headaches, irritability, extreme fatigue, swollen lymph nodes, and aching muscles and joints are common symptoms of sleeping sickness [31]. Progressive confusion, personality changes, slurred speech, seizures, and difficulty in walking and talking occur when infection has invaded the central nervous system [31]. The study of the duration of symptoms and the case fatality of *T. brucei rhodesiense* showed that the disease progressed to the stage of central nervous system involvement between three weeks to two months of infection [32]. Most deaths occurred within six months of illness [32]. According to the report of et al, the incidence of melarsoprol encephalopathy was 2.5% and case fatality due to this condition was 1.0% [32]. Gibson et al noted that the human serum resistance associated (SRA) gene is ubiquitous and conserved in *T. brucei rhodesiense* throughout East Africa [33]. They found that strain typing using minisatellite markers showed considerable genetic heterogeneity between *T. brucei rhodesiense* isolates, despite the presence of the conserved SRA gene [33].

C. Diagnosis

The diagnosis of *T. brucei rhodesiense* has the same manner as *T. brucei gambiense*. Parasitological examination is still the only method of definitive diagnosis. Blood smear interpretation is still a useful effective method for diagnosis. It should be noted that thresholds of trypanosome detection differ from one technique to another, such as 10,000 trypanosomes per millilitre (T/ml) for fresh blood smears, 5,000 T/ml for thick drop specimens stained with Giemsa, 500 T/ml for centrifugation in capillary tubes, less than 500 T/ml for the QBC test, and 100 T/ml for the ion exchange minicolumn system [34]. It should be noted that *T. brucei rhodesiense* cause more rapid fatal and posterior nucleate form than *T. brucei gambiense* when inoculated into the mice. Chappuis said that screening for *T. brucei rhodesiense* infection still relied on clinical features in the absence of serological tests available for field use [35].

D. Treatment and Prevention

Medication for East African sleeping sickness is similar to African sleeping sickness [24 – 25]. The control methods for African sleeping sickness can also be applied for East African sleeping sickness.

CHAGAS DISEASE

Chagas disease is a blood infection caused by *T. cruzi*. *T. cruzi* is not transmitted by tsetse fly but reduviid bug (*Panstrongylus megistus*). *T. cruzi* acute infections often go unperceived, but one third of chronically infected individuals die of Chagas disease, showing diverse manifestations affecting the heart, intestines, and nervous systems [36]. A common denominator of pathology in Chagas disease is the minimal rejection unit, whereby parasite-free target host cells are destroyed by immune system mononuclear effectors cells infiltrates [36]. Attention now turns to the future continuity of surveillance and control interventions - especially in regions where control has been so successful that the epidemiological significance of Chagas disease is in steep decline [37]. The effort and expenditure of the recent past cannot continue indefinitely, but a degree of surveillance and selective intervention will be required because of the risk of new infestations and infections resulting from adventitious silvatic vectors accidentally entering houses [37].

A. Pathogenesis

Chagas disease is found only in Latin America. It is named after Carlos Chagas, a Brazilian doctor who first described the disease in 1909 [38]. He also described the life cycle of the parasite, identified the insects that transmit the parasite, identified small mammals that act as reservoir hosts, and suggested means to help prevent its transmission [38]. Concerning the transmission of disease, reduviid bug plays an important role. An infected vector usually takes a blood meal and releases trypomastigotes in its feces near the site of the bite wound. Vectorial transmission (via the feces of Triatominae) is responsible for most of human infections. Direct skin penetration seems more difficult, and generally, the parasite enters via the biting site. It should be noted that there is no direct inoculation.. Trypomastigotes enter the host through the wound or through intact mucosal membranes, such as the conjunctiva [39]. Common triatomine vector species for trypanosomiasis belong to the genera *Triatoma*, *Rhodinius*, and *Panstrongylus*. One of the major problems confronting study of this zoonotic disease is the great biodiversity of the vector species; there are at least 30 different species, with at least 10 playing a major role in human infection [40]. The high variability of climates and biogeographic regions further complicate study and understanding of the dynamics of this disease [40]. Establishment of infection by *T. cruzi*, the agent of Chagas' disease, depends on a series of events involving interactions of diverse parasite molecules with host components [41]. Inside the host, the trypomastigotes invade cells, where they differentiate into intracellular amastigotes [39]. In *T. cruzi* isolates that enter host cells in gp82-mediated manner, parasite protein tyrosine kinase as well as phospholipase C are activated, and Ca2+ is released from I P3-sensitive stores, whereas in *T. cruzi* isolates that attach to target cells mainly through gp35/50, the signaling pathway involving adenylate cyclase appears to be stimulated, with Ca2+ release from acidocalciosomes [41]. In addition, T. cruzi isolate-dependent inhibitory signals, mediated by MT-specific gp90, may be triggered both in the host cell and the parasite [41]. The repertoire of TCT molecules implicated in cell invasion includes surface glycoproteins of gp85 family, with members containing binding sites for laminin and cytokeratin 18, enzymes such as cruzipain, trans-sialidase, and an oligopeptidase B that generates a Ca2+-agonist from a precursor molecule [41]. The amastigotes multiply by binary fission and differentiate into trypomastigotes, and then are released into the circulation as bloodstream trypomastigotes [39]. Trypomastigotes infect cells from a variety of tissues and transform into intracellular amastigotes in new infection sites [39].

A capacity to invade and replicate within many different cell types is a cornerstone of the remarkable fitness of this parasite [42]. Although invasion occurs independently of actin polymerization, the host cell still participates in the process, often in unexpected ways [42]. Clinical manifestations can result from this infective cycle [39]. It should be noted that the bloodstream trypomastigotes do not replicate, which is totally different from the African trypanosomes.

Table 1. Different stages of *T. cruzi* [42]

Stages	Details
Trypomastigote	This is the infective flagellate form of the parasite found in the blood of the mammalian host (blood trypomastigote) and in the terminal part of the digestive and urinary tracts of vectors (metacyclic trypomastigote).
Epimastigote	This is the replicative form of the parasite in the insect vector and in the acellular culture medium.
Amastigote	This is the intracellular replicative form of the parasite in the vertebrate host. It is a spherical form (with a diameter of 2-4 mm) devoid of a free flagellum that cannot move.
Spheromastigote	This is the intracellular replicative form of the parasite in the vertebrate host. It is a spherical form (with a diameter of 2-4 mm) devoid of a free flagellum that cannot move.

B. Clinical Manifestation

The incubation of Chagas disease is usually 7 – 10 days in cases of vectorial contamination and 20-40 days in cases of transmission by blood transfusion [42]. The latter, more prolonged incubation period is believed to be due to the weaker capacity of circulating blood trypomastigotes to invade cells, compared to the metacyclic trypomastigotes [42]. Transfusion is still important mode of this disease transmission in Latin America [43]. The acute phase, defined by the detection of blood parasites using direct classic parasitological techniques, usually affects children and young adults and remains asymptomatic in other patients [43]. The cytokines IFN-gamma and TNF-alpha and several chemoatractants molecules, which act on G protein-coupled serpentine receptors, are produced during the acute infection [44]. They play major roles in the induction of iNOS and in the NO production-dependent killing of *T. cruzi* by murine macrophages [44]. On the other hand, TGF-beta and IL-10, which are also produced during the infection, are negative regulators of NO production [44]. In addition to mediating resistance against the infection, NO can also suppress the immune response to *T. cruzi* via the induction of apoptosis of T cells [44]. Acute infection can produce the following signs and symptoms: acute signs and symptoms of initial bite lesions (Romana's sign), furuncle like skin lesions (Chagoma), and facial or body edema [45]. The manifestations of the acute disease resolve spontaneously within 3-8 weeks in approximately 90% of individuals who are infected [43]. However, life-threatening myocarditis or meningoencephalitis can occur during the acute phase. The death rate for infected cases in this phase is about 10%. A few patients progress into the next step of this disease, intermediate phase. This stage characterize by positive serological result but no pasitemia. More than half of the patients in intermediate phase of Chagas disease further develop chronic lesions and remain asymptomatic. The final stage of infection is the chronic symptomatic stage. The most common symptoms in chronic stage include cardiac and digestive symptoms. Heart involvement is the major feature of the disease because of its characteristics, frequency, and consequences, and is also the source of most controversies [46]. The cardiac involvement can lead to arrythmia, heart failure and thromboembolism. The indeterminate clinical form, despite its good prognosis on at least a medium-term basis (5-10 years), has acquired increasing importance due to the controversial meaning of the abnormality of some tests and the myocardial focal lesions found in many patients [46]. Simultaneous evaluation of the parasympathetic and of the sympathetic system in the heart should be done by spectral analysis of heart rate [46]. Chronic chagasic heart disease is the most common cause of cardiomyopathy in endemic areas of South and Central America and is the leading cause of cardiovascular death among middle age patients [43]. Considering the digestive manifestations, megaesophagus and megacolon are common. The basic mechanism is destruction of neurons of the enteric nervous system [44]. Whereas megaesophagus and megacolon are the most notable and most extensively studied expressions of the digestive form of Chagas' disease, involvement of the small intestine (Chagasic enteropathy) is less frequent and less known than involvement of the two above mentioned entities [47]. Chagasic enteropathy can be responsible for important clinical and laboratory manifestations resembling those of dyspeptic syndrome, intestinal pseudo-obstruction and bacterial overgrowth in the small intestine [47]. Chagasic enteropathy also involves peculiar functional changes, especially those related to motor activity of the organ and to intestinal absorption of carbohydrates [47].

C. Diagnosis

Demonstration of the causal agent is the diagnostic procedure in acute Chagas disease. The peripheral blood smear examination becomes a useful simple test for diagnosis of Chagas disease [48]. Trypomastigotes have a prominent subterminal kinetoplast that often distort the membrane of the cell, an elongated nucleus and an undulating membrane. In blood stream, trypomastigotes are 15-20 μm in lenght and appear with a typical C or S-shaped form. However, the blood smear examination is useful for diagnosis of acute stage of disease. For intermediate stage, the serological test is more useful. Indirect immunofluorescence for detecting IgG and IgM antibodies, hemagglutination and enzyme immunoassay are the widely used techniques [49 - 50]. The serologic testing is also the cornerstone of diagnosing chronic *T. cruzi* infections, and improved assays are needed [51]. Because diagnosis of individuals infected by Trypanosoma cruzi is performed mainly by serological tests using crude antigens, therefore, it might crossreact with other infections [52]. In recent years, many recombinant *T. cruzi* proteins and synthetic peptides have been described, to cope with this problem, and some are already on the market [52]. PCR diagnosis is the new technique for diagnosis of Chagas disease. Recently, a nested polymerase chain reaction (PCR)-based approach was recently developed to demonstrate preferential heart and skeletal muscle tropism in mice of a Mexican *T. cruzi* isolate [53].

D. Treatment and Prevention

Medication for Chagas disease is the best therapeutic method. There are two drugs available for the aetiological treatment of Chagas' disease: nifurtimox (Nfx) and benznidazole (Bz) [54]. Nfx is a nitrofurane and Bz is a nitroimidazole compound. The use of these drugs to treat the acute phase of the disease is widely accepted [54]. However, their use in the treatment of the chronic phase is controversial [54].

There is insufficient evidence to support the efficacy of nitrofurans or imidazolic drugs as recommended treatment in chronic Chagasic cardiopathy and chronic *T.. cruzi* infections, specifically if overt heart disease is present [55]. A well designed randomized controlled trial is necessary to establish if new drugs are suitable for treatment of cardiac patients with chronic Chagasic cardiopathy [55]. The undesirable side effects of both drugs are a major drawback in their use, frequently forcing the physician to stop treatment [54]. The most frequent adverse effects observed in the use of Nfx are: anorexia, loss of weight, psychic alterations, excitability, sleepiness, digestive manifestations such as nausea or vomiting, and occasionally intestinal colic and diarrhea [54]. In the case of Bz, skin manifestations are the most notorious including hypersensitivity, dermatitis with cutaneous eruptions, generalized oedema, fever, lymphoadenopathy, articular and muscular pain), with depression of bone marrow, thrombocytopenic purpura and agranulocytosis being the more severe manifestations [54]. Since the present drugs display undesirable toxic side effects and the emergence of drug-resistant trypanosomes has been reported, therefore, the development of new drugs in the treatment of Chagas' disease and sleeping sickness is urgently required [56].

For disease control, the Central American Initiative targeted the elimination of an imported triatomine bug and the control of a widespread native species (*Triatoma dimidiata*), and faced constraints such as a small scientific community, the difficulty in controlling a native species, and a vector control program that had fragmented under a decentralized health system [57]. Chagas disease control can now be readily demonstrated by the disappearance of acute cases and of new infections in younger age groups, as well as progressive reductions of mortality and morbidity rates in controlled areas [58]. In economic terms, the cost-benefit relationship between intervention and the reduction of Chagas disease is highly positive [58]. Effective control of Chagas disease is now seen as an attainable goal that depends primarily on maintaining political will, so that the major constraints involve problems associated with the decentralisation of public health services and the progressive political disinterest in Chagas disease [58].

References

[1] Nok AJ. Effective measures for controlling trypanosomiasis. *Expert Opin. Pharmacother.* 2005;6:2645-53.

[2] African sleeping sickness. Available online at http://www.emedicine. com/ med/topic2140.htm

[3] Trypanosoma cruzi. Available online at http://www.dbbm.fiocruz.br/ tropical/chagas/ chapter3.html

[4] Smith DH, Pepin J, Stich AH. Human African trypanosomiasis: an emerging public health crisis. *Br. Med. Bull.* 1998;54:341-55.

[5] Cattand P. The scourge of human African trypanosomiasis. *Afr. Health.* 1995;17:9-11.

[6] Tsetse flies. Available online at http://www.roberth.u-net.com/tsetse.htm

[7] Aksoy S. Tsetse--A haven for microorganisms. *Parasitol. Today.* 2000;16:114-8

[8] Dumas M, Bouteille B. Human African trypanosomiasis. *C. R. Seances Soc. Biol. Fil.* 1996;190:395-408.

[9] Rudenko G. Maintaining the protective variant surface glycoprotein coat of African trypanosomes. *Biochem. Soc. Trans.* 2005;33:981-2.
[10] Magez S, Stijlemans B, Baral T, De Baetselier P. VSG-GPI anchors of African trypanosomes: their role in macrophage activation and induction of infection-associated immunopathology. *Microbes Infect.* 2002;4:999-1006.
[11] Ortiz-Ordonez JC, Sechelski JB, Seed JR. Mechanism of lysis of Trypanosoma brucei gambiense by human serum. *J. Parasitol.* 1994;80:924-30.
[12] Diffley P. Trypanosoma brucei: immunogenicity of the variant surface coat glycoprotein of virulent and avirulent subspecies. *Exp. Parasitol.* 1985;59:98-107.
[13] Van der Ploeg LH. Control of antigenic variation in African trypanosomes. *New Biol.* 1991;3:324-30.
[14] Taiwo VO, Nantulya VM, Moloo SK, Ikede BO. Role of the chancre in induction of immunity to tsetse-transmitted Trypanosoma (Nannomonas) congolense in goats. *Vet. Immunol. Immunopathol.* 1990;26:59-70.
[15] Cochran R, Rosen T. African trypanosomiasis in the United States. Arch. *Dermatol.* 1983;119:670-4.
[16] Barry JD, Emergy DL. Parasite development and host responses during the establishment of Trypanosoma brucei infection transmitted by tsetse fly. *Parasitology.* 1984;88:67-84.
[17] Buguet A, Bisser S, Josenando T, Chapotot F, Cespuglio R. Sleep structure: a new diagnostic tool for stage determination in sleeping sickness. *Acta Trop.* 2005;93:107-17
[18] Courtioux B, Boda C, Vatunga G, Pervieux L, Josenando T, M'Eyi PM, Bouteille B, Jauberteau-Marchan MO, Bisser S. A link between chemokine levels and disease severity in human African trypanosomiasis. *Int. J. Parasitol.* 2006;36:1057-65
[19] Blum J, Schmid C, Burri C. Clinical aspects of 2541 patients with second stage human African trypanosomiasis. *Acta Trop.* 2006;97:55-64.
[20] Rifkin MR, Landsberger FR. Trypanosome variant surface glycoprotein transfer to target membranes: a model for the pathogenesis of trypanosomiasis. *Proc. Natl. Acad. Sci. U S A.* 1990;87:801-5.
[21] Inojosa WO, Augusto I, Bisoffi Z, Josenado T, Abel PM, Stich A, Whitty CJ. Diagnosing human African trypanosomiasis in Angola using a card agglutination test: observational study of active and passive case finding strategies. *BMJ.* 2006;332:1479
[22] Lutumba P, Robays J, Miaka C, Kande V, Simarro PP, Shaw AP, Dujardin B, Boelaert M. The efficiency of different detection strategies of human African trypanosomiasis by T. b. gambiense. *Trop. Med. Int. Health.* 2005;10:347-56.
[23] Jamonneau V, Solano P, Cuny G. Use of molecular biology in the diagnosis of human African trypanosomiasis. *Med. Trop. (Mars).* 2001;61:347-54.
[24] Doua F, Boa Yapo F. Current therapy of trypanosomiasis. *Bull. Soc. Pathol. Exot.* 1994;87:337-4.
[25] Docampo R, Moreno SN. Current chemotherapy of human African trypanosomiasis. *Parasitol. Res.* 2003;90 Supp 1:S10-3.
[26] Bouteille B, Oukem O, Bisser S, Dumas M. Treatment perspectives for human African trypanosomiasis. *Fundam. Clin. Pharmacol.* 2003;17:171-81.
[27] Oscherwitz SL. East African trypanosomiasis. *J. Travel. Med.* 2003;10:141-3.

[28] Hide G. History of sleeping sickness in East Africa. *Clin. Microbiol. Rev.* 1999;12:112-25.

[29] Tsuda A, Witola WH, Ohashi K, Onuma M. Expression of alternative oxidase inhibits programmed cell death-like phenomenon in bloodstream form of Trypanosoma brucei rhodesiense. *Parasitol. Int.* 2005;54:243-51.

[30] Milner JD, Hajduk SL. Expression and localization of serum resistance associated protein in Trypanosoma brucei rhodesiense. Mol Biochem Parasitol. 1999;104:271-83.

[31] East African trypanosomiasis. Available online at http://www.wrongdiagnosis.com/e/east_african_trypanosomiasis/symptoms.htm

[32] Odiit M, Kansiime F, Enyaru JC. Duration of symptoms and case fatality of sleeping sickness caused by Trypanosoma brucei rhodesiense in Tororo, Uganda. *East Afr. Med. J.* 1997;74:792-5.

[33] Gibson W, Backhouse T, Griffiths A. The human serum resistance associated gene is ubiquitous and conserved in Trypanosoma brucei rhodesiense throughout East Africa. *Infect. Genet. Evol.* 2002;1:207-14.

[34] Chappuis F, Loutan L, Simarro P, Lejon V, Buscher P. Options for field diagnosis of human african trypanosomiasis. *Clin. Microbiol. Rev.* 2005;18:133-46.

[35] Louis FJ, Buscher P, Lejon V. Diagnosis of human African trypanosomiasis in 2001. *Med. Trop. (Mars).* 2001;61:340-6.

[36] Teixeira AR, Nascimento RJ, Sturm NR. Evolution and pathology in chagas disease--a review. *Mem. Inst. Oswaldo Cruz.* 2006;101:463-91.

[37] Schofield CJ, Jannin J, Salvatella R. The future of Chagas disease control. *Trends Parasitol.* 2006;22:583-8.

[38] Chagas disease. Available online at http://www.who.int/tdr/diseases/chagas/default.htm

[39] American trypanosomiasis. Available online at http://www.dpd.cdc.gov/dpdx/HTML/TrypanosomiasisAmerican.htm

[40] Cruz-Reyes A, Pickering-Lopez JM. Chagas disease in Mexico: an analysis of geographical distribution during the past 76 years--a review. *Mem. Inst. Oswaldo Cruz.* 2006;101:345-54.

[41] Yoshida N. Molecular basis of mammalian cell invasion by Trypanosoma cruzi. *An. Acad. Bras. Cienc.* 2006;78:87-111.

[42] Chagas disease. Available online at http://www.emedicine.com/med/topic327.htm

[43] Smith LA, Wright-Kanuth MS. Transfusion-transmitted parasites. *Clin. Lab. Sci.* 2003;16:239-45, 251.

[44] Silva JS, Machado FS, Martins GA. The role of nitric oxide in the pathogenesis of Chagas disease. *Front Biosci.* 2003;8:s314-25.

[45] Goldsmith RS, Zarate RJ, Zarate LG, Morales G, Kagan I, Drickey R, Jacobson LB. Clinical and epidemiologic studies of Chagas' disease in rural communities of Oaxaca, Mexico, and an eight-year followup: II. Chila. *Bull. Pan. Am. Health Organ.* 1992;26:47-59.

[46] Prata A. Clinical and epidemiological aspects of Chagas disease. *Lancet Infect. Dis.* 2001;1:92-100.

[47] Meneghelli UG. Chagasic enteropathy. *Rev. Soc. Bras. Med. Trop.* 2004;37:252-60.

[48] Bianchini C, Cifarelli F. Laboratory methods for the diagnosis of Chagas's disease. Observations and clinical considerations. *Arch. Ital. Sci. Med. Trop. Parassitol.* 1967;48:307-22

[49] Cattand P, de Raadt P. Laboratory diagnosis of trypanosomiasis. *Clin. Lab. Med.* 1991;11:899-908.
[50] Ferreira AW, de Avila SD. Laboratory diagnosis of Chagas' heart disease. *Sao Paulo Med. J.* 1995r;113:767-71.
[51] Kirchhoff LV. Chagas disease. American trypanosomiasis. *Infect. Dis. Clin. North Am.* 1993;7:487-502.
[52] da Silveira JF, Umezawa ES, Luquetti AO. Chagas disease: recombinant Trypanosoma cruzi antigens for serological diagnosis. *Trends Parasitol.* 2001;17:286-91
[53] Andersson J. Molecular diagnosis of experimental Chagas disease. *Trends Parasitol.* 2004;20:52-3
[54] Castro JA, de Mecca MM, Bartel LC. Toxic side effects of drugs used to treat Chagas' disease (American trypanosomiasis). *Hum. Exp. Toxicol.* 2006;25:471-9.
[55] Reyes PA, Vallejo M. Trypanocidal drugs for late stage, symptomatic Chagas disease (Trypanosoma cruzi infection). *Cochrane Database Syst. Rev.* 2005;:CD004102.
[56] Steverding D, Tyler KM. Novel antitrypanosomal agents. *Expert Opin. Investig Drugs.* 2005;14:939-55.
[57] Yamagata Y, Nakagawa J. Control of Chagas disease. *Adv. Parasitol.* 2006;61:129-65.
[58] Dias JC, Silveira AC, Schofield CJ. The impact of Chagas disease control in Latin America: a review. *Mem. Inst. Oswaldo Cruz.* 2002;97:603-12.

Chapter VIII

NEOSPOROSIS

INTRODUCTION TO NEOSPOROSIS

Neosporosis is a parasitic infestation mainly caused by *Neospora caninum*, a coccidian parasite of animals [1 – 2]. *N. carninum* is a toxoplasma like parasite [2]. First it is misunderstand to be a variant of *Toxoplasma* spp. In analogy to *T. gondii*, three stages of N. caninum; asexually proliferating tachyzoites, tissue cysts harbouring slowly dividing bradyzoites; and oocysts containing sporozoites can be identified [1 – 2]. Since its first description in dogs in 1984, the protozoan parasite *Neospora caninum* has been found to infect a wide range of animals, worldwide [3]. It is a major pathogen for cattle and dogs and it occasionally causes clinical infections in horses, goats, sheep, and deer [1 – 2]. Domestic dogs are the only known definitive hosts for *N. caninum* [1 – 2]. The dog has recently been identified as the definitive host and the parasite may be transmitted through the ingestion of oocysts or congenitally from mother to fetus [4]. In addition, *N. caninum* is known to infect red foxes (*Vulpes vulpes*) and coyotes (*Canis latrans*) [4].

In cattle, *N. caninum* has particular significance as a cause of abortion in which persistence of infection in the mother, recrudescence of the parasite during pregnancy, and the vulnerability of the placenta and fetus to invasion are important features [3]. Dubey said that it is one of the most efficiently transmitted parasite of cattle and up to 90% of cattle in some herds are infected [1]. Evidence is accumulating that neosporosis is a major cause of reproductive failure in cattle all over the world [5]. Innes *et al* said that information on the rates of repeat abortion due to neosporosis were less well defined however current estimated put this at 5% suggesting that cattle might develop some form of protective immunity against *N. caninum*-induced abortion [4]. Transplacental transmission is considered the major route of transmission of *N. caninum* in cattle [1]. Anderson *et al* said that horizontal transmission utilized a two-host life cycle whereby the cow was infected from ingestion of coccidial oocyst stages shed by the definitive host [6]. There is epidemiological evidence that the dog has a role in the prevalence of the infection but, as yet, no confirmation that the dog is the source for natural infections in cattle [6]. Dubey noted that *N. caninum* was a major cause of abortion in cattle in many countries and said that to elicit protective immunity against abortion in cows that already harbor a latent infection is a major problem [1]. In addition, Innes *et al* said that CD4+ T-cells, interferon gamma and macrophages have all been found to significantly inhibit multiplication of *N. caninum* tachyzoites. Concerning the pathology, multifocal nonsuppurative encephalitis represents the most frequent pathohistological finding in *N. caninum*-associated abortions [7].

Diagnosis of the disease is based upon detection of the parasite in the tissues, most commonly using immunohistochemistry [4]. The causative agent can also be demonstrated by polymerase chain reaction [7]. Tachyzoites can be cultivated in vitro using similar techniques as previously described for *T. gondii* [8]. Methods for generating tissue cysts containing *N. caninum* bradyzoites in mice, and purification of these cysts, have also been developed [8]. However, although positive fetal serology is a strong indicator of exposure to the parasite, care should be taken in the interpretation of maternal serology [4]. Conraths and Schares concluded that serological techniques could be used for indirect diagnosis [7]. A number of studies have been undertaken to identify and characterise at the molecular level specific antigenic components of *N. caninum* in order to improve serological diagnosis [8 - 9].

Annually, neosporosis cause a considerably economical loss, responsible for a reduction in the value of female breeding cattle [10]. Although there are several attempts to develop the immunization to neosporosis, there is no effective vaccine for preventing Neospora-induced abortions in cattle or to prevent oocyst shedding in dogs [11].

Human Neosporosis, a Possible New Emerging Infectious Disease

Although the parasite is known to infect a range of warm blooded animals but the disease predominates in dogs and cattle it is not yet known if *N. caninum* can infect and cause disease in people [4]. There are some previous reports on the seroprevalence of neosporosis among human beings. In 1999, Tranas *et al* performed an interesting seroprevalence study on human neosporosis in USA [12]. According to their study, evidence of human exposure to this parasite was sought by screening for antibodies in blood donors by indirect fluorescent antibody (IFA) tests and immunoblotting [12]. Of 1,029 samples screened, 69 (6.7%) had titers of 1:100 by IFA testing and 50 of the 69 (72%) sera that were positive for *N. caninum* were also negative for a closely related protozoan pathogen of humans, *T. gondii* [12]. In addition, immunoblot analysis confirmed the specificity of the positive sera for N. caninum antigens, with several sera recognizing multiple Neospora antigens with molecular masses similar to those of antigens recognized by monkey anti-*N. caninum* serum [12]. Tranas *et al* concluded that the findings in this study provided evidence of human exposure to *N. caninum*, although the antibody titers in healthy donors were low [12]. A comparison between *N. caninum* and *T. gondii* is shown in table 8.1 [2].

Recently Petersen *et al* performed a study to determine whether N. caninum could cause repeated abortions in humans [13]. They retrospectively examined serum samples of 76 women with a history of abortions for evidence of *N. caninum* infection [13]. In this study, no antibodies to the parasite were detected by enzyme-linked immunosorbent assay, immunofluorescence assay, or Western blot [13]. However, Sargent proposed that neosposis might be one of the causal agents corresponding for pregnancy infection [14]. Hemphill and

Table 8.1. Comparison between Neospora caninum and Toxoplasma gondii

characteristics	*Neospora caninum*	*Toxoplasma gondii*
Definitive host	Dog	Cat
Pathology in humans	Not known	Lymphoreticular system
Cyst wall morphology	Thick	Thin
Specific antigen	43 kDa	30 kDa (SAG1), 22 kDa (SAG2)

Gottstein B placed neosporosis as a potential risk factor not only for animals, but also for human health [15]. Angwatcharaprakarn *et al* also proposed the possibility of neosporosis in human beings especially the immunodeficiency group [2]. Although there is no definite human neosporosis case there are evidence of past infection by serological investigaion and there are several expert ideas that N. carninum might be a possible human pathogen. Therefore, further studies to harvest the knowledge on this infection are recommended since there have been continuously new emerging zoonotic disease.

Epidemiology and Transmission [2]

The actual life cycle of *N.caninum* has never been discovered. Several animals can be infected with this pathogenic organism and cause several clinical manifestations. However, the confirmed definitive host for this infection is dog.

Transmission of disease can present in several modes with dog as definitive host. Generally, dog will pass unsporulated oocysts contaminating within its stool. Then the sporulation process will be occur externally. The intermediat hosts including cattle, goat, sheep and deer get the pathogenic organism during ingestion of food or water contaminated with infective stage of organism, tachyzoites. Basically, the stages include tachyzoites, tissue cysts and oocysts. The tachyzoites is the stage that can rapidly multiply and can invade into the cell causing the specific lesion of neosporosis. Then tachyzoites will transform into the latent form, tissue cysts with bradyzoite inside. Bradyzoite can also be seen in the central and peripheral nervous system tissues. When the wall of oocyst is destroyed, the sporozoites will be free and go into the external environment then multiply to reach the tachyzoites stage, which can be transmittable. However, the feco-oral route transmission is not problematic in veterinarian medicine because the amount of infected oocyst within the stool of dogs is not many [16].

The more problematic transmission is due to the transplancental route. This method of transmission is considered a vertical transmission. It can be found in cattle. There are many cases of infected cattle due to this mode of transmission. Similar to other infection, the transplacental transmission from mother to fetus follow the general rule of transmission, proper invasive mechanism. The tachizoites within infected mother can transmit to the fetus causing the infection of the recipient (fetus). This infection can result in abortion. In addition, neurological symptoms can be seen. However, some cases are asymptomatic infection. The aborted fetus can be the food source for other carnivore resulting in further horizontal transmission of disease. For the asymptomatic fetus, it might be survival and can be the reservoir for the disease. Finally, it can end up with the next round of transplacental transmission [17- 18]. Generally, horizontal transmission cause sporadic endemicity of infection in dogs while the infection in cattle is usually due to vertical transmission [19]. However, the exact mechanism and life cycle of the *N. carninum* is still not clarified at present.

PATHOPHYSIOLOGY

Neospora caninum is a coccidian belonging to apicomplexan group. It is a tissue cyst-forming parasite. CD4+ T-cells, interferon gamma and macrophages have all been found to significantly inhibit multiplication of *N. caninum* tachyzoites [25]. During neosporosis, IFN-γ induced by *N. caninum* tachyzoites plays a pivotal role in control of the acute phase of the disease [20 - 23]. It has been clearly shown that the complete lack of IFN-γ in the IFN-$\gamma^{-/-}$ mouse model renders the host highly susceptible to infection (often fatal) by *N. caninum* [24]. Continued production of *N. caninum*-elicited IFN-γ production during infection will lead to a chronic state of neosporosis in cows with no obvious acute symptoms of the disease [25]. Little is known about the range of parasite genotypes within the environment or the variation in virulence between different strains [25]. RAPD-PCR analysis of geographically distinct bovine and canine isolates has revealed little genetic variation [25].

It should be noted that the parasite can spread efficiently from mother to fetus over several generations, and naturally infected cattle do not appear to develop adequate protective immunity [26]. Modulation of the immune response during pregnancy favors parasite survival and multiplication [26]. However, induction of pro-inflammatory responses that are thought to be protective against *N. caninum* would be detrimental to the pregnancy [26]. Degenerative to inflammatory lesions could be found out in fetal tissues. Most commonly they are localized in the CNS, the heart, skeletal muscles and liver [27 – 30]. The characteristic CNS lesions are organized as a central necrotic zone, infiltrated by inflammatory cells (glial or mononuclear). Death fetus are usually autolyzed or mummified.

CLINICAL MANIFESTATION

This infection can cause abortion in several animals. The disorders of the neurological system of the fetus in utero are believed to be the major cause of abortion.

1. Canine Neosporosis

Barber and Trees a case series of neosporosis in European dogs [31]. In this work, the affected dogs were two days to seven years old, and of 13 different breeds [31]. Rigid hyperextension developed in approximately half of the cases [31]. Anorexia and pyrexia were rare. Other clinical signs included forelimb ataxia, head tremors with tetraparesis and sudden collapse due to myocarditis [31]. The dog can develop progressive paralysis and muscle atrophy, followed by cervical weakness, stiff jaws and dysphagia [32]. Death can be resulted [32].

Sometimes, at necropsy, tissue cysts can be seen in unstained smears and in histologic sections of their brains [33]. In addition, cutaneous symptoms can be a clinical manifestation of canine neosporosis. Cutaneous neosporosis manifested by pyogranulomatous ulcerative dermatitis is common [34]. Cutaneous neosporosis can be diagnosed by immunohistochemistry on skin biopsy specimens and a high serum antibody titer to Neospora caninum by Neospora agglutination test [35 – 36]. Electron microscopy examination of skin specimens further supported the diagnosis [36]. Histology revealed numerous intralesional protozoal tachysoites within macrophages and neutrophils [34]. Dermatitis is a finding rarely associated with juvenile neosporosis [35].

2. Bovine Neosporosis

Clinical signs are described only in congenitally infected calves, younger than 2 months. According to the study of Barr et al [37], the clinical signs are observed most commonly 3 to 5 days after birth but could also appear later 2 to 3 weeks after birth [37]. The calves infected with *N. caninum* are born with a lower body weight, unviable or without clinical signs of the disease [37]. The hindlimbs or/and the forelimbs could be bent or extremely extended [37]. The neurological examination shows ataxia, decreased patellar reflex and lack of orientation [37]. Sometimes, an exophtalmus, asymmetry of the eyes, hydrocephaly or narrowing can be seen [37]. Abortion is the common presentation of bovine neosporosis as previously mentioned. The pathogenesis of abortion due to Neospora is complex and only partially understood [38]. Losses occur after a primary infection during pregnancy but more commonly as the result of recrudescence of a persistent infection during pregnancy [38]. Parasitaemia is followed by invasion of the placenta and fetus [38]. Collantes-Fernandez performed a comparative study *N. caninum* distribution, parasite loads and lesions between epidemic and endemic bovine abortion cases [39]. A comparison of (a) *N. caninum* DNA- detectability by PCR, (b) N. caninum-associated lesions and (c) parasite loads in target organs was made between epidemic and endemic abortion cases [39]. This report confirms that the abortion herd pattern is an important factor that influences pathogenesis in natural *N. caninum* infections [39]. It is suggested that abortion occurs when primary parasite-induced placental damage jeopardises fetal survival directly or causes release of maternal prostaglandins that in turn cause luteolysis and abortion [38]. Fetal damage may also occur due to primary tissue damage caused by the multiplication of *N. caninum* in the fetus or due to insufficient oxygen/nutrition, secondary to placental damage [38].

Laboratory Diagnosis [2]

Laboratory investigation is required for the definitive diagnosis of neorsporosis. The main laboratory investigation is examination of histologic tissue lesions by immunohistochemical (IHC) technique. This technique is for detection of cyst or *N.caninum* tachyzoites. Other techniques include many serological tests to detect antibody in sera. These serological tests are indirect fluorescent antibody test (IFAT), enzyme linked immunosorbent assay (ELISA) and PCR [40]. Presently, the ELISA is widely used. The avidity of IgG antibodies directed to N. caninum is the new ELISA kit N. caninum proteins incorporated into immunostimulating complexes as antigen [41]. However, Bjorkman et al found that that avidity tests wee sometimes less robust than conventional ELISAs [42]. Therefore, it is essential that they are carefully standardised and their performance continuously evaluated [42]. These serological tests have a wide range of sensitivity and specificity. Some new diagnostic test as modified direct agglutination test (MAT), which can give very high sensitivity up to 100 %, are also developed [43].

Treatment and Prevention

There are no proven control methods for the prevention or treatment of neosporosis [44]. Therefore, prevention is better. Totltrazuril is the drug in trial for treatment of neosporosis. In 2001, Gottstein et al described the use of a mouse model for the evaluation of toltrazuril and ponazuril medication as a means of preventing parasite dissemination and subsequent formation of cerebral lesions [45]. In this work, chemotherapy using either toltrazuril or ponazuril, both applied in a drinking-water formulation (20 mg toltrazuril or ponazuril kg/body weight/ day) completely prevented the formation of cerebral lesions in all treated animals, as assessed by immunohistochemistry [45]. In addition, PCR analyses of these treated animals showed that DNA-detectability was reduced by 91% and 90% upon toltrazuril and ponazuril medication, respectively [45]. Kritzner et al performed another study to assess the efficacy of toltrazuril-sulfone in calves experimentally infected with *N. caninum* [46]. In this work, ponazuril chemotherapy of infected calves in comparison to non-treated infected animals reduced symptoms, but no differences were observed between treated and non-treated animals with regard to serum enzymes and metabolites [46]. Efficacy of a treatment was also reflected by significantly lower anti-Neospora antibody concentrations developed after infection, when compared to non-treated animals [46]. Based on their findings, a basic effectiveness of ponazuril against experimental *N. caninum* infection in calves can be seen [46]. Ammann et al proposed that treatment with toltrazuril appeared to act parasitostatically rather than parasitocidically [47]. This is supported bye the fact that: (1) although the lack of B-cells did not impair the effect of toltrazuril, (2) the lack of T-cells did not allow for a full efficacy of treatment [47]. Therefore, chemotherapy with toltrazuril against experimental infections with *N. caninum* requires the support of T-cell immunity in order to be successful [47].

Considering the economic and agricultural importance of neosporosis, there is the urgent need to develop biological control measures aimed at preventing its transmission, infection, as well as reducing severity of the disease [48]. For prevention of neosporosis, vaccination is the current focus. NcSAG1 and NcSRS2, the two major immunodominant tachyzoite surface antigens of the apicomplexan parasite Neospora caninum, were investigated for their potential as vaccine candidates in mice [49]. Cannas et al performed an animal model study on vaccination of mice against experimental *N. caninum* infection using NcSAG1- and NcSRS2-based recombinant antigens and DNA vaccines [49].They found that a combined DNA/recombinant antigen-vaccine, based on NcSAG1 and NcSRS2, respectively, exhibited a highly significant protective effect against experimentally induced cerebral neosporosis in mice [49]. In 2004, Jenkins et al performed a trial to evaluate the immunologic response of a killed tachyzoite vaccine against *N. caninum* and its effectiveness in preventing fetal loss associated with experimentally induced neosporosis in sheep [50]. The *N. caninum* tachyzoite vaccine used in this study appeared to provide protection against fetal loss associated with experimentally induced neosporosis in a high proportion of pregnant ewes [50].

REFERENCES

[1] Dubey JP. Review of Neospora caninum and neosporosis in animals. *Korean J. Parasitol.* 2003;41:1-16

[2] Angwatcharaprakarn V, Yamsuwan T, Wiwanitkit V, Soogarun S. *Neospora caninum* infection and neosporosis. *Songkla. Med.* J2004; 22: 131-135

[3] Buxton D, McAllister MM, Dubey JP. The comparative pathogenesis of neosporosis. *Trends Parasitol.* 2002;18:546-52

[4] Innes EA, Buxton D, Maley S, Wright S, Marks J, Esteban I, Rae A, Schock A, Wastling J. Neosporosis. Aspects of epidemiology and host immune response. *Ann. N. Y. Acad. Sci.* 2000;916:93-101

[5] Wouda W. Diagnosis and epidemiology of bovine neosporosis: a review. *Vet. Q.* 2000;22:71-4

[6] Anderson ML, Andrianarivo AG, Conrad PA. Neosporosis in cattle. *Anim. Reprod. Sci.* 2000;60-61:417-31

[7] Conraths FJ, Schares G. Diagnosis and epidemiology of Neospora caninum-associated abortions in cattle. *Tierarztl Prax Ausg G Grosstiere Nutztiere.* 1999;27:145-53

[8] Hemphill A, Fuchs N, Sonda S, Hehl A. The antigenic composition of Neospora caninum. *Int. J. Parasitol.* 1999;29:1175-88

[9] Bjerkas I, Jenkins MC, Dubey JP. Identification and characterization of Neospora caninum tachyzoite antigens useful for diagnosis of neosporosis. *Clin. Diagn. Lab. Immunol.* 1999;1:214-21

[10] Trees AJ, Davison HC, Innes EA, Wastling JM. Towards evaluating the economic impact of bovine neosporosis. *Int. J. Parasitol.* 1999;29:1195-200

[11] Dubey JP. Recent advances in Neospora and neosporosis. *Vet. Parasitol.* 1999;84:349-67

[12] Tranas J, Heinzen RA, Weiss LM, McAllister MM. Serological evidence of human infection with the protozoan Neospora caninum. *Clin. Diagn. Lab. Immunol.* 1999;6:765-7

[13] Petersen E, Lebech M, Jensen L, Lind P, Rask M, Bagger P, Bjorkman C, Uggla A. Neospora caninum infection and repeated abortions in humans. *Emerg. Infect. Dis.* 1999;5:278-80

[14] Sargent I. Infection in pregnancy. Report on the workshop held by the Materno-Fetal Immunology Group (MFIG) of the British Society for Immunology at the 6th Annual Congress of the BSI, December 4, 1998, in Harrogate, UK. *J. Reprod. Immunol.* 1999;44:81-3

[15] Hemphill A, Gottstein B. A European perspective on Neospora caninum. *Int. J. Parasitol.* 2000;30:877-924

[16] Lindsay DS, Dubey JP, Duncan RB. Confirmation that the dog is a definitive host for Neospora caninum. *Vet. Parasitol.* 1999;82:327-3.

[17] French NP, Clancy D, Davison HC, Trees AJ. Mathematical models of *Neospora caninum* infection in dairy cattle: transmission and options for control. *Int. J. Parasitol.* 1999;29:1691-704.

[18] Hemphill A. The host-parasite relationship in neosporosis. *Adv. Parasitol.* 1999;43:47-104.

[19] Anderson ML, Reynolds JP, Rowe JD, Sverlow KW, Packham AE, Barr BC, Conrad PA. Evidence of vertical transmission of Neospora sp infection in dairy cattle. *J. Am. Vet. Med. Assoc.* 1997;210:1169-72.

[20] Baszler, T. V., M. T. Long, T. F. McElwain, and B. A. Mathison. 1999. Interferon-gamma and interleukin-12 mediate protection to acute Neospora caninum infection in BALB/c mice. *Int. J. Parasitol.* 29:1635-1646.

[21] Long MT, Baszler TV. 2000. Neutralization of maternal IL-4 modulates congenital protozoal transmission: comparison of innate versus acquired immune responses. *J. Immunol.* 2000; 164:4768-4774.

[22] Nishikawa Y, Inoue N, Makala L, Nagasawa H. A role for balance of interferon-gamma and interleukin-4 production in protective immunity against Neospora caninum infection. *Vet. Parasitol.* 2003; 116:175-184.

[23] Nishikawa Y, Inoue N, Makala L, Nagasawa H. A role for balance of interferon-gamma and interleukin-4 production in protective immunity against Neospora caninum infection. *Vet. Parasitol.* 2003; 116:175-184.

[24] Tuo W, Fetterer R, Jenkins M, Dubey JP. Identification and characterization of Neospora caninum cyclophilin that elicits gamma interferon production. *Infect. Immun.* 2005;73:5093-100.

[25] Innes EA, Buxton D, Maley S, Wright S, Marks J, Esteban I, Rae A, Schock A, Wastling J. Neosporosis. Aspects of epidemiology and host immune response. *Ann. N. Y. Acad. Sci.* 2000;916:93-101.

[26] Innes EA, Andrianarivo AG, Bjorkman C, Williams DJ, Conrad PA. Immune responses to Neospora caninum and prospects for vaccination. *Trends Parasitol.* 2002;18:497-504.

[27] Barr BC, Anderson ML, Blanchard PC, Daft BM, Kinde H, Conrad PA. Bovine fetal encephalitis and myocarditis associated with protozoal infections. *Veterinary Patho.* 1990; 27: 354–361.

[28] Barr BC, Anderson ML, Dubey JP, Conrad PA. Neospora-like protozal infections associated with bovine abortions. *Vet. Patho.* 1991; 28:110–116.

[29] Wouda WA, de Gee L, Moen AR, van Knapen F. Laboratory experiences with bovine Neospora abortion in Dutch dairy herds. In: Proceedings of the Symposium Neospora abortus, 8 November 1995, Morra 2, Drachten, 3–9.

[30] Nietfeld JC, Dubey JP, Anderson ML, Libal MC, Yaeger JM, Nieger RD. Neospora - like protozoan infection as a cause of abortion in dairy cattle. *J. Vet. Diag. Invest.* 1992;4:223–226.

[31] Barber JS, Trees AJ. Clinical aspects of 27 cases of neosporosis in dogs. *Vet. Rec.* 1996;139:439-43.

[32] Basso W, Venturini MC, Bacigalupe D, Kienast M, Unzaga JM, Larsen A, Machuca M, Venturini L. Confirmed clinical Neospora caninum infection in a boxer puppy from Argentina. *Vet. Parasitol.* 2005;131:299-303.

[33] Dubey JP, Dorough KR, Jenkins MC, Liddell S, Speer CA, Kwok OC, Shen SK. Canine neosporosis: clinical signs, diagnosis, treatment and isolation of Neospora caninum in mice and cell culture. *Int. J. Parasitol.* 1998 ;28:1293-304.

[34] Perl S, Harrus S, Satuchne C, Yakobson B, Haines D. Cutaneous neosporosis in a dog in Israel. *Vet. Parasitol.* 1998;79:257-61.

[35] Boyd SP, Barr PA, Brooks HW, Orr JP. Neosporosis in a young dog presenting with dermatitis and neuromuscular signs. *J. Small Anim. Pract.* 2005;46:85-8.

[36] Ordeix L, Lloret A, Fondevila D, Dubey JP, Ferrer L, Fondati A. Cutaneous neosporosis during treatment of pemphigus foliaceus in a dog. *J. Am. Anim. Hosp. Assoc.* 2002;38:415-9.

[37] Barr BC, Anderson ML, Blanchard PC, Daft DM, Kinde H, Conrad PA. Bovine fetal encephalitis and myocarditis associated with protozoal infections. *Vet. Patho.* 1990; 27: 354–361.

[38] Dubey JP, Buxton D, Wouda W. Pathogenesis of bovine neosporosis. *J. Comp. Pathol.* 2006;134:267-89.

[39] Collantes-Fernandez E, Arnaiz-Seco I, Burgos BM, Rodriguez-Bertos A, Aduriz G, Fernandez-Garcia A, Ortega-Mora LM. Comparison of Neospora caninum distribution, parasite loads and lesions between epidemic and endemic bovine abortion cases. *Vet. Parasitol.* 2006;142:187-91.

[40] Jenkins M, Baszler T, Bjorkman C, Schares G, Williams D. Diagnosis and seroepidemiology of Neospora caninum- associated bovine abortion. *Int. J. Parasitol.* 2002; 32:631-6.

[41] Bjorkman C, Naslund K, Stenlund S, Maley SW, Buxton D, Uggla A. An IgG avidity ELISA to discriminate between recent and chronic Neospora caninum infection. *J. Vet. Diagn. Invest.* 1999;11:41-4.

[42] Bjorkman C, Alvarez-Garcia G, Conraths FJ, Mattsson JG, Ortega-Mora LM, Sager H, Schares G. Neospora caninum IgG avidity tests: an interlaboratory comparison. *Vet. Parasitol.* 2006;140:273-80.

[43] Packham AE, Sverlow KW, Conrad PA, Loomis EF, Rowe JD, Anderson ML, Marsh AE, Cray C, Barr BC. A modified agglutination test for *Neospora caninum*: development, optimiza tion, and comparison to the indirect fluorescent- antibody test and enzyme-linked immunosorbent assay. *Clin. Diagn. Lab. Immunol.* 1998;5:467-73.

[44] Anderson ML, Andrianarivo AG, Conrad PA. Neosporosis in cattle. *Anim. Reprod. Sci.* 2000 2;60-61:417-31.

[45] Gottstein B, Eperon S, Dai WJ, Cannas A, Hemphill A, Greif G. Efficacy of toltrazuril and ponazuril against experimental Neospora caninum infection in mice. *Parasitol. Res.* 2001;87:43-8.

[46] Kritzner S, Sager H, Blum J, Krebber R, Greif G, Gottstein B. An explorative study to assess the efficacy of toltrazuril-sulfone (ponazuril) in calves experimentally infected with Neospora caninum. *Ann. Clin. Microbiol. Antimicrob.* 2002;1:4.

[47] Ammann P, Waldvogel A, Breyer I, Esposito M, Muller N, Gottstein B. The role of B- and T-cell immunity in toltrazuril-treated C57BL/6 WT, microMT and nude mice experimentally infected with Neospora caninum. *Parasitol. Res.* 2004;93:178- 87.

[48] Nishikawa Y, Mikami T, Nagasawa H. Vaccine development against Neospora caninum infection. *J. Vet. Med. Sci.* 2002;64:1-5.

[49] Cannas A, Naguleswaran A, Muller N, Eperon S, Gottstein B, Hemphill A. Vaccination of mice against experimental Neospora caninum infection using NcSAG1- and NcSRS2-based recombinant antigens and DNA vaccines. *Parasitology.* 2003;126:303-12.

[50] Jenkins MC, Tuo W, Dubey JP. Evaluation of vaccination with Neospora caninum protein for prevention of fetal loss associated with experimentally induced neosporosis in sheep. *Am. J. Vet. Res.* 2004;65:1404-8.

Chapter IX

HISTOPLASMOSIS

INTRODUCTION TO HISTOPLASMOSIS

Histoplasmosis is a fungal infection caused by *Histoplasma capsulatum* [1 – 2]. It is a significant cause of respiratory and systemic disease in mammals including humans, especially immunocompromised individuals such as HIV-infected patients. *Histoplasma capsulatum* is a dimorphic fungus that remains in a mycelial form at ambient temperatures and grows as yeast at body temperature in mammals. The fungus can be found in temperate climates throughout the world. Soil contaminated with bird droppings or excrements of bats is the common natural habitat for this fungus [3]. Mycologically, the genus Histoplasma contains one species, *Histoplasma capsulatum*. *H. capsulatum* has two varieties: *H. capsulatum* var. capsulatum and *H. capsulatum* var. *duboisii*. It has a teleomorph referred to as *Ajellomyces capsulatus* [3]. As an environmental mold found in the soil, it is a successful member of a competitive polymicrobial ecosystem [4]. Its host-adapted yeast form is a facultative intracellular pathogen of mammalian macrophages [4]. *H. capsulatum* faces a variety of environmental changes during the course of infection and must survive under harsh conditions or modulate its microenvironment to achieve success as a pathogen [4]. Histoplasmosis may be considered the fungal homolog of the bacterial infection tuberculosis, since both *H. capsulatum* and *Mycobacterium tuberculosis* exploit the macrophage as a host cell and can cause acute or persistent pulmonary and disseminated infection and reactivation disease [4].

Considering the epidemiology of this fungus, the Mississippi-Ohio River Valley is the endemic area of this pathogen in USA [3]. Classical histoplasmosis caused by *H. capsulatum* var. capsulatum, and African histoplasmosis caused by H. capsulatum var. duboisii are both endemic in Africa [5]. In South Africa, only classical histoplasmosis caused by Histoplasma capsulatum var. capsulatum is known to occur and cases are seen frequently [5]. For Thailand, although there are reported cases of histoplasmosis for years the epidemiological studies usually show negative soil culture results [6 - 7].

PATHOGENESIS

H. capsulatum is the causative agent of a true systemic endemic mycosis namely hisotplasmosis. This fungus is well adapted to be infectious and pathogenic for humans [8]. As a soil fungus with no known requirement for interacting with a mammalian host as part of an obligate lifecycle, its plethora of strategies for successful pathogenesis is particularly remarkable [8]. These features include the dimorphic mold-yeast transition, entry into host macrophages, subcellular localization, intracellular survival and proliferation during active infection and persistence during clinically inapparent infection with the capacity for reactivation [8]. To thrive within the harsh environment of a professionally phagocytic and antimicrobial host cell, *H. capsulatum* displays mechanisms for modulating its microenvironmental pH level, resisting host reactive oxygen and nitrogen intermediates and degradative enzymes, and withstanding nutrient starvation conditions, including acquisition of iron and calcium and biosynthesis of nucleic acid precursors [8].

The spectrum of the disease is wide, varying from an acute benign pulmonary infection to a chronic pulmonary or fatal disseminated disease. Following acquisition of the conidia by inhalation, lungs are primarily involved. Macrophages initially serve as a protected environment in which the primary fungal pathogen *H. capsulatum* multiplies and disseminates from the lung to other organs [9]. Upon induction of cell-mediated immunity, cytokines activate macrophages to destroy the yeasts and thus remove them from the host [9]. In animal models, once phagocytosed, H. capsulatum is not killed by fusion of the phago-lysosomes, instead it multiplies within non-activated macrophages and destroys them [10]. Upon induction of cell-mediated immunity, cytokines activate macrophages and destroy the yeast cells [10]. Some aspects of the fungus-macrophage interaction have been elucidated, and it is clear that some of the mechanisms by which *H. capsulatum* escapes the lethal effects of this very hostile environment, involve the regulation of specific genes [10]. Gildea et al demonstrated that human dendritic cell can phagocytose and degrade a fungal pathogen and subsequently process the appropriate antigens for stimulation of lymphocyte proliferation [11]. In vivo, such interactions between dendritic cell and *H. capsulatum* may facilitate the induction of cell-mediated immunity [11]. The concerted action of several cytokines is necessary for resolution of both primary and secondary infection with Histoplasma capsulatum. Among the soluble factors that contribute to tissue sterilization, TNF-alpha stands as a central mediator of protective immunity to this fungus [12]. Recently Allendoerfer and Deepe demonstrated the pivotal influence of TNFR1 and -2 in controlling primary infection and highlighted the differences between these receptors for regulation reexposure histoplasmosis [12].

In cases of dissemination of *H. capsulatum* var. *capsulatum* infection, reticuloendothelial system (RES) is most frequently involved [3]. The fungus resides intracellularly in RES cells [3]. Watson et al said that impaired amplification of the immune response consequent to abnormal generation of IL 1 and IL 2 might be the important mechanism in dissemination of histoplasmosis [13]. Some reports indicate that, in humans, treatment with inhibitors of TNF-alpha is associated with disseminated histoplasmosis [14]. *H. capsulatum* may also rarely involve the thyroid glands and may be isolated in fungemia. Infection of the thyroid with Histoplasma capsulatum is rarely reported as part of disseminated disease, even in geographic areas where histoplasmosis is endemic [15].

Unlike var. *capsulatum*, var. *duboisii* rarely involves the lungs but commonly involves the bones and skin [3]. African histoplasmosis is the disease caused by var. *duboisii*. For this disease, direct examination of biopsy tissue showed numerous specimens of *H. capsulatum* var. duboisii. However, Okeke and Muller found that both elastolytic proteinases measured in the crude enzymes of v. duboisii and v. capsulatum after incubation in the pH ranges 4.5-8.0 and 4.0-7.0 respectively, at 4 degrees C for 24 hours had similar optimum pH (pH 8) and temperature (35 degrees C) [16].

Pathogenic Organism

H. capsulatum is called a thermal dimorph because it has two forms. In nature at room temperature about 25° C it takes on a mycelial (filamentous) form, forming the macroconidia as well as smaller microconidia [17]. At body temperature (37° C) it morphs into a yeast [17]. The two forms are grown in separate test tubes at different temperatures [17]. In culture below 35° it and on natural substrates it grows as a white to brownish mycelial fungus, with characteristic echinulate oval or pyriform macroconidia (8-16 um diameter) and microconidia (2-5 um diameter) [17]. When inhaled into the alveolar spaces it is primarily the microconidia that germinate and then transform into small budding yeasts 2-5 um diameter [17]. Yeast cells are found in reticuloendothelial system. The fungus also grows as a yeast in culture at 37° C [17]. Until recently, *H. capsulatum* was believed to harbour three varieties, var. *capsulatum* (chiefly a New World human pathogen), var. *duboisii* (an African human pathogen) and var. *farciminosum* (an Old World horse pathogen), which varied in clinical manifestations and geographical distribution [18]. However, Kasuka et al suggested that the three varieties of Histoplasma are phylogenetically meaningless [18].]. In 2002, Tamura et al noted that DNA sequence analysis of the internal transcribed spacer (ITS) region provided useful information to understand the epidemiology and evolution of *H. capsulatum* [19]. In 2005, Komori et al said that that analysis of the nucleotide sequence of the 28S rRNA gene was very effective for identification of *H. capsulatum* and that three varieties of *H. capsulatum* should be reclassified according to the phylogenetic relationship established from analysis of the D1/D2 region sequences [20].

Diagnosis of Histoplasmosis

Histoplasmosis is a common infection endemic in many regions of America, Asia, India and Africa, with sporadic cases also occurring throughout the world [21]. Although excellent laboratory methods for diagnosis are available; there are deficiencies that must be met by continued research. Clinicians and laboratory directors must be familiar with the uses and limitations of a battery of serologic and mycological tests to accurately diagnose histoplasmosis [21]. Understanding the uses and limitations of a battery of laboratory methods is essential to diagnose histoplasmosis [22]. Although excellent laboratory methods for diagnosis are available, diagnosis in many cases is missed or delayed because histoplasmosis is not considered in the differential. Physicians must be aware of the clinical syndromes and take advantage of epidemiologic clues [23].

Antigen detection and serology are valuable adjuncts to histopathology and culture [22]. Improvements incorporated into the second-generation Histoplasma antigen assay have increased its sensitivity and specificity for diagnosis of histoplasmosis [22 - 24]. More recently, the antigen assay has been modified to provide quantitation, which improves reproducibility and facilitates monitoring antigen clearance during treatment [22]. Furthermore, detection of antigen in bronchoalveolar lavage fluid increases the sensitivity for diagnosis of pulmonary histoplasmosis [22]. Serological tests for antibodies are also useful, but may be falsely negative in immunosuppressed patients [22]. In addition, elevated antibody titres persist for several years following initial infection, complicating their interpretation [22]. However, Wheat et al mentioned that demonstrate a wider range of cross-reactions in Histoplasma serology than has been previously recognized, and the cross-reactivity was greatest when observed by radioimmunoassay [25]. They noted that caution should be exercised in the interpretation of serologic data from patients with suspected fungal infections [25].

Histopathology is another method for diagnosis of histoplasmosis. Although histopathology may provide for rapid diagnosis, its sensitivity is < 50% in patients with disseminated disease and even lower in pulmonary histoplasmosis [22].

Polymerase chain reaction (PCR) has been described, but the cost of diagnosis is significantly higher that that of histopathology [26 - 27]. Culture, although highly specific, has notable limitations, including insensitivity, a need for invasive procedures and delayed growth [22].

Disseminated histoplasmosis in HIV-infected patients often presented with erythematous maculopapular eruption. Carbon dioxide laser can be used to ablate the epidermal layer of this lesion to identify the underlying pathogenic yeast cells by skin smear method [28]. This new method is safe and effective for diagnosis of this opportunistic fungal infection in HIV infected individuals [28]. In additional, a routine examination is also useful for diagnosis of disseminated histoplasmosis. Complete blood count is useful. Organism can be seen in blood. Wheat et al said that a search for Histoplasma capsulatum in peripheral blood smears from patients with AIDS was warranted, especially in endemic midwestern states [29]. Matulionyte et al also indicated for the possible usefulness of peripheral blood smear examination [30]. However, Wiwanitkit and Chaiwong found that the examination of blood smear might not be useful in diagnosis of histoplasmosis [31]. el Guedj et al said that the infection should be suspected in any febrile HIV-infected patient with CD4 blood cell count < 200/mm3, if he/she ever travelled in an endemic zone and direct examination of smear relating to clinical symptoms help guide diagnosis, while culture will confirm it after at least 4 weeks [32]. el Guedj et al also mentioned that efficient serologic techniques for HIV-infected patients were not available [32]. Lacson et al concluded that the peripheral blood smear in a patient with AIDS is an unexpected clue for diagnosis [33].

Clinical Manifestation

H. capsulatum is the etiological agent of histoplasmosis, a chronic respiratory infection that is generally asymptomatic in healthy individuals, but severe or fatal in patients who are immunosuppressed or otherwise debilitated [10]. Acute pulmonary infection, chronic pulmonary, and progressive disseminated histoplasmosis are the most commonly recognized clinical manifestations, pericarditis, rheumatologic syndromes, esophageal compression, and sarcoid-like manifestations are well-recognized complications of histoplasmosis [23]. When the AIDS epidemic spread around the world, histoplasmosis became recognized as a common and important opportunistic infection among the patients with AIDS. Clinicians must maintain a high level of suspicion for histoplasmosis in any HIV-infected patient who presents with unexplained fever, particularly if the patient has evidence of hepatosplenomegaly, generalized lymphadenopathy, pancytopenia, abnormal liver function tests, or bilateral pulmonary infiltrates [34]. The diagnosis of histoplasmosis can be established rapidly by observation of organisms on peripheral blood smear or bone marrow biopsy specimens or by Histoplasma Polysaccharide Antigen testing [34].

A. Pulmonary Histoplasmosis

Pulmonary histoplasmosis is a common lung infection [35]. The most frequent clinical forms observed in immunocompetent subjects are generally benign or silent and usually limited to a fortuitously discovered pulmonary nodule [36]. Massive exposure may lead to an acute primary invasion producing a miliary aspect. Chronic forms simulating tuberculosis are exceptional [36]. As previously mentioned, the infection can be either acute or chronic. However, most cases are chronic due to the nature of fungal infection. Generally, a history of recurrent episodes of respiratory infection and abnormal radiological lung lesions inducing a misdiagnosis of chronic pulmonary tuberculosis of the adults are common findings [37]. Ideally, mycelium should be isolated for diagnosis, a task which is easier in disseminated or operated nodular forms [36]. More often, the epidemiological context, clinical and radiological features, the elimination of differential diagnoses and, retrospectively, serology are sufficient for diagnosis [36]. The diagnosis of histoplasmosis, suggested by the immunodiffusion test and the detection of yeast-like cells in smeared and stained sputum, is confirmed by the isolation and identification of *H. capsulatum* var. *capsulatum* in selective media [37]. The treatment can be carried out with amphothericin B and ketoconazole or itraconazole [37]. For acute infection, the patient usually presents with a dry cough, fever and an abnormal chest X-ray [38]. Acute pulmonary histoplasmosis can be diagnosed after culture of *H. capsulatum* from bronchial washings [38]. A favorable response can also be seen upon treatment with antifungal drug [38]. The clinical course is usually favorable [36]. Itraconazole is the treatment of choice for symptomatic or complicated forms [36]. Inversely, opportunistic histoplasmosis in AIDS patients can produce a severe multiple organ disease [36].

B. Cutaneous Histoplasmosis

For African histoplasmosis, infected cases usually manifest by ulcers and cutaneous swellings [39]. Histology of a skin biopsy can reveal superficial colonization by numerous fungal elements described as spores and hyphae [40].Treatment with amphotericin B combined with ketoconazole is usually successful [39]. It is suggested that asymptomatic infections due to the duboisii variety of *H. capsulatum* may be common in the human population around the cave [41]. A diligent search with the help of local hospitals and public health officials may reveal clinical cases of histoplasmosis duboisii with cutaneous and systemic lesions [41].

Considering cutaneous histoplasmosis due to *H. capsulatum* var. *capsulatum*, it is usually a part of disseminated histoplasmosis. Cutaneous lesions as a manifestation of histoplasmosis, primarily a disease of the respiratory system, are rare and most commonly appear secondary to progressive dissemination [42]. Biopsy and cultures of the lesions are usually positive for *H. capsulatum* [42].

C. Disseminated Histoplasmosis

Disseminated histoplasmosis is a severe form of histoplasmosis. It usually occurs in the immunocompromised host. Disseminated histoplasmosis in HIV-infected patients is usually associated with advanced immunosuppression, with CD4+ lymphocyte counts of < 75/mm3 [43]. Currently, histoplasmin skin testing of HIV-infected patients does not seem to be useful in detecting previous exposure and therefore is not helpful in identifying groups of patients who are at risk for dissemination and who should be targeted for preventive efforts [43].

The infection usually begins in the lungs even though the chest X-ray may be normal [44]. Clinical findings are nonspecific; most patients present with symptoms of fever and weight loss of at least 1 month's duration. When untreated, many cases eventually develop severe clinical manifestations resembling septicemia [44]. Chest X-ray, when abnormal, show interstitial or reticulonodular infiltrates [44]. Many cases have been initially misdiagnosed as disseminated mycobacterial infection or Pneumocystis carinii pneumonia [44]. Patients are often concurrently infected with other opportunistic pathogens, supporting the need for a careful search for co-infections [44]. Useful diagnostic tests include serologic tests for anti-H. capsulatum antibodies, peripheral blood and bone marrow smear examination, silver stains of tissue sections or body fluids, and cultures using fungal media from blood, bone marrow, bronchoalveolar lavage fluid, and other tissues or body fluids suspected to be infected on clinical grounds [44]. It is important that all physicians who care for HIV-infected patients become thoroughly familiar with the clinical manifestation of this illness [45]. Timely diagnosis depends on a high degree of diagnostic suspicion since the illness seldom presents with primary respiratory symptoms [45]. It is prudent to consider PDH in the differential diagnosis of any systemic, wasting, febrile illness in HIV-infected individuals, especially if currently or in the past they have resided in areas endemic for the fungus [45]. Similarly, whenever progressive disseminated histoplasmosis is diagnosed in any patient who is in a high-risk group for HIV infection, prompt testing for HIV should be performed [45]. Treatment with amphotericin B is highly effective, reversing the clinical manifestations of infection in at least 80% of cases [44]. The current public health recommendation for HIV-infected patients is to avoid exposure to sites likely to harbor high levels of *H. capsulatum*, such as chicken coops and bird roosts [43]. The role of chemoprophylaxis is not clear [43].

There are some important specific patterns of organ involvement in disseminated histoplasmosis. Central nervous system manifestations occur in 10 to 20% of patients with disseminated histoplasmosis [46]. Additionally, histoplasmosis may be the cause of cases of chronic meningitis in patients with no other evidence for dissemination [46]. Histoplasmosis in the CNS may produce meningitis, single or multiple brain abscesses, and may present with either a clinical picture of obtundation or a deteriorating space-occupying CNS lesion [47].

Histoplasmosis may also cause spinal cord mass lesions resembling neoplasms or abscesses [46]. Diagnosis of chronic meningitis or mass lesions caused by *H. capsulatum* may be difficult and involves careful analysis of serologic tests for antibodies and cultures [46]. Amphotericin B remains the treatment of choice, but relapses occur in half of cases despite total courses of at least 35 mg/kg [46]. Adrenal histoplasmosis is another interesting manifestation.

This can be a cause of unusual adrenal mass [48]. Imaging features were variable [49]. The adrenal masses are usually hypoechoic, homogeneous or heterogeneous. The masses may be hypodense or hyperdense on CT scan [49].

D. Asymptomatic Infection

As previously mentioned, many cases of histoplasmosis are asymptomatic. These cases can be detected by histoplasmin skin test, a common skin test. A person can learn from a histoplasmin skin test whether he or she has been previously infected by *H. capsulatum* [50]. This test is similar to a tuberculin skin test. It is a delayed hypersensitivity skin testing is based on the reaction that occurs in response to the intradermal injection of an antigen [51]. The histoplasmin skin test reflects the frequency of asymptomatic forms of histoplasmosis [52]. A previous infection can provide partial immunity to reinfection [50]. Since a positive skin test does not mean that a person is completely immune to reinfection, appropriate exposure precautions should be taken regardless of a worker's skin test status whenever disturbances of materials that might be contaminated with *H. capsulatum* occur [50]. According to a recent study by Vernuil et al, no significative association was found between a positive skin test and diabetes, rural occupations or exposure to bats [52]. At present, histoplasmin skin test is not mainly used as a tool for diagnosis but a tool for epidemiology survey [53 – 55].

TREATMENT OF HISTOPLASMOSIS

Mild cases of histoplasmosis are usually resolved without treatment. For severe cases, special antifungal medications are needed to arrest the disease [50]. Disseminated histoplasmosis is fatal if untreated, but death can also occur in some patients even when medical treatment is received [50]. In most cases, amphotericin B is the initial drug of choice, followed by one of the azoles for lifelong maintenance therapy [56]. Itraconazole is the drug of choice for treatment of disseminated histoplasmosis in less severe cases, while fluconazole therapy for histoplasmosis is only moderately effective [56]. In HIV-infected cases, induction therapy consists of amphotericin B for acutely ill patients or itraconazole for patients with mild to moderately severe disease [57]. Subsequent lifelong maintenance therapy with itraconazole is recommended [57]. Detection of histoplasma polysaccharide antigen (HPA) in serum or urine may prove to be a promising approach for the rapid diagnosis and therapeutic monitoring of DH in AIDS patients [58]. In contrast to immunocompetent hosts, high relapse rates are reported after therapy in AIDS patients. Therefore, initial (induction) therapy is routinely followed by long-term (maintenance) therapy to prevent relapse [58]. Amphotericin

B is presently the drug of choice for induction therapy [58]. Maintenance therapy with either amphotericin B or an oral azole antifungal agent active against *H. capsulatum* is necessary to prevent relapse [58]. It appears that long-term suppression with 50 to 100 mg of amphotericin B weekly, after completion of initial therapy, has the best chance of maintaining a satisfactory functional status [59]. Itraconazole, a triazole antifungal agent, may provide effective alternative therapy for both induction and maintenance treatment of DH [58]. For prevention, in patients with CD4 counts of < or = 150/microL, itraconazole is effective primary prophylaxis [57].

Intolerance to therapy with amphotericin B and ketoconazole led its rapid replacement by surgical treatment. In addition, excessive inflammatory response may bring some patients to the attention of a thoracic surgeon to exclude malignancy of a noncalcified pulmonary or mediastinal mass or to relieve compression of specific structures [60]. Mediastinal granuloma or fibrosing mediastinitis may involve the superior vena cava, pulmonary vessels, heart and pericardium, tracheobronchial tree, or esophagus [60].

References

[1] Wheat LJ. Histoplasmosis: a review for clinicians from non-endemic areas. *Mycoses.* 2006;49:274-82.

[2] Adderson E. Histoplasmosis. *Pediatr. Infect. Dis. J.* 2006;25:73-4.

[3] Histoplasm species. Available online at www.doctorfungus.org/thefungi/Histoplasma.htm

[4] Woods JP. Histoplasma capsulatum molecular genetics, pathogenesis, and responsiveness to its environment. *Fungal. Genet. Biol.* 2002;35:81-97.

[5] Gugnani HC. Histoplasmosis in Africa: a review. *Indian J. Chest. Dis. Allied Sci.* 2000;42:271-7.

[6] Prijyanonda B. Epidemiological study of histoplasmosis in Thailanda survey at Pechburi. *J. Med. Assoc. Thai.* 1968; 51: 298-305.

[7] Prijyanonda B, Bovornkitti S, Thianprasit M, Dermat F, Mettiyawongse S, Chantarakul N, Skolphadungkhet B. Epidemiological study of histoplasmosis in Thailanda survey at Cholburi Province. *Siriraj Hosp Gaz.* 1967; 19: 289-297.

[8] Newman SL. Macrophages in host defense against Histoplasma capsulatum. *Trends Microbiol.* 1999;7:67-71.

[9] Woods JP, Heinecke EL, Luecke JW, Maldonado E, Ng JZ, Retallack DM, Timmerman MM. Pathogenesis of Histoplasma capsulatum. *Semin. Respir. Infect.* 2001;16:91-101.

[10] Gildea LA, Morris RE, Newman SL. Histoplasma capsulatum yeasts are phagocytosed via very late antigen-5, killed, and processed for antigen presentation by human dendritic cells. *J. Immunol.* 2001;166:1049-56.

[11] Porta A, Maresca B. Host response and Histoplasma capsulatum/macrophage molecular interactions. *Med. Mycol.* 2000;38:399-406.

[12] Allendoerfer R, Deepe GS Jr. Regulation of infection with Histoplasma capsulatum by TNFR1 and -2. *J. Immunol.* 2000;165:2657-64.

[13] Watson SR, Schmitt SK, Hendricks DE, Bullock WE. Immunoregulation in disseminated murine histoplasmosis: disturbances in the production of interleukins 1 and 2. *J. Immunol.* 1985;135:3487-93.

[14] Deepe GS Jr. Modulation of infection with Histoplasma capsulatum by inhibition of tumor necrosis factor-alpha activity. *Clin. Infect. Dis.* 2005;41 Suppl 3:S204-7.

[15] Goldani LZ, Klock C, Diehl A, Monteiro AC, Maia AL. Histoplasmosis of the thyroid. *J. Clin. Microbiol.* 2000;38:3890-1.

[16] Okeke CN, Muller J. In vitro production of extracellular elastolytic proteinase by Histoplasma capsulatum var. duboisii and Histoplasma capsulatum var. capsulatum in the yeast phase. *Mycoses.* 1991;34:461-7.

[17] Histoplasma capsulatum. Available online at http://botit.botany.wisc.edu/toms_fungi/jan2000.html

[18] Kasuga T, White TJ, Koenig G, McEwen J, Restrepo A, Castaneda E, Da Silva Lacaz C, Heins-Vaccari EM, De Freitas RS, Zancope-Oliveira RM, Qin Z, Negroni R, Carter DA, Mikami Y, Tamura M, Taylor ML, Miller GF, Poonwan N, Taylor JW. Phylogeography of the fungal pathogen Histoplasma capsulatum. *Mol. Ecol.* 2003;12:3383-401.

[19] Tamura M, Kasuga T, Watanabe K, Katsu M, Mikami Y, Nishimura K. Phylogenetic characterization of Histoplasma capsulatum strains based on ITS region sequences, including two new strains from Thai and Chinese patients in Japan. *Nippon Ishinkin Gakkai Zasshi.* 2002;43:11-9.

[20] Komori T, Sano A, Yarita K, Kitagawa T, Kamei K, Nishimura K. Phylogenetic analysis of Histoplasma capsulatum based on partial sequence of the D1/D2 region of the 28S rRNA gene. *Nippon Ishinkin Gakkai Zasshi.* 2005;46:291-5.

[21] Joseph Wheat L. Current diagnosis of histoplasmosis. *Trends Microbiol.* 2003;11:488-94.

[22] Wheat LJ. Improvements in diagnosis of histoplasmosis. *Expert Opin. Biol. Ther.* 2006;6:1207-21.

[23] Wheat LJ. Laboratory diagnosis of histoplasmosis: update 2000. *Semin Respir. Infect.* 2001;16:131-40.

[24] Wheat LJ, Garringer T, Brizendine E, Connolly P. Diagnosis of histoplasmosis by antigen detection based upon experience at the histoplasmosis reference laboratory. *Diagn. Microbiol. Infect. Dis.* 2002;43:29-37.

[25] Wheat J, French ML, Kamel S, Tewari RP. Evaluation of cross-reactions in Histoplasma capsulatum serologic tests. *J. Clin. Microbiol.* 1986;23:493-9.

[26] Bracca A, Tosello ME, Girardini JE, Amigot SL, Gomez C, Serra E. Molecular detection of Histoplasma capsulatum var. capsulatum in human clinical samples. *J. Clin. Microbiol.* 2003;41:1753-5.

[27] Rickerts V, Bialek R, Tintelnot K, Jacobi V, Just-Nubling G. Rapid PCR-based diagnosis of disseminated histoplasmosis in an AIDS patient. *Eur. J. Clin. Microbiol. Infect. Dis.* 2002;21:821-3.

[28] Chirachanakul P. Carbon dioxide laser-assisted epidermal ablation increases the yield of skin smear for the diagnosis of disseminated histoplasmosis in HIV-infected patient: A preliminary study. *Thai. J. Dermatol.* 2005; 21: 76-81

[29] Wheat LJ.Tomita T, Chiga M. Disseminated histoplasmosis in acquired immunodeficiency syndrome: light and electron microscopic observations. *Hum. Pathol.* 1988;19:438-41.

[30] Matulionyte R, Garbino J, Uckay I, Lambert JF, Hirschel B. Disseminated histoplasmosis in an HIV-infected patient discovered by routine blood smear staining. *Eur. J. Clin. Microbiol. Infect. Dis.* 200524:361-3.

[31] Wiwanitkit V, Chaiwong T. Blood smear examination for disseminated histoplasmosis in 50 HIV seropositive patients in Chulalongkorn Hospital. *Srinagarind. Med. J.* 2003 ; 1827-29.

[32] el Guedj M, Couppie P, Pradinaud R, Aznar C, Carme B, Clity E, Farge D. Histoplasmosis due to Histoplasma capsulatum capsulatum and HIV infection. *Rev. Med. Interne.* 2000;21:408-15.

[33] Lacson EK Jr, Al-Makki A, Caplan E, Zigel C. An unexpected clue: the peripheral blood smear in a patient with *AIDS. Md. Med. J.* 1996;45:482-4.

[34] McKinsey DS, Smith DL, Driks MR, O'Connor MC. Histoplasmosis in Missouri: historical review and current clinical concepts. *Mo. Med.* 1994;91:27-32.

[35] Forrest JV. Common fungal diseases of the lungs. II. Histoplasmosis. *Radiol. Clin. North Am.* 1973;11:163-8.

[36] Guigay J, Cuguilliere A, Miltgen J, Lonjon T, Jancovici R, Vaylet F, Natali E, Le Vagueresse R, Bonnet D, L'Her P. American pulmonary histoplasmosis caused by Histoplasma capsulatum. *Rev. Pneumol. Clin.* 1998;54:311-20.

[37] Capone D, Wanke B, Monteiro PC, Lazera MS, de Noronha Andrade G, do Valle AC, Moreno AM, Londero AT. Chronic pulmonary histoplasmosis in the State of Rio de Janeiro, Brazil. *Mycopathologia.* 1999;145:75-9.

[38] van Crevel R, van der Ven AJ, Meis JF, Kullberg BJ. Acute pulmonary histoplasmosis as an imported disease. *Ned Tijdschr Geneeskd.* 1997;141:1242-4.

[39] Akpuaka FC, Gugnani HC, Iregbulam LM. African histoplasmosis: report of two patients treated with amphotericin B and ketoconazole. *Mycoses.* 1998;41:363-4.

[40] Eichmann A, Schar G. African histoplasmosis in a patient with HIV-2 infection. *Schweiz. Med. Wochenschr.* 1996;126:765-9.

[41] Muotoe-Okafor FA, Gugnani HC, Gugnani A. Skin and serum reactivity among humans to histoplasmin in the vicinity of a natural focus of Histoplasma capsulatum var. duboisii. *Mycopathologia.* 1996;134:71-4.

[42] Studdard J, Sneed WF, Taylor MR Jr, Campbell GD. Cutaneous histoplasmosis. *Am. Rev. Respir. Dis.* 1976;113:689-93.

[43] Hajjeh RA. Disseminated histoplasmosis in persons infected with human immunodeficiency virus. *Clin. Infect. Dis.* 1995;21 Suppl 1:S108-10.

[44] Wheat LJ, Connolly-Stringfield PA, Baker RL, Curfman MF, Eads ME, Israel KS, Norris SA, Webb DH, Zeckel ML. Disseminated histoplasmosis in the acquired immune deficiency syndrome: clinical findings, diagnosis and treatment, and review of the literature. *Medicine.* (Baltimore). 1990;69:361-74.

[45] Sarosi GA, Johnson PC. Progressive disseminated histoplasmosis in the acquired immunodeficiency syndrome: a model for disseminated disease. *Semin. Respir. Infect.* 1990;5:146-50.

[46] Wheat LJ, Batteiger BE, Sathapatayavongs B. Histoplasma capsulatum infections of the central nervous system. A clinical review. Medicine (Baltimore). 1990;69:244-60.

[47] Anaissie E, Fainstein V, Samo T, Bodey GP, Sarosi GA. Central nervous system histoplasmosis. An unappreciated complication of the acquired immunodeficiency syndrome. *Am. J. Med.* 1988;84:215-7.

[48] Lerttumnongtum P, Muttarak M, Visrutaratna P, Ya-In C. Imaging features of unusual adrenal masses. *Australas Radiol.* 2004;48:107-13.

[49] Kumar N, Singh S, Govil S. Adrenal histoplasmosis: clinical presentation and imaging features in nine cases. *Abdom. Imaging.* 200328:703-8.

[50] Histoplasmosis. Available online at http://www.cdc.gov/niosh/97146eng.html

[51] Ahmed AR, Blose DA. Delayed-type hypersensitivity skin testing. A review. *Arch. Dermatol.* 1983;119:934-45.

[52] Verneuil L, Boisseau-Garsaud AM, Desbois N, Garsaud P, Helenon R, Cales-Quist D. Cutaneous sensitivity to histoplasmin in a Martinique hospitalized population. *Ann. Dermatol. Venereol.* 1999;126:405-7.

[53] Fava S di C, Netto CF. Epidemiologic surveys of histoplasmin and paracoccidioidin sensitivity in Brazil. *Rev. Inst. Med. Trop. Sao Paulo.* 1998 ;40:155-64.

[54] Wen FQ, Sun YD, Watanabe K, Yoshida M, Wu JN, Baum GL. Prevalence of histoplasmin sensitivity in healthy adults and tuberculosis patients in southwest China. *J. Med. Vet. Mycol.* 1996;34:171-4.

[55] Rodrigues MT, de Resende MA. Epidemiologic skin test survey of sensitivity to paracoccidioidin, histoplasmin and sporotrichin among gold mine workers of Morro Velho Mining, Brazil. *Mycopathologia.* 1996;135:89-98.

[56] Bregani ER, Van Tien T, Ceraldi T, Delfitto C, Figini G. Histoplasmosis: not only a tropical disease. *Recenti Prog. Med.* 2000; 91:396-401.

[57] McKinsey DS. Histoplasmosis in AIDS: advances in management. *AIDS Patient Care STDS.* 1998 ;12:775-81.

[58] Drew RH. Pharmacotherapy of disseminated histoplasmosis in patients with AIDS. *Ann. Pharmacother.* 1993;27:1510-8

[59] Johnson PC, Hamill RJ, Sarosi GA. Clinical review: progressive disseminated histoplasmosis in the AIDS patient. *Semin. Respir. Infect.* 1989;4:139-46.

[60] Garrett HE Jr, Roper CL. Surgical intervention in histoplasmosis. *Ann. Thorac. Surg.* 1986;42:711-22.

Chapter X

TOXOPLASMOSIS

INTRODUCTION TO TOXOPLASMOSIS

Toxoplasmosis is a parasitic infestation mainly caused by *Toxoplasma* spp. parasite of animals [1 – 2]. It is classified as an obligate intracellular parasite [1]. The main pathogenic protozoan was first observed in the North African rodent (*Ctenodactylus gundi*) by Nicolle and Manceaux in 1908 therefore it was later given the name "*Toxoplasma gondii*". Since the first discovery, there have been continuously reported on detection of disease in other animals including rabbut, squirrel, dog, monkey and pegion. Finally, it has been reported in humans. A complete life cycle for the ubiquitous protozoan parasite Toxoplasma was proposed over 30 years ago [3]. Since that time, despite attempts to make the genus polyspecific, there has been only one clinically important species, *T. gondii*, consistently recognised in the genus. Recent studies on taxa in genera closely related to Toxoplasma such as Neospora, Hammondia, Frenkelia, Isospora and Sarcocystis, have convincingly showed the need for a reclassification of many of the species in these genera [3].

Based on Taxonomy, this parasite is placed in the apicomplexan family Eimeriidae. Until present, at least 7 species of Toxoplasma are recognized: *T. gondii* (problematic species) from about 200 species of mammals and birds, with oocysts in felids; *T. alencari* (Da Costa and Pereira) from the frog *Leptodactylus ocellatus*; *T. brumpti Coutelen* from the iguana *Iguana tuberculata*; *T. colubri Tibaldi* from the snakes *Coluber melanoleucus* and *Coluber viridiflavus*; *T.hammondi* (Frenkel and Dubey) (a new combination for *Hammondia hammondi*) from the house mouse with oocysts in the domestic cat; *T. ranae Levine* and *Nye* from the leopard frog *Rana Pipiens*; and *T. serpai Scorza, Dager*t and *Iturriza Arocha* from the toad *Bufo marinus* [4]. Published results already clearly indicate that the population can be divided into two distinct groups that are genetically and biologically distinct [5]. The more virulent group, as defined by their LD50 in mice, is apparently a single, clonal line [5].

Epidemiology

T. gondii has been found worldwide in many species, including carnivorous and herbivorous mammals and birds. It has also been found in every population group of humans investigated [6]. However, the definitive host was shown to be cats, which have been associated with transmission of the parasite in every population investigated [6]. At present, this disease can be seen all over the world. In addition, it becomes an emerging for humans in the era of human immunodeficiency virus (HIV) infection.

A. Asia

For Southeast Asia, toxoplasmosis is an important tropical infection for a long time. This food borne parasitic zoonosis hits all countries in this region. Many newborn children in Indonesia have congenital anomalies attributable to T. gondii [7]. The parasite is widespread, with seroprevalence rates of 2-63% in humans, 35-73% in cats, 75% in dogs, 11-36% in pigs, 11-61% in goats, and less than 10% in cows [7]. In Malaysia, the prevalence rates of Toxoplasma antibody were consistently foundhighest among Malays, followed by Indians, Orang Aslis (Aborigines) and lowest among Malays, followed by Indians, Orang Aslia (Aborigines) and lowest among Chinese, the 4 major ethnic groups living in Malaysia [8]. Positive titres, present in all age groups, showed an increase with age but no difference due to sex [8]. For Thailand, an interesting picture of this zoonosis can be seen. Dog becomes an interesting reservoir for this disease. According to a recent report by Wiwanitkit et al, abandoned dogs within the Buddhist temple was the main source of infection to the monks living in the templ [9]. Fan et al also performed another interesting seroepidemiological survey of Toxoplasma gondii infection among Chinese refugees, including Akka and Yau aborigines and Han people living in mountainous areas at elevations of 1,100-1,400 m in Chiang-Rai Province of northern Thailand [10]. Ethnically, Yau aboriginal populations had a significantly higher seroprevalence than did the Akka aborigines and Han people [10]. This is corresponding to the nature that the Yau aboriginal populations generally feed a dog within their house.

In East Asia, China also faces up with this emerging disease. According to a recent study by Zhang et al [11] on serologic prevalence of T. gondii in field mice, Microtus fortis, from Yuanjiang, Hunan Province, People's Republic of China, very high prevalence of infection could be seen. Sun et al studied the prevalence in pregnant and newborns in Chengdu. They found that sera prevalence of toxoplasma IgG antibodies and IgM antibodies of pregnant women were 39.14% and 4.21% respectively and seraprevalence of toxoplasma IgM antibodies of newborn infants was 1.07% [12]. This result confirms the existence of the toxoplasmosis as important problem in China.

In India, high prevalence of this infection can be detected. Akoijam et al reported that 41.75% of pregnant visiting a secondary hospital in North India were seropositive for *T. gondii* infection [13]. These results indicate that a large number of the study subjects were vulnerable to toxoplasma infection. If these infections had occurred during the pregnancy, their fetuses would have been at high risk of infection [13]. According to another study by Murdha et al, *T. gondii*-antibodies were found in 21 (19.6%), 10 (25%), 26 (52%), goat, sheep and cow sera respectively [14]. These results indicate that Toxoplasma gondii antibodies are widespread in animal populations which supports that toxoplasmosis is a widely spread zoonotic infection in this country [14].

B. Africa

In Africa, the high prevalence of toxoplasmosis is noted. High prevalence of HIV also contributes to high prevalence of toxoplasmosis in Africa. Toxoplasmosis seems to be more frequent in AIDS patients in Africa than those from Europe or America [15]. According to a recent seroepidemiological survey in Northren Tunisia, the rate of seroconversion seems the highest between ten and 20 years of age and the majority of women were infected before reaching childbearing age [16]. According to the data reported from Institut Pasteur de Bangui, the seroprevalence did not vary significantly according to sex or age [17]. Risks of acute infections during pregnancy and of opportunistic infections in HIV-infection patients are high [17]. A control of toxoplasmosis is justifiable (screening during pregnancy, sanitary education) [17].

C. Europe

In Europe, the highest seroprevalences have been reported from France, both among women of reproductive age and the general population [18]. There is a higher seroprevalence in Central Europe than in Scandinavia or the United Kingdom [15]. Previously, the prevalence of toxoplasmosis in Europe is not as high as tropical Asia. However, the change of the epidemiology according to the abrupt emerging of HIV infection is observed. As a consensus, the European experience does not permit conclusions either in favor of or against a programme for the systematic screening of congenital toxoplasmosis [19]. However, cost-benefit analysis plays a very important role in determining whether such a programme should be implemented. Parameters such as the security of diagnosis (standardization of methods, quality and experience of the laboratories) and the monitoring of cases (definition, multidisciplinary approach to the surveillance and long-term treatment of patients, national collection of case reports, evaluation of the programme) are indispensable for the implementation of an effective surveillance system [19].

D. USA

Similar to Europe, the problem of toxoplasmosis becomes new emerging problem in the AIDS booming era. *T. gondii*-specific antibodies are common in serum samples of clinically ill cats from all regions of the USA [20]. Seroprevalence increases as cats age and is higher in male and domestic shorthair cats, compared with females and other breeds [20]. McQuillan et al reported the racial/ethnic differences in the seroprevalence of *T. gondii* in analyses stratified according to risk categories to identify patterns and to determine whether demographic, socioeconomic, and behavioral characteristics explain these differences [21]. In this work, stratification and adjustment for socioeconomic factors reduced or eliminated racial/ethnic differences in the prevalence of infection in the high-risk but not the low-risk group, wherein race/ethnicity remained significant and might have been a surrogate for unmeasured risk factors [21]. Jones et al noted that except for the risk of transmission from cats, knowledge among pregnant women about toxoplasmosis was low however toxoplasmosis-preventive practices are generally good, suggesting that providers should continue to offer education about practices that help prevent this foodborne disease [22]

PATHOGENIC ORGANISM

The pathogenic organism of toxoplasmosis is mainly *T. gondii*. The morphology of this parasite varies during its developmental cycle. Banana- or crescent-shaped forms of the parasite are ingested with food and enter the body via the pharyngeal and intestinal mucosa [23]. In intermediate hosts and humans these multiply during the acute phase of infection by cell division within a fine network of cells. At this stage of their development the protozoa are known as tachyzoites [23]. These 4–7 microns x 2–4 microns forms of the pathogen with a nucleus in the lower half of the cell are distributed via the blood and lymph to the entire body, where they cause lysis of host cells and go on to infect adjacent cells [23]. This process gradually gives rise to tissue damage in the form of necrotic foci surrounded by inflammation [23].

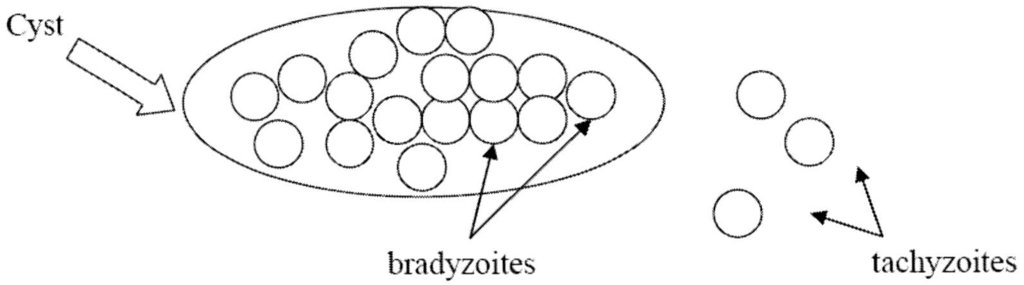

Figure 10.1 Diagram showing tachyzoites and bradyzoites of *T. gondii*.

Concerning the pathogenesis of *Toxoplasma* spp, the main pathogenesis process focuses on selected aspects of penetration into host cells followed by the biogenesis of specialized host cell compartment, parasitophorus vacuole, in which the parasite resides [24 - 26]. The invasive process involves six steps: a) cellular recognition, b) parasite movements by means of a subpellicular microtubule cytoskeleton, c) cell to cell adhesion, d) rhoptry secretion of penetrating enhancing factor (PEF) with Ca++ and Ca++ activated ATPase dependence, e) conoid penetration, f) induction of a parasitophorous vacuole, a protective and exchange site, interiorization of the parasite [27]. The invasion is an active, oriented and specific process depending on chemical factors as energy sources, cations, as well as microviscosity and membrane structures [27]. *T. gondii* stimulates T cell subsets and induces lymphokine (IFN gamma, IL2) release [27]. T. *gondii* potently stimulates IFN-gamma production by both the innate and adaptive immune system as part of its host adaptation [28]. This response is known to be dependent on Myeloid Differentiation factor 88 signaling pathway used by Toll-like receptors (TLRs), a family of proteins involved in the recognition of microbial molecular patterns [28]. TLR11 may have evolved as a general pattern recognition receptor for apicomplexan protozoa and that as highly conserved proteins associated with actin- based motility, profilins are logical ligand targets for this form of pathogen detection [28]. According to the study of Zimmerman et al, the inhibitory effects of *T. gondii* on IFN-gamma were diminished in macrophages from SOCS-1-/- mice [29]. The results suggest that induction of SOCS proteins within phagocytes due to infection with *T. gondii* contributes to the parasite's immune evasion strategies [29]. Subauste and Wessendarp noted that CD40 stimulation restricted *T. gondii* replication independently of STAT1, p47 GTPases, and nitric oxide. In vivo CD40 ligation enhanced TNF-alpha production by *T. gondii*-infected macrophages [30]. In addition, CD40 stimulation required the presence of TNF receptor 2 to reduce parasite load in vivo [30].

The tachyzoite lytic cycle begins with active invasion of host cells involving the release of adhesive proteins from apical secretory organelles called micronemes [31]. A protein complex consisting of the transmembrane adhesin MIC2 and a tightly associated partner, M2AP, is abundantly released from the micronemes [31]. Similar to many proteins in a regulated secretory pathway, *T. gondii* proteins destined for micronemes and rhoptries (another secretory organelle associated with invasion) undergo proteolytic maturation [31]. The vacuole membrane is the interface between host and parasite, playing a role in nutrient acquisition by the parasite from the host cells [32]. The parasitophorus vacuole phenomenon is regarded as a generalized host cells response to the introduction of alien bodies (microorganisms), which eventually reflects the evolutionary established host-parasite relationships at cellular, subcellular and molecular levels [32]. The parasite actively recruits host microtubules, resulting in selective attraction of endo-lysosomes to the parasitophorus vacuole [33]. Microtubule-based invaginations of the parasitophorus vacuole membrane serve as conduits for the delivery of host endo-lysosomes within the parasitophorus vacuole [33]. These tubular conduits are decorated by a parasite coat, including the tubulogenic protein GRA7, which acts like a garrote that sequesters host endocytic organelles in the vacuolar space [33].

LIFE CYCLE OF *TOXOPLASMA* SPP

T. gondii is a widespread protozoan parasite that can infect all nucleated cell types of warm-blooded vertebrates [34]. Parasite motility is regulated by polymerization of new actin filaments that provide a substrate for the small myosin TgMyoA [34]. Interaction between the cytoplasmic tails of parasite adhesins and the actin-binding protein aldolase links these cell surface proteins with the cytoskeleton. Translocation of adhesins coupled to extracellular receptors allows the parasite to glide across the substrate [34]. Concerning the life cycle of this parasite, cat is the definitive host of this parasite. The definitive host can be infected by ingestion of the cysts of *T. gondii* that are contained in the tissues of intermediate hosts. Cysts then disintegrate within the stomach and small intestine. After multiplication and reproduction within the walls of the intestines, egg-like “oocysts” are passed in the feces [35]. Oocysts can survive in the environment for several months and are extremely resistant to disinfectants, freezing, and drying [35].

It can be seen that the contamination of Toxoplasma spp eggs in the environment becomes an important public health threaten for many cities. The infection is still the important problem in many urban areas. Wiwanitkit [36] found that the frequency rate of Toxocara species contamination in soil samples from public yards in an urban area "Payathai", Bangkok, Thailand. In addition, the rate of contamination in the public yard of the hospital is also high [37]. Human toxocariasis develops by ingesting embryonated eggs in contaminated soil. From the reviewed literature, the contaminated soil with *Toxocara* spp. of urban and suburban area was 63.6% [38]. High crowding index, latrines shared with other families and no piped water inside the household, are more common in urban areas as compared with rural settlements and also associated with a higher intensity of infection by soil-transmitted helminths. The trend toward urbanization seems to have caused deterioration of living conditions and sanitation standards in some areas of the city, with the most vulnerable people experiencing an increase in intestinal parasitic infections [38].

Generally, cysts can be formed in the tissue of intermediates hosts. The common sites are muscles and nervous tissues. Sometimes, cysts can be found at the lungs, liver and renal tissues. These cysts may persist in the intermediate hosts for years. The intermediate hosts for *Toxoplasmosis* spp can be either herbivores/omnivores or carnivores and result in distinctive differences in the life cycle stages [39]. For herbivore/omnivore (type 1 intermediate host), hosts usually get infected by eating sporulated oocysts [39]. Each oocyst contains 2 sporocysts with 4 sporozoites. The liberated sporozoites infect extra-intestinal sites, initially in the acute phase mesenteric lymph nodes and liver, but as the infection becomes more chronic the others visceral organs especially brain become infected [39]. For carnivore (Type 2 intermediate host), both the pseudocyst and tissue cysts require the host for the life cycle to continue [39]. If the tissue cysts are eaten by a carnivore other than a cat, the released merozoites once again penetrate extra intestinal cells and form pseudocysts which produce more merozoites or bradyzoites, as they are called when the appear in carnivore tissue [39]. It should be noted that vertical transmission can be detected in both types of intermediate hosts [39].

The continuity of the cycle can occur when when a cat consumes meat contaminated with cysts [35]. Tachyzoites, bradyzoites (in tissue cysts), and sporozoites (in oocysts) are the three infectious stages of *T. gondii* [40]. The prepatent period (time to shedding of oocysts after primary infection) varies with the stage of *T. gondii* ingested by the cat (table 1) [39 - 40]. The prepatent period (pp) after ingesting bradyzoites is short (3-10 days) while it is long (18 days or longer) after ingesting oocysts or tachyzoites [40]. Dubey noted that the pp in cats is stage and not dose dependent, and that transmission of *T. gondii* is most efficient when cats consume tissue cysts or when intermediate hosts consume oocysts (fecal-oral transmission) [40]. As previously mentioned, human usually gets infection by ingestion of food or water contaminated by cat feces. However, consuming meat contaminated with cysts can also bring infection to human. In addition to domestic animals and human, infections are also common in wild carnivores, including pigs, bears, felids, fox, raccoons, and skunks [41].

Table 1. Time to appearance of oocyst in stool when the cat is infected with different stages [39 – 40]

Stages	Time (days)
Tissue cyst	3 – 5
Pseudocyst	9 – 12
Oocyst	20 -24

PATHOGENESIS

In general most of the human population infected with Toxoplasma is asymptomatic carriers [40]. Epidemiological surveys in which serum antibodies to Toxoplasma are measured has demonstrated a wide prevalence of this parasite [40]. Studenicova et al found that an increased prevalence of *T. gondii* was observed in the age group over 40 years and in women who consume raw meat, vegetables, or fruit [42]. Cavalcante et al found that Home-grown vegetable consumption and origin of drinking water (well or river) were the independent variables that displayed significant association [43]. They noted that higher values of occurrence were found in people with consumption of home-grown vegetables and people that drink well water compared with people that did not consume this type of food and drink river water [43]. Clinical cases are less common. Studenicova et al found that there was no difference in clinical symptoms between serologically positive and negative patients. They found that lymphadenopathy with or without other symptoms (influenza, arthralgia, ocular symptom, dermatosis), was the most common clinical symptom in seropositive patients [42].

However, emerging in number of the infected human cases are reported in the AIDS era. Nissapatorn et al found that half of HIV infected patients were seropositive for toxoplamosis [44]. They also noted for statistically significance in the association between CD4 count and toxoplasmic encephalitis [44]. Meisheri et al performed another interesting prospective study of seroprevalence of Toxoplasmosis in general population, and in HIV/AIDS patients in Bombay [45]. According to this work, the seroprevalence in the HIV infected group is about two times higher than general non-infected population [45].

There are a number of factors which determine whether an infected host will express disease symptoms. These factors include the strain of the pathogen, the susceptibility of the host, age of the host and degree of acquired immunity

A. Strain of Pathogen

Toxoplasma has an unusual population structure with a few clonally reproducing strains apparently dominating in many of its hosts, which include humans [46]. In mice, the various strains of the parasite differ enormously in their virulence and disease presentation [46]. Analysis of independent recombinant progeny identified several quantitative trait loci that contributed to acute virulence [47]. A major quantitative trait locus located on chromosome VII accounted for approximately 50% of the virulence phenotype, whereas a minor locus on chromosome IV, linked to the ROP1 gene, accounted for approximately 10% [47]. These loci are conserved in other type I strains, indicating that acute virulence is controlled by discrete genes common to the type I lineage [47]. In humans, disease manifestations are highly variable, ranging from asymptomatic to severe, especially in cases of brain and eye infection [46]. Recent data suggest that, as with mice, at least part of this variability in human infection may be tied to the type of strain that causes the infection [46].

B. Susceptibility of the Host

The protozoan parasite *T. gondii* is capable of infecting all warm blooded animals; however, the consequences of infection are very variable between different species of animal [48]. Marsupials and New World monkeys, which have evolved largely separately from the cat, the definitive host of the parasite, are among the most vulnerable species where infection with *T. gondii* can prove fatal [48]. In more resistant species such as humans and sheep, infection is generally unapparent, provoking only mild symptoms; thereafter the host remains infected for life [48]. For human, the determinants which appear to influence directly the outcome of intracellular infection include: a. the magnitude of the phagocyte's respiratory burst capacity; b. the ability to respond specifically and effectively to microbial ingestion with the generation of O2- and H2O2; c. susceptibility to H2O2; and d. the presence of and susceptibility to oxygen-independent mechanisms [49]. For brain infection in humans, the HLA-DQ1 and -DQ3 genes are involved in regulating the resistance and susceptibility [50]. Since these genes are a part of the major histocompatibility complex, which regulates the immune responses, the regulation of the responses by these genes appears to be important for determining host resistance to this disease [50].

C. Age of the Host

Louria et al said that infections due to *Listeria monocytogenes*, *Salmonella typhimurium*, and *T. gondii* all appear to be worse in senescent mice; each of these organisms is dealt with primarily by the lymphocyte-macrophage system [51]. According to the seroprevalence study, positive titres, present in all age groups, showed an increase with age but no difference due to sex [52].

D. Degree of Acquired Immunity

Immunity is the main determinant for getting toxoplasmosis. As previously mentioned, high prevalence of toxoplasmosis can be seen in HIV infected patients.

In addition, the patients with other immune defects disorder such as SLE are also pose high seropositivity rate. Noel et al said that Toxoplasma infection may enhance the production of autoantibodies which, when combined with the high titres characteristic of SLE, might interfere in the dye test and other serological tests [53]. They also noted that immunoblotting could prove useful in the immunocompromised for confirming the presence of specific toxoplasma antibodies and for the staging of infection in those with positive serology [53]. Zamir et al noted that cerebral toxoplasmosis was a rare complication of SLE that may be misdiagnosed as lupus cerebritis [54].

Basically, *T. gondii* is an intracellular obligate parasite that enters the host via the gastrointestinal tract [55]. Both the infected enterocytes as well as the CD4 T cells from the lamina propria produce chemokines and cytokines that are necessary to clear the parasite whereas CD8 intraepithelial lymphocytes secrete transforming growth factor beta that reduces the inflammation [56]. The parasite is able to evade or subvert the immune response of its host via various mechanisms [55]. Lymphocytes and cytokines they produce play a crucial role in determining the outcome of parasitic infection in terms of both protective immunity and immunopathology [57]. The intracellular protozoan Toxoplasma gondii exerts profound effects on nuclear factor-kappaB (NF-kappaB)- and mitogen-activated protein kinase (MAPK)-signaling cascades in macrophages [58]. During early infection, nuclear translocation of NF-kappaB is blocked, and later, the cells display defects in lipopolysaccharide (LPS)-induced MAPK phosphorylation after undergoing initial activation in response to Toxoplasma itself [57]. *T. gondii* is a potent stimulus for cell-mediated immunity, and IL-12-dependent IFN-gamma induction is vital in resistance to the parasite [58]. Infected macrophages that are subjected to triggering through Toll-like receptor 4 (TLR4) with LPS display defective production of tumor necrosis factor-alpha and IL-12 (IL-12) that likely reflects interference with NF-kappaB- and MAPK-signaling cascades [59 – 60].Dendritic cells, neutrophils and macrophages are important sources of IL-12 during infection. T. gondii possesses two mechanisms for triggering IL-12 [58]. One is dependent upon the common adaptor protein MyD88, and is likely to involve Toll-like receptors [58]. The other is a more unusual pathway that involves triggering through CCR5 by a parasite cyclophilin molecule [58]. Nevertheless, *T. gondii* possesses molecules that themselves induce eventual proinflammatory cytokine synthesis [59 – 60]. After parasite proliferation has been contained by interferon-gamma-dependent responses, the onset of the chronic phase of infection is characterized by continuous cell-mediated immunity [61]. Such potent responses are kept under tight control by a class of anti-inflammatory eicosanoid, the lipoxins [61].

Diagnosis of Toxoplasma Infection

The diagnosis of toxoplasma infection is usually by serological study [62].

Identification of specific immunoglobulins G, M, A, and E can be done (table 2) [63]. The serological diagnosis should be confirmed by the clinical picture of the patient and possibly by finding the parasite or its genome, even using molecular methods [64]. Furthermore, since the presence of specific antibodies can reveal an acquired infection, but not necessarily a disease, it is particularly helpful, in addition to a qualitative evaluation, a quantitative one, by determining the serum antibody titre [64]. After recovery, the antibody levels decrease, however, they may persist for long periods, for this reason they do not help in evaluating the treatment outcome [64]. Basically, the immunodominance of tachyzoites is responsible for the induction of a strong humoral immune response leading to the formation of antibodies specifically directed against tachyzoite antigens [65]. In contrast, the bradyzoite stage which is associated with inactive/chronic infection, seems not to be a strong inducer of specific antibodies [65]. However, since the humoral antibody response is also directed against antigens that are expressed in both stages, serodiagnosis cannot always adequately discriminate between active and inactive/chronic infection [65]. Contrary to the most infectious diseases, however, the high specific IgM level has not proved to be a reliable marker of the acute infection in the case of toxoplasmosis [66]. Therefore, in the case of infections discovered in the "plateau" period (with persistent IgM and/or persistent high level of IgG antibody), the acute and the "chronic phases can be distinguished more reliably by the detection with ELISA of the IgA antibody response to the so called P30 protein of *T. gondii* [66]. The anti-P30 IgA antibody response appears very early and generally disappears in 3-9 months [66]. Interpretation of serological results may be difficult when the patients originate from areas where the suspected infection is endemic, in that case, serum positivity could reflect an old exposition to the parasite, and therefore it is not related to the present clinical status [64]. Furthermore, serology may frequently result falsely negative in not immunocompetent subjects [64].

Table 2. Examples of serological tests for toxoplasmosis diagnosis

Examples	Detected antibody
Sabin-Feldman test	IgG + IgM
Immunofluorescence assay (IFA)	Total antibodies or IgG or IgM
Agglutination test	IgG
Immunosorbent agglutination assay (ISAGA)	IgM
Enzyme-linked immunosorbent assay (ELISA)	IgG or IgM

In additional to serological method, there are also other methods for diagnosis of toxoplasmosis. In vitro culture and mouse inoculation are two classical methods. The animal inoculation can provide a confirmative diagnosis. The dose for mice for intraperitoneal inoculation is 0.1 mL of fresh exudate or 0.5 mL of 10 % suspension of mouse brain. Usually, death of animal occurs during 7 – 14 days and the parasites can be seen microscopically in the omentum tissue smears. However, these old methods are presently replaced by the serological tests. For blood film determination, it is hard to detect the organism. From complete blood count, lymphocytosis and moderate leukocytosis can be seen. The advanced diagnostic method is based on the molecular biology technique. Diagnosis based on clinical appearance and serology is not always easy, however, molecular methods do not depend on an immune response, and allow direct detection of the parasite in biological samples [67]. Thus they can be used to establish a diagnosis when serological tests are not definitive [67]. In the past decade, the use of the polymerase chain reaction (PCR) has made a significant improvement in both the prenatal diagnosis of congenital toxoplasmosis and the detection of acute disease in the immunocompromised patient [68]. Nevertheless, like many 'in-house' PCR assays, the PCR-Toxoplasma suffers from lack of standardization and variable performance according to the laboratory [68]. Multicopy sequences specific for *T. gondii*, e.g., the B1 gene or the 529-bp sequence, are especially useful in molecular tests [67]. Molecular methods are also used for genotypic characterisation of *T. gondii* isolates [67]. Analysis of polymorphic sequences determines the precise strain [67]. The choice of sequence is critical when undertaking studies on the correlation between clinical signs and symptoms of disease and the *T. gondii* genotype [67]. According to a recent comparative study by Fricker-Hidalgo et al [69], the PCR sensitivity was higher than that of cell culture and mouse inoculation but the number of PCR positive results in definitely or probably non-infected fetuses patients was also higher. Fricker-Hidalgo et al concluded that the detection of IgM by ELISA and ISAGA and the detection of neosynthesized Ig by immunoblotting were more satisfactory to diagnose congenital toxoplasmosis but the placenta analysis was important to improve the sensitivity of the diagnosis at birth, especially when the prenatal diagnosis was negative or not performed [69].

Clinical Manifestation of Toxoplasmosis

A. Feline Toxoplasmonsis

Feline toxoplasmosis is a classical infection of this parasite. As previously mentioned, cats acquire Toxoplasma infection by eating any of the three infective stages of the parasite: cyst, oocyst, or tachyzoite. Most cats show no clinical signs of infection with Toxoplasma. Occasionally, however, clinical disease occurs, kittens and young adult cats being more often affected than older animals. When disease does occur, it may develop either following primary infection (where an inadequate immune response fails to arrest the invasive tachyzoites), or as a result of reactivated infection (where compromised immunity allows the reactivation of infection from encysted bradyzoites with the formation of invading, multiplying tachyzoites) [70 – 71]. Lethargy, depression, loss of appetite, and fever are typical early nonspecific signs. Pneumonia, manifested by respiratory distress of gradually increasing severity, is the outstanding sign in many cats [70]. Hepatitis (inflammation of the liver) may cause vomiting, diarrhea, prostration, and jaundice (yellowing of the mucous membranes) [70]. Inflammation of the pancreas and enlargement of lymph nodes also occur [70]. Clinical disease appears to be most common in young cats (less than 2 years of age), and this may be due, in part, to a poorly developed immune response in these cats [71]. Reactivation of infection in older cats may be linked to co-infection with feline leukemia virus or feline immunodeficiency virus in some cats [71]. Fecal samples may be examined for the presence of *T. gondii* oocysts, although this test is both technically difficult and requires experience to correctly identify the oocysts. Serological diagnosis is more favorable [71].

B. Human Toxoplasmosis

Humans can become infected with *T gondii* by ingesting either material contaminated with infectious oocysts or tissue cysts contained in raw or undercooked meat from another intermediate host. Similar to feline toxoplasmosis, the infection in human is usually asymptomatic. The most severe symptoms occur in the congenitally acquired form and in immunocompromised hosts [72]. In the immunocompetent host, toxoplasmosis is classified as congenital, acquired, or ocular [72].

Congenital Toxoplasmosis

Congenital toxoplasmosis is an important congenital infection. Toxoplasma is an important member of the well-known TORCH agents. Pregnant women who acquire infection from *T. gondii* usually remain asymptomatic, although they can still transmit the infection to their fetuses with severe consequences [73]. Given the asymptomatic nature of most Toxoplasma infections, primary prevention in pregnant women may lower the risk of congenital toxoplasmosis [73]. Both consumption of undercooked meat and unprotected contact with soil are independent risk factors for *T. gondii* seroconversion during pregnancy, while contact with cat litter may pose a risk in certain situations [73]. Serologic tests are used to diagnose acute *T. gondii* infection in pregnant women [74]. Because false-positive tests occur frequently, serologic diagnosis must be confirmed at a Toxoplasma reference laboratory before treatment with potentially toxic drugs is considered [74]. In many instances, congenital toxoplasmosis can be prevented by educating pregnant women and other women of childbearing age about not ingesting raw or undercooked meat, using measures to avoid cross-contamination of other foods with raw or undercooked meat, and protecting themselves against exposure to cat litter or contaminated soil [74]. Congenital toxoplasmosis remains important causes of deafness, vision loss, and behavioral or neurologic disorders among children worldwide [75]. Chorioretinitis, hydrocephalus, intracranial calcifications, and convulsions are the typical presentation of classic congenital toxoplasmosis. Serology is the most common method of diagnosing neonatal infection, but more complex tests are also utilized. The prognosis for the untreated infant is poor; however, when antibiotic therapy is started early, the rate of sequelae is reduced significantly [76]. In general, prenatal therapy of congenital toxoplasmosis is beneficial in reducing the frequency of infant infection. Therapies are based primarily on spiramycin because of the relative lack of toxicity and high concentrations achieved in the placenta [77]. Clindamycin is the standard drug for chemoprophylaxis in newborn infants, and is directed at preventing the occurrence of retinochoroiditis as a late sequel to congenital infection [77].

Acquired Toxoplasmosis

Acquired toxoplasmosis in immunocompetent host is not common. Patients with acquired infection can present with a range of manifestations, from subclinical lymphadenopathy (the most common presentation) to fatal, fulminant disease [72]. The standard treatment for acquired toxoplasmosis in both immunocompetent and immunodeficient patients is the synergistic combination of pyrimethamine and sulphonamides [77].

Ocular Toxoplasmosis

Ocular toxoplasmosis occurs from activation of cysts deposited in or near the retina. Focal necrotizing retinitis is the characteristic lesion [72, 78]. Approximately 35% of all cases of retinochoroiditis can be attributed to ocular toxoplasmosis [72]. The appearance of toxoplasmic retinochoroiditis lesions varies with duration of active retinal infection and intensity of inflammation [78]. Severe ocular disease occurs in immunocompromised hosts [78]. Older patients who are recently infected with *T. gondii* may have a higher prevalence of ocular involvement and more severe ocular disease because of altered host defenses [78]. Since most cases of ocular toxoplasmosis are the result of congenital infection, clinical manifestation later in life usually represents reactivation of latent infection [72]. Many observational studies suggest a benefit of short-term antimicrobial therapy for toxoplasmic retinochoroiditis in immunocompetent patients, although the efficacy of these treatments has not been proven in randomized clinical trials [78]. Intermittent trimethoprim/sulfamethoxazole treatment was associated with fewer recurrences than placebo during a 20-month randomized clinical trial [78]. The risk of recurrent ocular disease appears to be greater during the first year after an episode of toxoplasmic retinochoroiditis than during subsequent years [79].

Considering the immunocompromised host, the clinical manifestation of toxoplasmosis is usually severe and involves the neurological system. A tumor like lesion in the imaging of brain is a classical sign of central nervous system (CNS) infection in the HIV infected patients. Before highly active antiretroviral therapy (HAART), up to 50% of all HIV-infected patients in Europe developed cerebral toxoplasmosis, an encephalitis caused by reactivation of infection [80]. Diagnosis is made on the basis of clinical presentation and brain imaging study findings and confirmed by demonstration of tachyzoites and/or cysts in tissues obtained by needle aspiration or brain biopsy [81]. MRI is the best imaging technique for detection of CNS toxoplasmosis since some lesions could not not visualized on CT scan. The common findings are single or multiple ring-enhancing lesions, most often in the basal ganglia or corticomedullary junction [72]. Cerebrospinal fluid may show mononuclear pleocytosis, elevated protein and normal glucose. Response to therapy with pyrimethamine and sulphadiazine is usually prompt but therapy has to be continued for the lifetime of AIDS patients with CNS toxoplasmosis [81]. To date, no alternative regimens of single or combination drugs appear to be effective in patients who fail, or are unable to tolerate pyrimethamine and sulphadiazine therapy. Relapse rate is high [81].

Treatment of Toxoplasmosis

Pharmacological treatment for toxoplasmosis is recommended. Combination of pyrimethamine and a sulfonamide is effective against acute toxoplasmosis in immunocompetent adults. These two drugs act synergistically against the tachyzoite form of *T gondii*. As an alternative to sulfonamides, clindamycin may be used in combination with pyrimethamine. In patients who are HIV negative, treatment is with pyrimethamine at an initial dose of 100 mg PO, followed by a dose of 25 mg/d, plus sulfadiazine 4-6 g/d PO for 4-5 weeks [72]. Folinic acid 5 mg/d PO reduces incidence of pyrimethamine-induced bone marrow suppression [72]. Postpartum treatment of congenital toxoplasmosis with sulfadiazine and pyrimethamine has remained almost unchanged for 50 years [82]. However, limited data are available on the use of pyrimethamine in the first trimester of pregnancy. More recently, sulfadiazine has been substituted by sulfadoxine, which has a much longer half-life and provides a basis for a dose schedule with higher compliance [82]. Treatment is recommended for all infected newborns with different strategies for infants with or without clinical symptoms [83]. Newer drugs with potential effects against *T. gondii*, such as azithromycin, atovaquone and clindamycin, require further evaluation in animal models and human studies [82].

Patients with AIDS are treated with pyrimethamine 200 mg PO initially, followed by 50-75 mg/d PO plus folinic acid 10 mg/d PO plus sulfadiazine 4-8 g/d PO for as long as 6 weeks, followed by lifelong suppressive therapy [72]. Suppressive therapy for patients with AIDS is pyrimethamine 50 mg/d PO plus sulfadiazine 1-1.5 g/d PO plus folinic acid 10 mg/d PO for life [72]. Treatment of toxoplasmic meningoencephalitis has been relatively successful in comparison to other opportunistic infections [84]. Prior to the introduction of HAART, a median survival of over a year was reported for patients who could tolerate the toxicity of toxoplasmic meningoencephalitis treatment [84]. However, this rate is dramatically improved after the easier availability of HAART. Trimethoprim-sulfamethoxazole appears to be an effective alternative therapy for toxoplasmic meningoencephalitis in resource-poor settings where pyrimethamine and sulfonamide are not available [84].

REFERENCES

[1] Dlugonska H. Toxoplasma gondii--intracellular parasite. *Wiad. Parazytol.* 2002;48:23-8.

[2] Dodds EM. Toxoplasmosis. *Curr. Opin. Ophthalmol.* 2006;17:557-61.

[3] Johnson AM. Is there more than one species in the genus Toxoplasma?? *Tokai J. Exp. Clin. Med.* 1998;23:383-9.

[4] Levine ND. Tazonomy of Toxoplasma. *J. Protozool.* 1977;24:36-41.

[5] Boothroyd JC. Population biology of Toxoplasma: clonality, virulence, and speciation (or not). *Infect. Agents Dis.* 1993;2:100-2.

[6] Toxoplasmosis. Available on http://www.stanford.edu/class/humbio103/ParaSites2006/Toxoplasmosis/epidemiology.h

[7] Gandahusada S. Study on the prevalence of toxoplasmosis in Indonesia: a review. *Southeast Asian J. Trop. Med. Public Health.* 1991;22 Suppl:93-8

[8] Saleha AA. Observations on some epidemiological aspects of toxoplasmosis in Malaysia. *Int. J. Zoonoses.* 1984;11:75-83.

[9] Wiwanitkit V, Soogarun S, Suwansaksri J. Platelet parameters in Toxoplasma gondii IgG-seropositive subjects. *Lab. Hematol.* 2003;9:248-9.

[10] Fan CK, Liao CW, Wu MS, Su KE, Han BC. Seroepidemiology of Toxoplasma gondii infection among Chinese aboriginal and Han people residing in mountainous areas of northern Thailand. *J. Parasitol.* 2003;89:1239-42.

[11] Serologic prevalence of Toxoplasma gondii in field mice, Microtus fortis, from Yuanjiang, Hunan Province, People's Republic of China. *J. Parasitol.* 2004;90:437-8.

[12] Sun RG, Liu ZL, Wang DC. The prevalence of Toxoplasma infection among pregnant women and their newborn infants in Chengdu. *Zhonghua Liu Xing Bing Xue Za Zhi.* 1995;16:98-100.

[13] Akoijam BS, Shashikant, Singh S, Kapoor SK. Seroprevalence of toxoplasma infection among primigravid women attending antenatal clinic at a secondary level hospital in North India. *J. Indian Med. Assoc.* 2002;100:591-2, 594-6, 602.

[14] Mirdha BR, Samantaray JC, Pandey A. Seropositivity of Toxoplasma gondii in domestic animals. *Indian J. Public Health.* 1999;43:91-2.

[15] Holliman RE. Toxoplasmosis and the acquired immune deficiency syndrome. *J. Infect.* 1988;16:121-8.

[16] Bouratbine A, Siala E, Chahed MK, Aoun K, Ben Ismail R. Sero-epidemiologic profile of toxoplasmosis in northern Tunisia. *Parasite.* 2001;8:61-6.

[17] Morvan JM, Mambely R, Selekon B, Coumanzi-Malo MF. Toxoplasmosis at the Pasteur Institute of Bangui, Central African Republic (1996-1998): serological data. *Bull. Soc. Pathol. Exot.* 1999;92:157-60.

[18] Zuber P, Jacquier P. Epidemiology of toxoplasmosis: worldwide status. *Schweiz. Med. Wochenschr. Suppl.* 1995;65:19S-22S.

[19] Raeber PA, Biedermann K, Just M, Zuber P. Prevention of congenital toxoplasmosis in Europe. *Schweiz. Med. Wochenschr. Suppl.* 1995;65:96S-102S.

[20] Vollaire MR, Radecki SV, Lappin MR. Seroprevalence of Toxoplasma gondii antibodies in clinically ill cats in the United States. *Am. J. Vet. Res.* 2005;66:874-7.

[21] McQuillan GM, Kruszon-Moran D, Kottiri BJ, Curtin LR, Lucas JW, Kington RS. Racial and ethnic differences in the seroprevalence of 6 infectious diseases in the United States: data from NHANES III, 1988-1994. *Am. J. Public Health.* 2004;94:1952-8.

[22] Jones JL, Ogunmodede F, Scheftel J, Kirkland E, Lopez A, Schulkin J, Lynfield R. Toxoplasmosis-related knowledge and practices among pregnant women in the United States. *Infect. Dis. Obstet. Gynecol.* 2003;11:139-45.

[23] Toxoplasmosis. Available online at http://www.roche.com/pages/ facets/2/ toxoplasmosis.htm

[24] Goncharov DB. The role of Toxoplasma gondii persistence in human clinical pathology. *Zh. Mikrobiol. Epidemiol. Immunobiol.* 2006;(4):92-7.

[25] Dlugonska H. Invasiveness and intracellular parasitism of Toxoplasma gondii. *Wiad. Parazytol.* 2005;51:213-7.

[26] Dlugonska H. Toxoplasma gondii--intracellular parasite. *Wiad. Parazytol.* 2002;48:23-8.

[27] Bonhomme A, Pingret L, Pinon JM. Review: Toxoplasma gondii cellular invasion. *Parassitologia.* 1992;34:31-43.

[28] Yarovinsky F, Sher A. Toll-like receptor recognition of Toxoplasma gondii. *Int. J. Parasitol.* 2006;36:255-9.

[29] Zimmermann S, Murray PJ, Heeg K, Dalpke AH. Induction of suppressor of cytokine signaling-1 by Toxoplasma gondii contributes to immune evasion in macrophages by blocking IFN-gamma signaling. *J. Immunol.* 2006;176:1840-7.

[30] Subauste CS, Wessendarp M. CD40 restrains in vivo growth of Toxoplasma gondii independently of gamma interferon. *Infect. Immun.* 2006;74:1573-9.

[31] Huynh MH, Harper JM, Carruthers VB. Preparing for an invasion: charting the pathway of adhesion proteins to Toxoplasma micronemes. *Parasitol. Res.* 2006;98:389-95.

[32] Beier TV, Svezhova NV, Radchenko AI, Sidorenko NV. Formation and diversity of parasitophorous vacuoles in parasitic protozoa. The Coccidia (Sporozoa, Apicomplexa). *Tsitologiia.* 2003;45:339-56

[33] Coppens I, Dunn JD, Romano JD, Pypaert M, Zhang H, Boothroyd JC, Joiner KA. Toxoplasma gondii sequesters lysosomes from mammalian hosts in the vacuolar space. *Cell.* 2006;125:261-74.

[34] Sibley LD. Toxoplasma gondii: perfecting an intracellular life style. *Traffic.* 2003;4:581-6.

[35] Toxoplasmosis. Available online at http://www.unbc.ca/nlui/ wildlife_diseases_bc/ toxoplasmosis.htm

[36] Wiwanitkti V. The frequency rate of Toxocara species contamination in soil samples from public yards in a urban area "Payathai", Bangkok, Thailand. *Rev. Inst. Med. Trop. Sao Paulo.* 2004 ;46:113-4.

[37] Wiwanitkit V, Waenlor W. Contamination of soil with parasites in a Thai hospital. *Am. J. Infect. Control.* 2005;33:374-5.

[38] Nakipoglu Y, Erturan Z, Buyukbaba-Boral O, Aksozek A, Aydin S, Derbentli S. Evaluation of the contaminant organisms of humidifier reservoir water and investigation of the source of contamination in a university hospital in Turkey. *Am. J. Infect. Control.* 2005;33:62-3.

[39] Toxoplasmosis. Available online at http://martin.parasitology.mcgill.ca/ jimspage/biol/ TOXOPLAS.HTM

[40] Dubey JP. Comparative infectivity of oocysts and bradyzoites of Toxoplasma gondii for intermediate (mice) and definitive (cats) hosts. *Vet. Parasitol.* 2006;140:69-75.

[41] Hill DE, Chirukandoth S, Dubey JP. Biology and epidemiology of Toxoplasma gondii in man and animals. *Anim. Health Res. Rev.* 2005;6:41-61.

[42] Studenicova C, Bencaiova G, Holkova R. Seroprevalence of Toxoplasma gondii antibodies in a healthy population from Slovakia. *Eur. J. Intern. Med.* 2006;17:470-3.

[43] Cavalcante GT, Aguilar DM, Camargo LM, Labruna MB, de Andrade HF, Meireles LR, Dubey JP, Thulliez P, Dias RA, Gennari SM. Seroprevalence of Toxoplasma gondii antibodies in humans from rural Western Amazon, Brazil. *J. Parasitol.* 2006;92:647-9.

[44] Nissapatorn V, Lee CK, Khairul AA. Seroprevalence of toxoplasmosis among AIDS patients in Hospital Kuala Lumpur, 2001. *Singapore Med. J.* 2003;44:194-6.

[45] Meisheri YV, Mehta S, Patel U. A prospective study of seroprevalence of Toxoplasmosis in general population, and in HIV/AIDS patients in Bombay, India. *J. Postgrad. Med.* 1997;43:93-7.

[46] Boothroyd JC, Grigg ME. Population biology of Toxoplasma gondii and its relevance to human infection: do different strains cause different disease? *Curr. Opin. Microbiol.* 2002;5:438-42.

[47] Su C, Howe DK, Dubey JP, Ajioka JW, Sibley LD. Identification of quantitative trait loci controlling acute virulence in Toxoplasma gondii. *Proc. Natl. Acad. Sci. U S A.* 2002;99:10753-8.

[48] Innes EA. Toxoplasmosis: comparative species susceptibility and host immune response. *Comp. Immunol. Microbiol. Infect. Dis.* 1997;20:131-8.

[49] Murray HW. Survival of intracellular pathogens within human mononuclear phagocytes. *Semin. Hematol.* 1988;25:101-11.

[50] Suzuki Y. Host resistance in the brain against Toxoplasma gondii. *J. Infect. Dis.* 2002;185 Suppl. 1:S58-65.

[51] Louria DB, Sen P, Buse M. Age-dependent differences in outcome of infections, with special reference to experiments in mice. *J. Am. Geriatr. Soc.* 1982;30:769-73.

[52] Saleha AA. Observations on some epidemiological aspects of toxoplasmosis in Malaysia. *Int. J. Zoonoses.* 1984;11:75-83.

[53] Noel I, Balfour AH, Wilcox MH. Toxoplasma infection and systemic lupus erythematosus: analysis of the serological response by immunoblotting. *J. Clin. Pathol.* 1993;46:628-32.

[54] Zamir D, Amar M, Groisman G, Weiner P. Toxoplasma infection in systemic lupus erythematosus mimicking lupus cerebritis. *Mayo Clin. Proc.* 1999;74:575-8.

[55] Buzoni-Gatel D, Werts C.Toxoplasma gondii and subversion of the immune system. *Trends Parasitol.* 2006;22:448-52.

[56] Kasper L, Courret N, Darche S, Luangsay S, Mennechet F, Minns L, Rachinel N, Ronet C, Buzoni-Gatel D. Toxoplasma gondii and mucosal immunity. *Int. J. Parasitol.* 2004;34:401-9.

[57] Lipska A, Wysocka J, Turowski D. Immune response and diagnostic aspects during Toxoplasma gondii infection. *Wiad. Parazytol.* 2000;46:315-25.

[58] Denkers EY. From cells to signaling cascades: manipulation of innate immunity by Toxoplasma gondii. *FEMS Immunol. Med. Microbiol.* 2003;39:193

[59] Denkers EY, Butcher BA, Del Rio L, Kim L. Manipulation of mitogen-activated protein kinase/nuclear factor-kappaB-signaling cascades during intracellular Toxoplasma gondii infection. *Immunol. Rev.* 2004;201:191-205.

[60] Dlugonska H, Dytnerska K. Identification of Toxoplasma gondii antigens recognized by specific T lymphocytes. *Wiad. Parazytol.* 2000;46:455-8.

[61] Aliberti J. Host persistence: exploitation of anti-inflammatory pathways by Toxoplasma gondii. *Nat. Rev. Immunol.* 2005;5:162-70.

[62] Makioka A. Immunologic tests: Toxoplasma Nippon Rinsho. 2005;63 Suppl. 7:274-6

[63] Pashanina TP, Napalkova GM, Korsakova II, Manankov VV. Prevalence of toxoplasmosis and methods for its laboratory diagnosis. *Med. Parazitol.* (Mosk). 2005;(1):51-4.

[64] Bruschi F, Castagna B. The serodiagnosis of parasitic infections. *Parassitologia.* 2004;46:141-4.

[65] Gross U, Holpert M, Goebel S. Impact of stage differentiation on diagnosis of toxoplasmosis. *Ann. Ist. Super Sanita.* 2004;40:65-70.

[66] Szenasi Z, Nagy E, Ozsvar Z, Szabo J, Gellen J, Jeszenszky M, Vegh M. Serodiagnosis of toxoplasmosis. *Orv. Hetil.* 1997;138:3241-7.

[67] Switaj K, Master A, Skrzypczak M, Zaborowski P. Recent trends in molecular diagnostics for Toxoplasma gondii infections. *Clin. Microbiol. Infect.* 2005;11:170-6.

[68] Bastien P. Molecular diagnosis of toxoplasmosis. *Trans. R. Soc. Trop. Med. Hyg.* 2002;96 Suppl. 1:S205-15.

[69] Fricker-Hidalgo H, Pelloux H, Racinet C, Grefenstette I, Bost-Bru C, Goullier-Fleuret A, Ambroise-Thomas P.Detection of Toxoplasma gondii in 94 placentae from infected women by polymerase chain reaction, in vivo, and in vitro cultures. *Placenta.* 1998;19:545-9.

[70] Toxoplasmosis in cat. Available online at www.vet.cornell.edu/fhc/brochures/toxo.html

[71] Toxoplasmosis. Available online at www.fabcats.org/toxoplasmosis.html

[72] Toxoplasmosis. Available online at www.emedicine.com/emerg/topic601.htm

[73] Kravetz JD, Federman DG. Kravetz JD, Federman DG. Toxoplasmosis in pregnancy. *Am. J. Med.* 2005;118:212-6.

[74] Jones J, Lopez A, Wilson M. Congenital toxoplasmosis. *Am. Fam. Physician.* 2003;67:2131-8.

[75] Bale JF Jr. Congenital infections. *Neurol. Clin.* 2002;20:1039-60, vii.

[76] Martin S. Congenital toxoplasmosis. *Neonatal. Netw.* 2001;20:23-30.

[77] Georgiev VS. Management of toxoplasmosis. *Drugs.* 1994;48:179-88.

[78] Holland GN. Ocular toxoplasmosis: a global reassessment. Part II: disease manifestations and management. *Am. J. Ophthalmol.* 2004;137:1-17.

[79] Holland GN. Ocular toxoplasmosis: a global reassessment. Part I: epidemiology and course of disease. *Am. J. Ophthalmol.* 2003;136:973-88.

[80] Happe S, Fischer A, Heese Ch, Reichelt D, Gruneberg U, Freund M, Kloska S, Evers S, Husstedt IW. HIV-associated cerebral toxoplasmosis -- review and retrospective analysis of 36 patients. *Nervenarzt.* 2002 ;73:1174-8.

[81] Tuazon CU. Toxoplasmosis in AIDS patients. *J. Antimicrob. Chemother.* 1989;23 Suppl A:77-82z

[82] Petersen E, Schmidt DR. Sulfadiazine and pyrimethamine in the postnatal treatment of congenital toxoplasmosis: what are the options? *Expert Rev. Anti Infect. Ther.* 2003;1:175-82.

[83] Christoph J, Kattner E, Seitz HM, Reiter-Owona I. Strategies for the diagnosis and treatment of prenatal toxoplasmosis - a survey. *Z. Geburtshilfe Neonatol.* 2004;208:10-6.

[84] Dedicoat M, Livesley N. Management of toxoplasmic encephalitis in HIV-infected adults (with an emphasis on resource-poor settings. *Cochrane Database Syst. Rev.* 2006;3:CD005420.

Chapter XI

Human Immunodeficiency Virus Infection

Introduction to the Most Problematic Sexually Transmitted Disease, Human Immunodeficiency Virus Infection

Human Immunodeficiency Virus (HIV) presents a complex knot for scientists to unravel [1 – 2]. HIV begins its infection of a susceptible host cell by binding to the CD4 receptor on the host cell [1 – 2]. CD4 is present on the surface of many lymphocytes, which are a critical part of the body's immune system. Recent evidence indicates that a coreceptor is needed for HIV to enter the cell [1 – 2]. After initial contact and attachment to a cell of the immune system (including lymphocytes, monocytes), there is a cascade of intracellular events [1 – 2]. The endproduct of these events is the production of massive numbers of new viral particles, death of the infected cells, and ultimate devastation of the immune system. Affected individuals with what had come to be known as the acquired immune deficiency syndrome (AIDS) have a high mortality [1 – 2].

Presently, several modes of HIV infection are identified. However, sexual contact is the most common mode of transmission and it can be said that "HIV infection is the most a most problematic sexually transmitted disease at present [3]".

In this article, the author reviews the roles of laboratory investigations in HIV medicine.

Screening for HIV Infection

The first role of laboratory investigation in HIV medicine is the role in screening. The U.S. Preventive Services Task Force (USPSTF) strongly recommends that clinicians screen for HIV all adolescents and adults at increased risk for HIV infection [4]. Since 1996, the USPSTF recommended routine counseling and screening for all persons at increased risk for HIV infection and routine counseling and screening for high-risk pregnant women, as well as those residing in communities where the prevalence of seropositive newborns is increased [4]. It is accepted that benefits of HIV screening appear to outweigh harms and the yield from screening higher-prevalence populations would be substantially higher than that from screening the general population [5]. In addition, identification and treatment of asymptomatic HIV infection in pregnant women can greatly decrease mother-to-child transmission rates [6]. However, Lurie et al This analysis provides no justification for testing inpatients to prevent HIV infection of health care workers [7]. They found that screening inpatients to detect HIV infection might be justified at seroprevalences exceeding 1%, but issues of medical or social discrimination, false-positive results, informed consent, and logistics must be resolved first [7].Universal precautions should be applied for all cases as principle.

According to the recommendation of USPSTF, clinicians should take a complete sexual and drug use history on all adolescent and adult patients [8]. Sexually active patients should be advised that abstaining from sex or maintaining a mutually faithful monogamous sexual relationship with a partner known to be uninfected are the most effective strategies to prevent infection with HIV or other sexually transmitted diseases [8]. All patients should be offered testing in accordance with recommendations on screening for syphilis, gonorrhea, chlamydial infection, genital herpes, hepatitis B and HIV infection [8]. In addition to individual screening, mass screening for HIV is also recommended as in the blood bank [9].

HIV test kits used both to screen donor blood, blood components and cellular products, and to diagnose, treat and monitor persons with HIV and AIDS. Many tests to detect antibodies, antigens or RNA in serum, plasma, oral fluid, dried blood spot, body fluid or urine have been approved by FDA for donor and individual screening, diagnosis, prognosis and patient monitoring [10]. For screening purpose, antibody tests are specifically designed for the routine screening testing of HIV, are inexpensive, and are very accurate. These tests will be not necessary in cases that do not have not a realistic risk of HIV infection [4 – 5]. The most technical problems for antibody tests is that most of the tests give false negative results during the window period of between three weeks and six months from the time of HIV infection until the immune system produces detectable amounts of antibodies [10]. It should be noted that many patients frequently visit ambulatory care settings with acute HIV seroconversion illness, but the illness is often misdiagnosed [11]. This acute viral syndrome, or seroconversion illness, occurs after initial exposure to the HIV virus; it is often resolved before the development of HIV-specific antibodies [11]. During this window period an infected person can transmit HIV to others, without their HIV infection being detectable using an antibody test. However, all the early seroconversions must be recognized as positive and less than 0.5% false positive results must be found in blood donors [12].

The ELISA was usually the first screening commonly used. It has a high sensitivity but low specificity [13]. The low specificity of the test is because antibodies attach to antigens in the test kits "by accident", even though the person has never been exposed to HIV [10]. About 80% of positive ELISA tests are followed by a negative confirmation, Western-Blot test, and therefore regarded as false positive [10]. As the ELISA results are reported as a number, the most controversial aspect of this test is deciding the "cut off" point between positive and negative [10]. According to the study of Goguel, the percentage of correct results varies depending on the method and specimen from 98% to 99% for anti-HIV [14]. It should be noted that tests for the detection of anti-HIV antibodies that show promise for adaptation to screening (such as the ELISA with recombinant antigen) also are discussed, as is the alternative of testing for HIV antigens or HIV-specific DNA [15].

Consequently, conventional testing doesn't always provide information on HIV status quickly enough to be clinically useful [16]. This limitation has led to the development of rapid HIV test kits, which can provide results in 20 minutes or less [16]. Presently, rapid or point-of-care tests are the new trends of HIV screening test at present. Basically, rapid Antibody Tests are qualitative immunoassays intended for use as a point-of-care test to aid in the diagnosis of HIV infection [10]. These tests should be used in conjunction with the clinical status, history, and risk factors of the person being tested [10]. Examples of new point-of-care tests for Anti HIV are OraQuick and Orasure. Rapid HIV tests can be used for testing pregnant women in labor whose HIV status is unknown (to reduce vertical transmission from mother to fetus or infant) and for testing source individuals after occupational exposures (to help with drug treatment decisions) [16 - 17]. Additionally, the use of rapid test kits for screening high-risk individuals (especially those who may not return for results) is expected to increase the number of individuals who know their HIV status [16 - 17].

In the U.S.; two are approved for use at point-of-care sites outside a traditional laboratory [18]. All four tests are interpreted visually. Sites offering rapid HIV testing must periodically run external controls (known HIV-positive and HIV-negative specimens) and provide persons who undergo rapid testing a subject information sheet [18].

Another important fact that should be concerned in the screening of HIV is there are many types and subtypes of HIV, which can bring the false negative of Anti-HIV test. An improvement of both sensitivity and specificity was obtained by using artificial proteins, which have been selected for having the most immuno-dominant epitopes [12]. Luckily, the combined HIV1 + HIV2 assays allow to screen simultaneously the subjects infected by HIV1 or by HIV2 [12, 19]. However, HIV1 variants, temporarily named sub-type O have brought a new difficulty to the HIV serology, due to a weak homology, especially in "env" domains, between these variants and the reference HIV1 strains [12]. In addition, there is an interesting report on the HIV-1, subtype F infection in case that. ELISA tests and also rapid tests were all negative [20].

Diagnosis of HIV Infection

There are many commercially available tests for HIV diagnosis [21]. How use of them in HIV diagnosis is dependent on which kind of test was used, when the proper technique can to be used and how to interpret the results [21]. A person exposed to HIV would be expected to produce antibodies that specifically bind to HIV [10]. The development of antibody tests for HIV has been complicated because all human blood has large quantities of antibodies that bind to components of the antibody test kits [10]. Manufacturers of all these kits state that, "There is no single recognised standard for establishing the presence or absence of antibodies to HIV in human blood [10]." Due to the limitation of the simple antibody test, ELISA, more specific test is introduced for diagnostic purpose. Modifications to conventional methods have introduced new assays, such as sensitive/less sensitive (detuned) assays that can estimate when someone was infected, thereby providing a useful tool for epidemiologic incidence estimates and enrollment into specific intervention programmes for recently infected persons

[22]. The following diagnostic techniques are described: antibody related Western blot, viral protein estimation (p24 Ag), cell and viral culture, and genetic test (PCR), [22 - 23].

The Western blot test uses the general Western blot procedure [10]. The Western blot test is usually performed after a positive ELISA test, because many samples that are ELISA negative have antibodies to one or more of the proteins in the Western blot test, and would give inaccurate results [10]. There no universal criteria for interpreting the Western blot test: the numbers of viral bands which must be present vary from definition to definition [10]. If no viral bands are detected, the result is negative and if at least one viral band for each of the GAG, POL, and ENV gene-product groups are present, the result is positive [10]. The Association of State and Territorial Public Health Laboratory Directors (ASTPHLD) and CDC standard interprets the presence of gp41 and gp120/160 bands as a positive result [10]. Presently, Western blot analysis detects antibodies to specific HIV antigens and is one of the best used as a confirmatory test [24]. However, variability in the profile of antigen-reactive bands in Western blot for serodiagnosis of HIV infection may result in disagreement regarding interpretation of positive result, due to lack of consensus in the interpretive criteria laid down by various organisations [25]. It is felt that before selecting any criterion for Western blot positivity, it should be evaluated in the local population at risk for HIV-1 infection with additional or follow-up tests [25].

Concerning p24Ag detection, the yield of HIV p24Ag positive: antibody negative is estimated to be about 1 : 90,000 in actual practice [26]. Prado et al found that signal amplification of a heat-dissociated p24Ag had a positive association with current HIV RNA assays in a population-based analysis [27]. However, it might not be sensitive enough to monitor longitudinal intrapatient viremia in patients with high CD4+ counts potentially due to the production of high-affinity anti-p24 antibodies and clearance of immune complexes by erythrocytes [27]. However, quantitative determination of p24 antigen by enzyme immunoassay still has a weakness due to its relatively poor sensitivity.

Concerning cell and viral culture for HIV, this technique is very hard to perform and limited used. In addition, quantitative culture is time consuming, cumbersome and requires appropriate laboratory safety equipment. For PCR test, detection of infection of newborn babies, characterisation of individual strains for subtyping and forensic identification, and therapeutic monitoring are the domain of nucleic-acid-based assays [10]. Nucleic-acid-based assays narrow the serological diagnostic window period in early HIV infection and, when quantified, give some indication of clinical status [10]. However, due to the fact that PCR test is a very expensive test, the usage is limited in the setting with limited resources.

FOLLOWING UP OF HIV INFECTION

There are many laboratory tests using in following up of HIV infection. The most frequently used laboratory test in following up of the patient is the determination of CD4+ count, which is usually performed by flow cytometry analysis. The CD4+ count is recommended as a basic test for following up of the progression of the disease in the HIV infected patients. Basically, The CD4+ T lymphocytes are the crucial cells in the orchestral events in forming immune response to the foreign antigen and it is also the primary target cells for HIV [28]. The progressive loss of these cells eventually results in the loss of an ability to mount desirable immune response to any pathogen and death of the patients in the terminal stage of HIV infection [28]. In additional to monitoring of progression of disease, CD4+ T cell count is also accepted as a tool to monitor effectiveness of anti-retroviral therapy [28]. Importance of maintaining both internal and external quality control systems in every laboratory performing CD4 count estimation should also be mentioned [28].

Another tests for following up of the disease progression in HIV infected patients is the viral load test. This test is performed based on nucleic-acid-based assays. quantitative determination of viral load using nucleic acid amplification techniques is the most accurate, prognostic marker for HIV type 1 infection, independently of the CD4+ cell count [29]. Overall, the different methods for HIV-1 RNA determination (RT-PCR, nucleic acid sequence-based amplification, branched DNA) show a good reproducibility (0.5 log), however for low copy numbers and in HIV-1-infected children the variability may exceed 0.7 log [30].

Another important groups of test for following up of HIV infected patients is those tests for monitoring of drug resistance. HIV drug resistance is one of the major limitations in the successful treatment of HIV-infected patients using currently available antiretroviral combination therapies [31]. When appropriate, drug susceptibility profiles should be taken into consideration in the choice of a specific combination therapy [31]. Specifically, the following recommendations can be made: (i) genotypic and phenotypic HIV-1 drug resistance analyses; (ii) HIV-1 drug resistance testing on plasma samples obtained before starting, stopping or changing therapy, on samples that have a viral load above the detection limit of the resistance test; (iii) all test must be performed in a certified laboratory under strict quality control and quality assurance standards; and (iv) resistance reports must include a list of drug-related resistance mutations (genotype) and/or a list of drug-related fold resistance values (phenotype) [31].

In addition to the laboratory tests for monitoring of the progression of disease and effectiveness of anti-retroviral therapy, there are also tests, which are useful for monitoring of the complication of disease. These tests are used for monitoring of opportunistic infections and malignancy. For general practitioner, the basic tests for monitoring of the chest complications is chest X ray [32] and for monitoring of gastrointestinal complication is stool examination [33].

PREDICTION OF HIV INFECTION

Prediction of prognosis of HIV is another important role of laboratory test in HIV medicine [34]. The progression of a HIV seropositive patient from an asymptomatic infection or persistent generalised lymphadenopathy to AIDS is dependent on many factors [35]. The most useful prognostic indicators appear to be CD4 + lymphocyte count, beta 2-microglobulin level, anti-p24 antibody titre and p24 antigenemia [35]. The use of a combination of prognostic indices can enhance the accuracy of the prediction [35].

REFERENCES

[1] Durack DT. The acquired immune deficiency syndrome. *Adv. Intern. Med.* 1984;30:29-51.

[2] Rezza G, Padian N. AIDS 2000. Epidemiology: overview. *AIDS.* 2000;14 Suppl 3:S45-6.

[3] Krowchuk DP. Sexually transmitted diseases in adolescents: what's new? *South Med. J.* 1998;91:124-31.

[4] Agency for Healthcare Research and Quality. U.S. Preventive Services Task Force. *Screening for HIV: Recommendation Statement.* AHRQ Publication No. 05-0580-A, July 2005. Available on http://www.ahrq.gov/clinic/uspstf05/hiv/hivrs.htm

[5] Chou R, Huffman LH, Fu R, Smits AK, Korthuis PT; US Preventive Services Task Force. Screening for HIV: a review of the evidence for the U.S. Preventive Services Task Force. *Ann. Intern. Med.* 2005;143:55-73.

[6] Chou R, Smits AK, Huffman LH, Fu R, Korthuis PT; US Preventive Services Task Force. Prenatal screening for HIV: A review of the evidence for the U.S. Preventive Services Task Force. *Ann. Intern. Med.* 2005;143:38-54.

[7] Lurie P, Avins AL, Phillips KA, Kahn JG, Lowe RA, Ciccarone D. The cost-effectiveness of voluntary counseling and testing of hospital inpatients for HIV infection. *JAMA.* 1994;272:1832-8.

[8] Counseling to prevent HIV infection and other sexually transmitted diseases. The U.S. Preventive Services Task Force. *Am. Fam. Physician.* 1990;41:1179-87.

[9] Lackritz EM. Prevention of HIV transmission by blood transfusion in the developing world: achievements and continuing challenges. *AIDS.* 1998;12 Suppl A:S81-6.

[10] HIV test. Available at *tp://www.reference.com/browse/wiki/HIV_test*

[11] Santangelo J. Acute seroconversion of HIV infection in the ambulatory care setting. Acute seroconversion of HIV infection in the ambulatory care setting. *Nurse Pract.* 2001;26:48, 51-4, 56.

[12] Courouce AM. Anti-HIV antibody screening kits and the difficulties of serology. Retrovirus Working Group of the Societe Francaise de la Transfusion Sanguine. *Transfus. Clin. Biol.* 1994;1:387-95.

[13] Farzadegan H. HIV-1 antibodies and serology. *Clin. Lab. Med.* 1994 ;14:257-69.

[14] Goguel AF. HBV and HIV serological markers: the National External Quality Assessment Scheme in France. *Ann. Ist Super Sanita.* 1991;27:511-5.

[15] Gauthier DK, Turner JG. Anti-HIV antibody testing: procedures and precautions. *Am. J. Infect. Control.* 1989;17:213-25.

[16] Rapid HIV test kits. *Health Devices.* 2006;35:157-77.

[17] Dewsnap CH, McOwan A. A review of HIV point-of-care tests. *Int. J. STD AIDS.* 2006;17:357-9.

[18] Greenwald JL, Burstein GR, Pincus J, Branson B. A rapid review of rapid HIV antibody tests. *Curr. Infect. Dis. Rep.* 2006;8:125-31.

[19] Fujii T. Diagnostic tests: Human immunodeficiency virus type 1, type 2 (HIV-1, HIV 2). *Nippon Rinsho.* 2005; 63 Suppl 7:434-7.

[20] Apetrei C, Gramada D, Stanciu V, Diculencu D, Panzaru C, Coman G, Carasievici E, Duca M. HIV infection in a seronegative child diagnosed by isolation of the virus. The

significant immunological and epidemiological signs. *Rev. Med. Chir. Soc. Med. Nat. Iasi.* 1996;100:125-30.
[21] Lipniacki A, Piasek A. Laboratory tests for HIV infection. Przegl Lek. 2003;60:478-84.
[22] Iweala OI. HIV diagnostic tests: an overview. *Contraception.* 2004;70:141-7.
[23] Constantine NT, Zink H. HIV testing technologies after two decades of evolution. *Indian J. Med. Res.* 2005;121:519-38.
[24] Cordes RJ, Ryan ME. Pitfalls in HIV testing. Application and limitations of current tests. *Postgrad. Med.* 1995;98:177-80, 185-6, 189.
[25] Chattopadhya D, Aggarwal RK, Kumari S. Profile of antigen-specific antibody response detectable by western blot in relation to diagnostic criteria for human immunodeficiency virus type-1 (HIV-1) infection. *Clin. Diagn. Virol.* 1996;7:35-42.
[26] Wendel S, Fachini RM, Levi JE, Ghaname JN, Mendonca MC, de Almeida Neto C, de Carvalho Braga M, Di Pietro AE. A single window-period donation detected by human immunodeficiency virus p24 antigen after 5 years of routine screening in a group of Brazilian blood banks. *Vox Sang.* 2002;83:309-12.
[27] Prado JG, Shintani A, Bofill M, Clotet B, Ruiz L, Martinez-Picado J. Lack of longitudinal intrapatient correlation between p24 antigenemia and levels of human immunodeficiency virus (HIV) type 1 RNA in patients with chronic hiv infection during structured treatment interruptions. *J. Clin. Microbiol.* 2004;42:1620-5.
[28] Pattanapanyasat K, Thakar MR. CD4+ T cell count as a tool to monitor HIV progression and anti-retroviral therapy. *Indian J. Med. Res.* 2005;121:539-49.
[29] Berger A, Preiser W, Doerr HW. The role of viral load determination for the management of human immunodeficiency virus, hepatitis B virus and hepatitis C virus infection. *J. Clin. Virol.* 2001;20:23-30.
[30] Berger A, Braner J, Doerr HW, Weber B. Quantification of viral load: clinical relevance for human immunodeficiency virus, hepatitis B virus and hepatitis C virus infection. *Intervirology.* 1998;41:24-34.
[31] Vandamme AM, Houyez F, Banhegyi D, Clotet B, De Schrijver G, De Smet KA, Hall WW, Harrigan R, Hellmann N, Hertogs K, Holtzer C, Larder B, Pillay D, Race E, Schmit JC, Schuurman R, Schulse E, Sonnerborg A, Miller V. Laboratory guidelines for the practical use of HIV drug resistance tests in patient follow-up. *Antivir. Ther.* 2001;6:21-39.
[32] How to detect and diagnose TB. *Child Health Dialogue.* 1996;Suppl:6-7.
[33] Wiwanitkit V. Intestinal parasite infestation in HIV infected patients. *Curr. HIV Res.* 2006;4:87-96.
[34] Low N, Egger M. Can we predict the prognosis of HIV infection? How to use the findings of a prospective study. *Sex Transm. Infect.* 1998;74:149-54.
[35] Cooper EH, Lacey CJ. Laboratory indices of prognosis in HIV infection. *Biomed. Pharmacother.* 1988;42:539-45.

Chapter XII

Cytomegalovirus Infection

Introduction to Cytomegalovirus

Cytomegalovirus (CMV) is a well-known virus. Human CMV can infect hematopoietic progenitor cells from normal cord blood directly, researchers have suggested. It is a member of DNA virus in the group Herpesviridae. It is in the same group as Latency common. Includes herpes simplex type 1 and 2, varicella zoster virus (chicken pox, shingles) and Epstein Barr virus (infectious mononucleosis).

The target cells of CMV are epithelia, monocytes, lymphocytes as previously mentioned. The latency can be found in monocytes, lymphocytes and possibly others. There are several mode of transmission of this virus including contact, blood transfusions, transplantation, congenital. During the past several years, studies have indicated that CMV genes can be grouped into two broad categories; those essential for replication in cell culture and those dispensible for virus replication [1]. The latter group of genes is likely to be important for pathogenesis and host-virus interactions [1]. Human CMV clinical isolates display genetic polymorphisms in multiple genes [2]. Some authors have suggested that those polymorphisms may be implicated in HCMV-induced immunopathogenesis, as well as in strain-specific behaviours, such as tissue-tropism and ability to establish persistent or latent infections [2]. However, the gene complement of wild-type human CMV is incompletely understood, on account of the size and complexity of the viral genome and because laboratory strains have undergone deletions and rearrangements during adaptation to growth in culture [3]. Cha et al said that that wild-type virus carries more than 220 genes, some of which are lost by large-scale deletion and rearrangement of the UL/b' region during laboratory passage [4].

Pathogenesis

Human CMV causes serious disease in immunocompromised individuals [5]. CMV persists as a subclinical, lifelong infection in the normal human host, maintained at least in part by its carriage in the absence of detectable infectious virus--the hallmark of latent infection [6]. Normally, anti-CMV immune response controls virus replication following reactivation from latency [5 - 8]. Reactivation from latency in immunocompromised individuals, in contrast, often results in serious disease [6]. Accumulating evidences suggest that reactivation of human CMV from latency appears to be linked intrinsically to the differentiation status of the myeloid cell [6 - 8]. Dosa et al found that human CMV latency is associated with the state of differentiation of the host cells [7]. In human CMV-infected differentiated NTera2 cells, the MIEP becomes associated with hyperacetylated histones, which results in an open structure of chromatin, enhancing the access of DNA-binding factors which positively regulate MIE gene expression and viral replication [7]. CMV infection of endothelial cells and macrophages plays an important role in the establishment of latency and persistence, which appears critical for the maintenance of CMV within the host [9]. CMV infection is profoundly influenced by endothelial cell origin and the specific pathway of macrophage differentiation [9]. The specific human CMV genes involved in endothelial cell and macrophage tropism are unknown [10]. However, studies in the closely related murine cytomegalovirus (MCMV) model have provided considerable insight into viral genes that enable replication in these cell types [10]. Multiple CMV genes appear to be involved in enabling virus replication in these two cell types [9]. In addition, infectious virus and productive cycle transcripts, such as transcripts of early-phase gene M55 (gB) and ie3 transcripts specifying the essential transactivator protein IE3, can be found to be absent during mCMV latency in the lungs [11]. Understanding how HCMV persists has clinical relevance in that its transmission to seronegative recipients might be more easily prevented, and the mechanisms by which it produces disease in the neonate and immunocompromised hosts more easily understood, if we knew more about the cells in which the virus is latent and the way in which it reactivates [12].

For reactivation, Hummel et al proposed that induction of IE-1 gene expression was the first step in reactivation of the virus in an immunocompromised transplant recipient, and that occurs as a result of the allogeneic response, which induces expression of TNF and subsequent activation of NFkappaB, and ischemia/reperfusion injury, which induces activation of AP-1 [13]. Previous studies have shown that allogeneic stimulation induces reactivation of human HCMV in vitro [13 - 14]. Hummel et al speculated that the natural stimulus for reactivation in an immunocompetent host was an inflammatory immune response to infection and that allogeneic transplantation mimics this process [13 - 14]. Hummerl et al found that transplantation of vascularized allogeneic kidneys induced murine CMV (MCMV) and HCMV immediate-early (ie) gene expression and this induction is accompanied by increased expression of transcripts encoding inflammatory cytokines, including tumor necrosis factor (TNF), interleukin-2, and gamma interferon, and by activation of NF-kappaB [14].

However, CMV, like other large herpesviruses, encodes immune evasion proteins that allow the virus to replicate, for a time or in specific tissues, and produce viral progeny in the face of robust host immunity [5]. CMV glycoproteins unique short(US)2, US3, US6 and US11 all inhibit different stages of the MHC class I antigen presentation pathway and can reduce recognition by CD8+ [5]. Human CMV can elude CTL as well as NK cells by modulating surface expression of MHC class I molecules. This strategy would be most efficient if the virus would selectively down-regulate viral Ag-presenting alleles, while at the same time preserving other alleles to act as inhibitors of NK cell activation [15]. US2 binds to newly synthesized MHC class I H chains and supports their dislocation to the cytosol for subsequent degradation by proteasomes [15]. The kinetics of MHC class I down-regulation by US2-11 genes observed at early and late phases postinfection with wild-type virus correlated with increased susceptibility to NK lysis [16]. Thus, the influence of HCMV genes on NK reactivity follows a hierarchy dominated by the US2-11 region, which encodes all viral genes capable of down-modulating expression of classical and non-classical MHC class I molecules [16]. Barel et al found that the MHC class I endoplasmic reticulum-lumenal domain alone was not sufficient for degradation by US2, as illustrated by the stability of soluble HLA-G1 in the presence of US2. Furthermore, they showed that the membrane-bound HLA-G1 isoform, but also tailless HLA-A2, were targeted for degradation [15]. This indicates that the cytoplasmic tail of the MHC class I H chain is not required for its dislocation to the cytosol by US2 [15]. Human CMV US3 and US6 down-regulate the cell-surface expression of both HLA-G and HLA-C by two different mechanisms [17]. HCMV US3 physically associates with both trophoblast class I MHC species, retaining them in the endoplasmic reticulum [17]. In contrast, human CMV US6 inhibits peptide transport by TAP and thus specifically the intracellular trafficking of class I molecules. Therefore, these findings suggest for the first time a possible molecular mechanism underlying human CMV-related spontaneous pregnancy loss [17].

Dysfunctional T-cell immunity contributes to susceptibility to infectious disease in the elderly [18]. A characteristic feature of this immunosenescence is the predominance of clonal expansions of CD8 cells and decreased diversity of the T-cell antigen receptor repertoire [18]. It is hypothesized that for that majority of elderly people infected with CMV, which seems to act as the dominant chronic stressor, anti-viral strategies would be of benefit in abrogating some of the detrimental clinical manifestations of immunosenescence [18]. The fraction of CMV-specific T cells able to secrete interferon-gamma after specific antigenic stimulation is significantly lower in the elderly than in the young, although the total number of functional cells is comparable [19]. Therefore, the majority of the clonally expanded virus-specific CD8+ cells in the elderly are dysfunctional; therefore, T cell responses are altered in the aged by an accumulation of replicatively senescent dysfunctional T cells carrying receptors for persistent herpes viruses [19]. The presence of clonal expansions of such virus-specific cells may shrink the available repertoire for other antigens and contribute to the increased incidence of infectious disease in the elderly [19].

MHC/peptide multimer staining indicated that the frequency of CMV-specific T cells was higher in nonagenarians than in the middle-aged, but the ratio of functionally intact cells was significantly lower [20]. The number of different CD8 T cell clonal expansions increases as the individual ages, possibly, as a compensatory mechanism to control CMV but eventually a point is reached where clonal exhaustion leads to shrinkage of the CD8 clonal repertoire, associated with decreased survival [20].

Furthermore, it has also been shown that the combination of virus-specific CD4 and CD8 T-cell responses are critical components of the immune response in the control of virus replication [21]. Although complete CMV eradication is unusual even in immunocompetent hosts, its morbidity can be limited by CMV-specific CD8+ cytotoxic lymphocytes supported by CD4+-mediated T lymphocyte helper activity [22]. In patients with congenital or acquired deficiencies of cell-mediated immunity, recovery of CD4+ lymphocyte numbers and/or function coincides with cessation of CMV-associated morbidity [22].

CLINICAL MANIFESTATION

Cytomegalovirus infection can produce a variety of clinical manifestations. The important groups are hereby presented.

A. Congenital Cytomegalovirus Infection

CMV is a member of TORCH agent. The vertical transmission of this virus is confirmed [23]. The congenital CMV infection is the most common intrauterine transmitted viral infection [23]. Since the first description in 1904 a lot of knowledge on epidemiology has been gained [23]. Concerning the interaction of CMV and placental cells, reactions of the host immune system have a dual effect - protection against the virus on the one hand, and supporting of virus production and release of CMV on the other hand [23].Basically, CMV infection is mainly related to a primary maternal infection [24]. The placenta should be considered the most important site of both the protection of the fetus from CMV infection and the transmission of CMV from mother to fetus [24]. The control of the passage of CMV across the placenta probably involves a cascade of regulatory events [24]. Roles are played by factors relating to the host immune-selective pressures, such as local cytokines and maternal CMV-specific neutralizing antibodies. The presence of other pathogens at the maternal-fetal interface also influences the outcome of CMV infection [24]. Up to 90% of infants with congenital infection have no signs or symptoms at birth. The other 10% will be symptomatic and about half of the will have the classic stigmata of CMV inclusion disease [24]. It is estimated that 10 to 30 % of the severely affected infants will die; more then 90% of survivors will have neurological handicaps, sensorineural hearing loss, and chorioretinitis [24]. It is also estimated that 10 to 15% of children asymptomatic at birth have a risk of abnormal development and 10% develop hearing loss during the first years of life [24]. It should also be noted that symptomatic congenital CMV infection can occur after a nonprimary or recurrent maternal infection [25 - 26]. However, the exact incidence of symptomatic congenital CMV infection among children born to women with preexisting immunity remains to be defined [25 - 26].

The gold standard for diagnosing congenital CMV infection is isolation of the virus from infants within the first 2 weeks of life through conventional or rapid cell culture techniques [27]. Prenatal detection of congenital disease by ultrasound examination is not sufficient, but prenatal diagnosis can be confirmed by amniocentesis (culture of amniotic fluid and detection of virus DNA by quantitative polymerase chain reactions) [24]. Prenatal diagnosis is based on the direct detection of the virus by culture (CMV), of its antigens (CMV) or of its genome, essentially by PCR [28]. This direct detection can be done either on fetal blood or on amniotic fluid. Prenatal diagnosis can also be performed by detection of specific IgM in fetal blood (rubella). Non specific markers of viral infections can also help diagnosis [28]. Newer molecular diagnostic methods to diagnose congenital CMV infection, including the nucleic acid amplification of viral DNA from the peripheral blood of infants, are being investigated, and the preliminary results show promise [27]. However, more work must be done to standardize and validate these methods before they can be used routinely in establishing the diagnosis of congenital CMV infection [27]. At present, CMV is accepted as the most important pathogen to be screen in TORCH agent group [29]. Collinet et al proposed that 5 different preventive methods for congenital CMV infection are possible: (1) Routine CMV screening at the beginning of pregnancy for primary prevention. (2) Secondary prevention by antenatal diagnosis of congenital CMV infection complications. (3) Tertiary prevention by serological testing during pregnancy. (4) Tertiary prevention by serological screening at birth. (5) Tertiary prevention: Hearing loss screening at birth [30].

B. Cytomegalic Inclusion Disease

This is a variety of congenital CMV infection. Cytomegalic inclusion disease (CID) is characterized by intrauterine growth retardation, hepatosplenomegaly, hematological abnormalities (particularly thrombocytopenia), and a variety of cutaneous manifestations, including petechiae and purpura (blueberry muffin baby) [31]. However, the most significant manifestations of CID are those involving the central nervous system. Microcephaly, ventriculomegaly, cerebral atrophy, chorioretinitis, and sensorineural hearing loss are the most common neurological consequences of CID [31].

C. CMV Pneumonitis

CMV pneumonitis is a common form of CMV infection. It usually occurs in the immunocompromised host. CMV pneumonia is a major cause of morbidity and mortality in allogeneic bone marrow transplant and lung transplant recipients [32]. The clinical presentations of these patients were nonspecific, including fever, shortness of breath, cough, and Pao2 of < 75 mm Hg [33]. A high correlation in the degree of viral burden in lung biopsy specimens was demonstrated by histologic examination, immunohistochemical analysis, and in situ hybridization [33]. However, its role as a cause of lung disease in patients with the human HIV is controversial [32]. Although CMV can be isolated from lung specimens in patients with HIV-associated respiratory illness, it is rarely the causative pathogen [32]. Millar et al said that CMV was not a pathogen in the lungs of patients with HIV infection, and suggested that its presence at this site does not warrant specific therapy in these patients [34]. Most adults with HIV infection have latent CMV infection of many tissues including the lung, and most cases of CMV pneumonia are believed to be caused by reactivation secondary to severe immunocompromise [32]. The clinical presentation of pneumonia caused by CMV pneumonia is similar to that of Pneumocystis carinii, with fever, cough, hypoxemia, and diffuse radiographic opacities [32]. Although approximately 60% of cases respond initially to anti-CMV therapy, the disease is associated with progression and high early mortality, probably related to severe underlying immunosuppression [32].

D. CMV Retinitis

CMV retinitis is emerging at present due to the emerging of HIV infection. CMV retinitis is the important cause of blindness in AIDS [35]. It is is the commonest opportunistic ocular infection in patients with HIV infection/AIDS, typically occurs when CD4+ T cell counts fall below 50/mm3 [36]. CMV infection usually produces a necrotic rapidly progressing retinitis with characteristic white perivascular infiltrate with hemorrhage (brushfire retinitis) [31]. The diagnosis of CMV retinitis is a clinical one and it is important for physicians to be familiar with the clinical features of the disease [37]. The characteristic appearance of the infection is distinctive enough that recourse to ancillary tests or diagnostic procedures is rarely needed [38]. However, atypical cases of CMV retinitis or infections with other organisms in individuals at high risk for CMV retinitis may require invasive diagnostic testing of ocular fluids or tissues using comparative antibody titers, amplification of organismal DNA or RNA, culture, or histology [38]. Ophthalmic screening of AIDS sufferers should be undertaken at regular intervals, and this is dictated, in part, by the patient's CD4+ T-lymphocyte (CD4) counts. CMV retinitis may be treated with systemic ganciclovir, foscarnet or cidofovir, or with local (intravitreal) therpy. CMV-related retinal detachment is treated surgically [38]. The aggressive multidrug regimen of highly active antiretroviral therapy (HAART) has offered some degree of promise of immune reconstitution in AIDS patients, a phenomenon that theoretically would impact positively on the incidence and severity of opportunistic infections [39]. Some studies already have noted complete regression of CMV retinitis without specific use of anti-CMV agents in patients undergoing HAART [39]. Initial therapy must be based on characteristics of the CMV retinitis and patient conditions [40]. However, the role of HAART in CMV retinitis remains controversial among investigators [39]. There is also the question of whether CMV retinitis progression in any way represents failure of HAART in those patients receiving this type of combination therapy [39]. HAART is seen as an encouraging development in the treatment of AIDS and opportunistic infection, but its more specific therapeutic effect on CMV retinitis requires further research with controlled prospective clinical trials [39]. Long term therapy of HAART must be pursued, even in patients with increased CD4 and undetectable HIV viral load, until results from large controlled studies are available [40].

E. CMV Gasrtrohepatoenterology

GI tract disease caused by CMV can include esophagitis, gastritis, gastroenteritis, pyloric obstruction, hepatitis, pancreatitis, colitis, and cholecystitis [31]. Characteristic signs and symptoms may include nausea, vomiting, dysphagia, epigastric pain, icterus, and watery diarrhea [31]. CMV gastroenteritis is another important form of CMV infection. CMV colitis is rare in patients with an intact immune system [41]. Advanced age, male gender, presence of immune-modulating comorbidities, and need for surgical intervention are factors negatively influencing survival. Conversely, young healthy patients have a good prognosis with no intervention [41]. CMV hepatitis is another type of hepatitis. Although CMV is not a hepatitis virus it can cause hepatitis. The pattern of liver cell pathology is similar to that of other hepatitis viruses. Concerning ulcerative colitis, a clear association between complicated courses of ulcerative colitis and the presence of CMV has been established [42]. However, the exact pathogenic role of CMV in these patients remains unclear despite a great number of published reports [42].

DIAGNOSIS

For general laboratory investigation, the change in complete blood count can be seen in the patients infected with CMV virus. The monocytosis and atypical lymphocytosis can be seen. The cytopathic effects of CMV include both nuclear and cytoplasmic inclusions. CMV inclusions can be demonstrated in infected cell by special PAS staining. Both nucleus and cytoplasmic inclusions can be seen. At the edge of the viral inclusion, a rounded clump of peripheral chromatin may be seen extending into the clear region of the halo, which is the hallmark pathology of CMV infection. The diagnosis of CMV infection can base on the virological technique. The variety of available test methods - mostly not standardized - with their different test characteristics, sample types etc. is often confusing for the clinician [43]. There is often great uncertainty as to whether a given laboratory results is pathognomonic [43]. In addition, not only is the diagnostic repertoire growing constantly - for instance through genome quantification and measurement of virus-specific T lymphocytes - but also the available antiviral therapeutic options with the need for adequate surveillance [43]. Recently developed techniques have greatly increased the sensitivity and speed of detection of CMV and of host antibody responses to it [44]. Newer serologic assays such as enzyme immunoassay or latex agglutination assay are accurate and efficient for screening donors and recipients and for determining susceptibility to primary infection [44]. IgM antibody assays have occasional utility in recognition of recent infection [44 - 45]. The technique of detection of early fluorescent antigen foci (DEAFF) has for some time been available as a diagnostic service to immunocompromised patients [46]. Although it requires cell culture and immunofluorescent techniques it is capable of detecting most patients with productive infection [46]. The slow process of isolating CMV in cell culture has prompted development of effective rapid techniques that utilize CMV-specific monoclonal antibodies and DNA sequences [44]. Immediate-early viral antigen can be detected in infected cell cultures within hours of specimen inoculation [44]. CMV antigens can also be detected directly in cells within clinical specimens [44]. DNA hybridization has been used for CMV analysis in dot-blot, Southern blot, and in situ hybridization assays; the use of the latter is increasing for the detection of virus in fixed, paraffin-embedded tissue sections [44]. In recent years, quantitative PCR assays are increasingly being utilized in the clinical setting to (1) identify individuals at risk of developing CMV disease(determination of clinical threshold), (2) monitor viral response to antiviral treatment, (3) predict individuals at risk of clinical relapse, and (4) serve as an early indicator of antiviral resistance [47].

TREATMENT

Considering the treatment for CMV infection, antiviral drug treatment is available. There are three systemic drugs approved for CMV treatment: ganciclovir, or its prodrug valganciclovir, foscarnet, and cidofovir [48]. Valganciclovir is an orally administered prodrug of the standard anti- CMV drug ganciclovir. Valganciclovir is as effective as intravenous ganciclovir for the treatment of AIDS-related CMV retinitis, and oral ganciclovir for the prophylaxis of CMV infection and disease in high-risk solid organ transplant recipients [49]. Ganciclovir is a nucleoside analogue which is used to treat and prevent CMV infection [50].

Most recent clinical studies of ganciclovir in transplant recipients have focused on preventive approaches [50]. Two strategies had emerged: prophylaxis for all patients or early treatment started after detection of asymptomatic CMV infection [50]. Subsequently, a large double-blind study has shown that ganciclovir prophylaxis is more effective than early treatment in preventing early CMV disease after allogeneic bone marrow transplantation and is not associated with an increased incidence of neutropenia [50]. The efficacy of prophylactic intravenous ganciclovir in liver transplant recipients, including high risk donor seropositive/recipient seronegative (D+/R-) or antilymphocyte-treated patients, is now well established [50]. Foscarnet sodium, a pyrophosphate analog active against both CMV and the HIV, may be an effective alternative to ganciclovir in the management of CMV retinitis [51]. Trials with intravenous foscarnet in CMV retinitis have reported favorable results using initial daily doses of 180-230 mg/kg/d given as intermittent infusions every eight hours, followed by maintenance regimens of 60-90 mg/kg/d given as single daily one- or two-hour infusions [51]. Foscarnet therapy may result in renal impairment, and indefinite intravenous maintenance therapy may be required to prevent recurrence of CMV infection [51]. Cidofovir [(S)-1-(3-hydroxy-2-phosphonylmethoxypropyl)cytosine, HPMPC] has since 1996 been licensed for clinical use in the treatment of cytomegalovirus (CMV) retinitis in AIDS patients [52]. Cidofovir also has broad-spectrum activity against virtually all DNA viruses, including herpes-, adeno-, polyoma-, papilloma- and poxviruses [52]. The drug is generally well tolerated and has a similar tolerability profile to that of oral or intravenous ganciclovir, but is devoid of adverse events related to intravenous or indwelling catheter access associated with the use of intravenous ganciclovir, cidofovir and foscarnet [49]. The simple and convenient once-daily valganciclovir regimen offers potential for improved patient compliance [49]. An anti-sense therapeutic, ISIS 2922, is also approved specifically as in intravitreal treatment for CMV retinitis [48]. Ganciclovir, and more recently, valganciclovir, have been useful in proactive approaches of CMV disease management; in both prophylactic and preemptive regimens in HSCT and SOT populations [48]. The major anti-herpes agent valacyclovir has also been approved for prophylaxis of renal transplant recipients, or SOTs outside of the USA [48]. These drugs have provided major advances in CMV disease management, although they are limited by intolerable toxicities, oral bioavailability and efficacy, and risk of drug resistance with extended use [48]. Clinical resistance of cytomegalovirus against the currently licensed antiviral drugs is becoming an increasingly recognized problem [53]. The molecular basis of resistance and describes mutations in the UL54 DNA polymerase leading to resistance against cidofovir, foscarnet and ganciclovir is described [53]. There are two important developments in our appreciation of resistance [53]. Firstly, the use of more rapid molecular based assays to detect genotypic resistance and secondly, the relationship between resistance profiles in multiple organ systems of the same host [53]. Finally, the changing face of CMV disease in the era of highly active antiviral chemotherapy is considered with respect to its impact on the frequency of CMV resistance in the clinic [53].

References

[1] Stenberg RM, Kerry JA. Cytomegalovirus genes: their structure and function. *Scand. J. Infect. Dis. Suppl.* 1995;99:3-6.

[2] Pignatelli S, Dal Monte P, Rossini G, Landini MP. Genetic polymorphisms among human cytomegalovirus (HCMV) wild-type strains. *Rev. Med. Virol.* 2004;14:383-410.

[3] Davison AJ, Dolan A, Akter P, Addison C, Dargan DJ, Alcendor DJ, McGeoch DJ, Hayward GS. The human cytomegalovirus genome revisited: comparison with the chimpanzee cytomegalovirus genome. *J. Gen. Virol.* 2003;84:17-28.

[4] Cha TA, Tom E, Kemble GW, Duke GM, Mocarski ES, Spaete RR. Human cytomegalovirus clinical isolates carry at least 19 genes not found in laboratory strains. *J. Virol.* 1996;70:78-83.

[5] Johnson DC, Hegde NR. Inhibition of the MHC class II antigen presentation pathway by human cytomegalovirus. *Curr. Top. Microbiol. Immunol.* 2002;269:101-15.

[6] Sinclair J, Sissons P. Latency and reactivation of human cytomegalovirus. *J. Gen. Virol.* 2006;87:1763-79.

[7] Dosa R, Burian K, Gonczol E. Human cytomegalovirus latency is associated with the state of differentiation of the host cells: an in vitro model in teratocarcinoma cells. *Acta Microbiol. Immunol. Hung.* 2005;52:397-406.

[8] Eizuru Y. Latency and reactivation of HCMV. Nippon Rinsho. 2006;64 Suppl 3:435-9

[9] Reddehase MJ, Podlech J, Grzimek NK. Mouse models of cytomegalovirus latency: overview. *J. Clin. Virol.* 2002;25 Suppl 2:S23-36.

[10] Jarvis MA, Nelson JA. Mechanisms of human cytomegalovirus persistence and latency. *Front Biosci.* 2002;7:d1575-82.

[11] Jarvis MA, Nelson JA. Human cytomegalovirus persistence and latency in endothelial cells and macrophages. *Curr. Opin. Microbiol.* 2002 Aug;5(4):403-7.

[12] Sissons JG, Bain M, Wills MR. Latency and reactivation of human cytomegalovirus. *J. Infect.* 2002;44:73-7.

[13] Hummel M, Abecassis MM. A model for reactivation of CMV from latency. *J. Clin. Virol.* 2002;25 Suppl 2:S123-36.

[14] Hummel M, Zhang Z, Yan S, DePlaen I, Golia P, Varghese T, Thomas G, Abecassis MI. Allogeneic transplantation induces expression of cytomegalovirus immediate-early genes in vivo: a model for reactivation from latency. *J. Virol.* 2001;75:4814-22.

[15] Barel MT, Ressing M, Pizzato N, van Leeuwen D, Le Bouteiller P, Lenfant F, Wiertz EJ. Human cytomegalovirus-encoded US2 differentially affects surface expression of MHC class I locus products and targets membrane-bound, but not soluble HLA-G1 for degradation. *J. Immunol.* 2003;171:6757-65.

[16] Falk CS, Mach M, Schendel DJ, Weiss EH, Hilgert I, Hahn G. NK cell activity during human cytomegalovirus infection is dominated by US2-11-mediated HLA class I down-regulation. *J. Immunol.* 2002;169:3257-66.

[17] Jun Y, Kim E, Jin M, Sung HC, Han H, Geraghty DE, Ahn K. Human cytomegalovirus gene products US3 and US6 down-regulate trophoblast class I MHC molecules. *J. Immunol.* 2000;164:805-11.

[18] Pawelec G, Gouttefangeas C. T-cell dysregulation caused by chronic antigenic stress: the role of CMV in immunosenescence? *Aging Clin. Exp. Res.* 2006;18:171-3.

[19] Ouyang Q, Wagner WM, Voehringer D, Wikby A, Klatt T, Walter S, Muller CA, Pircher H, Pawelec G. Age-associated accumulation of CMV-specific CD8+ T cells expressing the inhibitory killer cell lectin-like receptor G1 (KLRG1). *Exp. Gerontol.* 2003;38:911-20.

[20] Hadrup SR, Strindhall J, Kollgaard T, Seremet T, Johansson B, Pawelec G, thor Straten P, Wikby A. Longitudinal studies of clonally expanded CD8 T cells reveal a repertoire shrinkage predicting mortality and an increased number of dysfunctional cytomegalovirus-specific T cells in the very elderly. *J. Immunol.* 2006;176:2645-53.
[21] Harari A, Zimmerli SC, Pantaleo G. Cytomegalovirus (CMV)-specific cellular immune responses. *Hum. Immunol.* 2004;65:500-6.
[22] Weinberg A. The role of immune reconstitution in cytomegalovirus infection. *BioDrugs.* 2002;16:89-95.
[23] Halwachs-Baumann G. The congenital cytomegalovirus infection: virus-host interaction for defense and transmission. *Curr. Pharm. Biotechnol.* 2006;7:303-12.
[24] Pusztai R, Lukacsi A, Kovacs I. Mother-to-fetus transmission of cytomegalovirus. A review. *Acta Microbiol. Immunol. Hung.* 2004;51:385-401.
[25] Boppana SB, Fowler KB, Britt WJ, Stagno S, Pass RF. Symptomatic congenital cytomegalovirus infection in infants born to mothers with preexisting immunity to cytomegalovirus. *Pediatrics.* 1999;104:55-60.
[26] Milewska-Bobula B. Congenital cytomegalovirus infection--clinical characteristics including prenatal diagnosis. *Med. Wieku. Rozwoj.* 2003;7(3 Suppl 1):123-7.
[27] Ross SA, Boppana SB. Congenital cytomegalovirus infection: outcome and diagnosis. *Semin. Pediatr. Infect. Dis.* 2005;16:44-9.
[28] Grangeot-Keros L. Routine CMV screening during pregnancy. *Eur. J. Obstet. Gynecol. Reprod. Biol.* 2004 ;114:3-11.
[29] Abdel-Fattah SA, Bhat A, Illanes S, Bartha JL, Carrington D. TORCH test for fetal medicine indications: only CMV is necessary in the United Kingdom. *Prenat Diagn.* 2005;25:1028-31.
[30] Collinet P, Subtil D, Houfflin-Debarge V, Kacet N, Dewilde A, Puech F. Routine CMV screening during pregnancy. *Eur. J. Obstet. Gynecol. Reprod. Biol.* 2004;114:3-11.
[31] Cytomegalovirus infection. Available online at http://www.emedicine.com/ped/topic544.htm.
[32] Salomon N, Perlman DC. Cytomegalovirus pneumonia. *Semin. Respir. Infect.* 1999;14:353-8.
[33] Rodriguez-Barradas MC, Stool E, Musher DM, Gathe J Jr, Goldstein J, Genta RM, Yoffe B. Diagnosing and treating cytomegalovirus pneumonia in patients with AIDS. *Clin. Infect. Dis.* 1996;23:76-81.
[34] Millar AB, Patou G, Miller RF, Grundy JE, Katz DR, Weller IV, Semple SJ. Cytomegalovirus in the lungs of patients with AIDS. Respiratory pathogen or passenger? *Am. Rev. Respir. Dis.* 1990;141:1474-7.
[35] Wiegand TW, Young LH. Cytomegalovirus retinitis. *Int. Ophthalmol. Clin.* 2006;46:91-110.
[36] Li HY, Ye JJ. Progress in the studies on cytomegalovirus retinitis. *Zhongguo Yi Xue Ke Xue Yuan Xue Bao.* 2003;25:223-7.
[37] Au Eong KG, Beatty S, Charles SJ. Cytomegalovirus retinitis in patients with acquired immune deficiency syndrome. *Postgrad. Med. J.* 1999;75:585-90
[38] Davis JL. Differential diagnosis of CMV retinitis. *Ocul. Immunol. Inflamm.* 1999;7:159-66.

[39] Reed JB, Morse LS. CMV retinitis and the controversies associated with highly active antiretroviral therapy and the immune recovery hypothesis. *AIDS Patient Care STDS.* 1998;12:181-5.

[40] Jouan M, Katlama C. Management of CMV retinitis in the era of highly active antiretroviral therapy. *Int. J. Antimicrob. Agents.* 1999;13:1-7.

[41] Galiatsatos P, Shrier I, Lamoureux E, Szilagyi A Meta-analysis of outcome of cytomegalovirus colitis in immunocompetent hosts. *Dig. Dis. Sci.* 2005;50:609-16.

[42] Hommes DW, Sterringa G, van Deventer SJ, Tytgat GN, Weel J. The pathogenicity of cytomegalovirus in inflammatory bowel disease: a systematic review and evidence-based recommendations for future research. *Inflamm. Bowel. Dis.* 2004;10:245-50.

[43] Preiser W, Fleckenstein C, Doerr HW. New methods for the diagnosis of cytomegalovirus. *Dtsch. Med. Wochenschr.* 2004;129:1509-12.

[44] Chou S. Newer methods for diagnosis of cytomegalovirus infection. *Rev. Infect. Dis.* 1990;12 Suppl 7:S727-36.

[45] Tong CY. Diagnosis of cytomegalovirus infection and disease. *J. Med. Microbiol.* 1997;46:717-9.

[46] Griffiths PD. Rapid diagnosis of cytomegalovirus infection. *J. Hosp. Infect.* 1985;6 Suppl C:35-41.

[47] Toyokawa M, Nishi I. Cytomegalovirus infection. *Rinsho Byori.* 2002 ;Suppl 123:71-8.

[48] Biron KK. Antiviral drugs for cytomegalovirus diseases. *Antiviral. Res.* 2006;71:154-63.

[49] Cvetkovic RS, Wellington K. Valganciclovir: a review of its use in the management of CMV infection and disease in immunocompromised patients. *Drugs.* 2005;65:859-78.

[50] Noble S, Faulds D. Ganciclovir. An update of its use in the prevention of cytomegalovirus infection and disease in transplant recipients. *Drugs.* 1998;56:115-46

[51] Minor JR, Baltz JK. Foscarnet sodium. *DICP.* 1991;25:41-7

[52] De Clercq E. Cidofovir in the treatment of poxvirus infections. *Antiviral Res.* 2002;55:1-13.

[53] Emery VC. Cytomegalovirus drug resistance. *Antivir. Ther.* 1998;3:239-42.

Chapter XIII

Filariasis and Dirofilariasis

Introduction to Filariasis and Dirofilariasis

Filariasis and dirofilariasis are important tropical mosquito-borne parasitic infections. Filariasis is the name of name for a group of tropical diseases caused by various thread-like parasitic roundworms and their larvae. Filariasis presents with fever, chills, headache, and skin lesions in the early stages and, if untreated, it can progress to include gross enlargement of the limbs and genitalia in a condition called elephantiasis. Several different types of worms are mentioned as causes of filariasis but the common species include the following: *Wucheria bancrofti, Brugia malayi, Onchocerca volvulus, Loa loa, Mansonella streptocerca, Dracunculus medinensis*, *Mansonella pustans*, and *Mansonella ozzardi*. However, it should be noted that not all human filariasis diseases are mosquito-borne. Concerning dirofilariasis, it is described as infection with roundworms of the genus dirofilaria, usually in animals, especially dogs, but occasionally in man [2]. Cats and dogs are the main hosts suffering from dirofilariasis.

Dhanda *et al* said that dengue was becoming increasingly recognized as one of the world's major infectious diseases due to the increased incidence and geographical distribution of filariasis in the recent years [3]. In India, Dhanda *et al* said that Filariasis, once considered to be more associated with urban areas and urbanization, was rapidly emerging as a major problem in rural areas [3]. They noted for the need to delimit the endemic areas through a new rapid assessment procedure and the possible control methods of rural filariasis [3]. Raccurt said that dirofilariasis was an emerging and underestimated zoonoses [4]. Raccurt noted that data concerning canine heartworm in France was available but the extent of human infestation was probably underestimated and would require further study [4]. In addition, Raccurt also mentioned that data on other animal reservoirs should be updated [4]. Ault said that vector control might be accomplished by environmental management (EM), which consists of permanent or long-term modification of the environment, temporary or seasonal manipulation of the environment, and modifying or changing populations' life styles and practices to reduce human contact with infective vectors [5].

Infections with the filarial nematodes affect more than 150 million people mainly in the tropics [6]. The very successful efforts to control filarial infections, however, have to be sustained by new tools that require long-term commitment to research [6]. It should be noted that according to the globalization at present, the filariasis becomes an emerging infectious problem not only to the tropical but also to the non-tropical countries [7]. Hochberg and Ryan noted that many infections associated with long-term overseas deployment might include dermatologic manifestations, including filariasis and leishmaniasis [8]. In additional to filariasis, dirofilariasis becomes an interesting zoonosis at present. Muso *et al* said that infection with immature worms had been found in humans, who developed nodules, mainly in subcutaneous tissue or in lung parenchyma arising from branches of the pulmonary artery [9]. They noted that the parasites did not usually reach the adult stage and microfilaremia is absent in human, as has been shown by diagnosis using invasive methods for removing the nodules [9]. Schlotthauer *et al* noted that dirofilariais should be considered as an important emerging zoonosis in public health [10]. The knowledge on the filariasis and dirofilariasis is, therefore, an interesting topic for general practitioners all over the world.

FILARIASIS

Filaria worm, a parasite in Superfamily Filariodea is an important blood parasite. Up to billion of people around the world is the population at risk for filariasis [11]. As previously mentioned, there are many nematodes that can be the pathogens for the filariasis. The summative details for important species are described in the following text.

1. Bancroftian Filariasis

1.1. Introduction

Bancroftian filariasis is the term used for the filariasis that is caused by *Wucheria bancrofti.* This lymphatic filariasis has been identified as the second leading cause of permanent and long-term disability [12]. Melrose said that lymphatic filariasis had afflicted people in the tropical areas of the world for thousands of years but even up to comparatively recent times it had been poorly understood and its importance under recognised [13]. Melrose noted that there had been a flurry of activity in filariasis research, which had provided new insights into the global problem of filariasis, the pathogenesis of filarial disease, diagnosis and control [13].

1.2. Worldwide Epidemiology of Bancroftian Filariasis

de Almeida and Freedman said that human lymphatic filariasis affected 120 million people worldwide [14]. They noted that although the disease is considered to be potentially erradicable by the World Health Organization, comprehensive studies on epidemiological aspects as well as mechanisms of pathology development are still premature [14]. Bancrofti filariasis is endemic in Asia, especially Southeast Asia. There are many reports from Asia concerning the epidemiology of this disease. In Southeast Asia, Kron *et al* said that lymphatic filariasis caused by *Wuchereria bancrofti* was endemic throughout most of the southern half of the Philippine archipelago [15]. Kron *et al* noted that analysis of cumulative prevalence data on filariasis indicates the persistence of filariasis in each of the three major island groups - Luzon, Visayas and Mindanao - including 45 out of 77 provinces [15]. Kazura and Bockarie noted that bancroftian filariasis is a major public health problem in Papua New Guinea, where the level of transmission by the mosquito vector, human infection rates and clinical morbidity were among the highest in the world [16]. They said that coordinated research efforts within the country, involving the disciplines of epidemiology, vector biology, immunology and genetics, had led to new insights into the ecology and pathogenesis of human lymphatic filariasis [16]. They also noted that recent work using this knowledge base should be helpful in assessing local and global strategies aimed at eliminating *Wuchereria bancrofti* and in guiding research that will facilitate achievement of this goal [16].

In South America, the bancroftian filariasis is also common. Rocha and Fontes recently performed a review on the distribution of Bancroftian filariasis in Brazil [17]. They noted that the autochthonous transmission of Wuchereria bancrofti having been found only in 11 places in the country as follows, with the corresponding prevalences; Ponta Grossa, 14.5% Belem, 9.8%; Barra de Laguna, 9.4%; Recife, 6.9%; Castro Alves, 5.9%; Florianopolis, 1.4%; Sao Luis, 0.6%; Salvador, 0.4%; Maceio (AL), 0.3%; Manaus 0.2% and Porto Alegre, 0.1% [17]. They also noted that distribution of infection was urban and focal, occurring mainly along the coast [17]. They proposed that recent studies showed the active transmission of filariasis with higher prevalences than those observed in the past, in Maceio, considered to be free from infection [17].

Bancroftian is also endemic in tropical Africa. In 2000, Njenga *et al* performed an interesting study In Kenya to determine the prevalence of *Wuchereria bancrofti* infection in an area designated for filariasis control trial [18]. According to this study, the overall prevalence of microfilaraemia in the population was 16.4% and the prevalence of microfilaraemia was age-dependent and significantly higher in males than in females [18]. They noted that the prevalence of clinical signs of infection was also age-dependent with elephantiasis being significantly higher in females than in males [18]. Njenga *et al* concluded from their findings that there was high prevalence of bancroftian filariasis in Kwale district and this warranted similar studies followed by implementation of intervention measures to reduce transmission in all areas of endemicity in the Coast Province [18]. In 2002, Gyapong *et al* performed another study to document the geographical distribution of human infection with *Wuchereria bancrofti* in four West African countries (Benin, Burkina Faso, Ghana and Togo), using a commercial immunochromatographic test for filarial antigen [19]. The results, which were subjected to an independent random validation in Burkina Faso and Ghana, revealed that prevalence in the adult population of some communities exceeded 70% and that, over large areas of Burkina Faso, community prevalences were between 30% and 50%. Most of Togo, southern Benin and much of southern Ghana appeared completely free of the infection [19]. The results also indicated that bancroftian filariasis was more widely distributed in arid areas of Burkina Faso than hitherto recognized and that the prevalences of infection had remained fairly stable for at least 30 years [19]. Gyapong *et al* noted that the campaign to eliminate lymphatic filariasis as a public-health problem in Africa would require significantly more resources (human, financial, and logistic) than previously anticipated [19].

1.3. Vector and Transmission

Bancroftian filariasis is an important nematode infection. The causative worm is *Wuchereria bancrofti*. As previously mentioned, bancroftian filariasis is a mosquito-borne infection. Culcicine or anopheline mosquitoes are the main vectors of the nocturnally periodic forms of *Wuchereria bancrofti*, while day biting *Aedes polynesiensis* transmit the subperiodic form in various pacific islands [20]. Concerning the life cycle, once the microfilariae have entered an appropriate mosquito host through its blood meal they penetrate the insect's gut wall and move to the thoracic muscles where they mature, through two life stages, into third-stage infective larvae (L3i) [20]. Then the L3i enter the blood through the wound made by the vector mosquito [20]. They then migrate to the nearest lymph gland where they mature into the thread like adult worms about 3 months to 1 year later [20]. The average incubation time before patency is about 15 months [20]. The mature adults can survive for 5 to 10 years and the damage of the lymphatic vessels they cause and the immune system's response to their presence and that of microfilaria and newly innoculated L3i can result in the various clinical manifestations (figure 1) [20].

Similar to other mosquito-borne diseases, the three factors affecting the transmission are a) the nature of mosquito-man contacts, b) the susceptibility of the mosquito to the pathogen and multiplication of the latter, and c) the transmission.

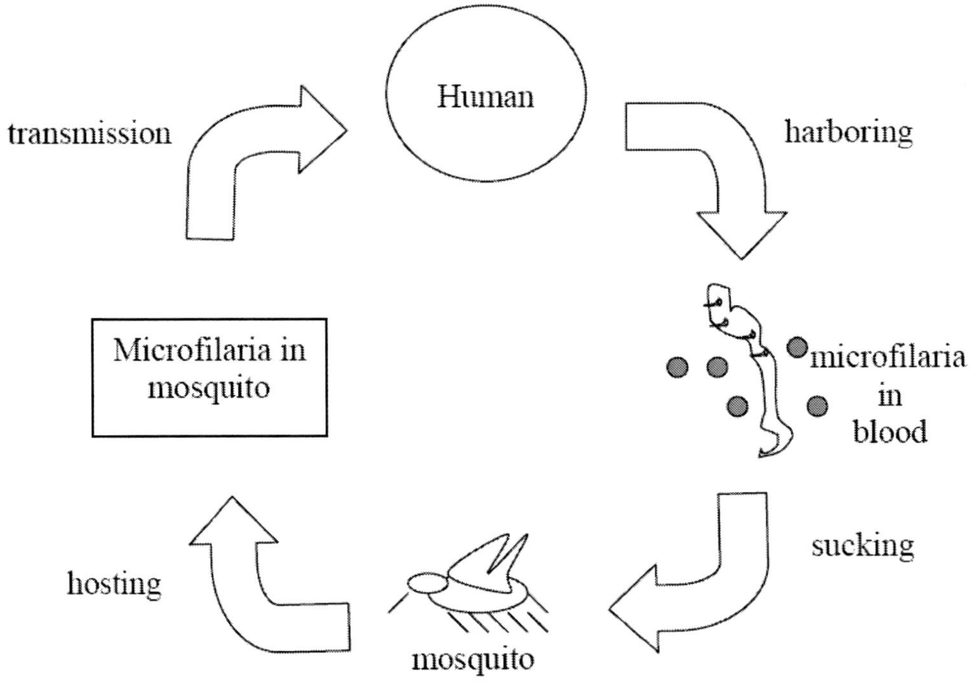

Figure 1. Life cycle of *Wuchereria bancrofti.*

There are some recent previous reports concerning the transmission of bancroftian filariasis. Triteeraprapab *et al* proposed that it was possible that an urban cycle of transmission could become established in Thailand [21]. Triteeraprapab *et al* said that the Myanmar immigrants are infected with the nocturnal periodic (urban) type *Wuchereria bancrofti* for which *Culex quinquefasciatus* serves as the main vector, however, the Thai strains of *Culex quinquefasciatus* had never been reported to transmit Bancroftian filariasis [21]. Triteeraprapab *et al* performed feeding experiments and found that the Thai *Culex quinquefasciatus* were permissive for the development of Myanmar *Wuchereria bancrofti* to infective third-stage larvae thus establishing the potential for establishing an urban cycle of transmission in Thailand [21]. Calheiros *et al* performed a study to determine the susceptibility of local strains of *Culex quinquefasciatus* and *Aedes aegypti* to infection with the strain of *Wuchereria bancrofti* that occurred in Brazil [22]. They found that survival rates of both species of insects living for 21 days after blood feeding on microfilaraemic patients were not significantly different from the survival rates of mosquitoes that blood fed on amicrofilaraemic individuals [22]. They noted that *Wuchereria bancrofti* parasites underwent normal development in *Culex quinquefasciatus*, with third stage larvae first being recorded on the 11th day post infection, and their numbers increasing thereafter while development of filariae in *Aedes aegypti* did not proceed beyond the first larval stage, and there was a progressively increasing number of non-viable larvae with the passage of time [22]. Calheiros *et al* concluded that *Aedes aegypti* was not involved in the transmission of *Wuchereria bancrofti* in Maceio [22].

In addition to vector transmission, other modes of transmission for bancroftian filariasis are also documented. Rao *et al* first reported the transplacental transmission in bancroftian filariasis in India in 1984 [23]. Recently, Pires *et al* investigated the occurrence of circulating *Wuchereria bancrofti* microfilariae in 304 pregnant women in Brazil [24]. According to this study, the filtration technique was employed to detect microfilaraemia during pregnancy, and 13 women were found to be positive (4.2%) [24]. They found that microfilariae in the cord blood of their children was negative, and also in venous blood samples collected up to 72 hours after birth and with 6 months of life [24]. In addition, they found that milk samples from these mothers also had no microfilariae [24]. Pires *et al* suggested that the occurrence of placentary lesions may be a possible factor involved in the transplacental transfer of microfilariae, and that in utero exposure to microfilariae and/or filarial antigens may influence the response to a filarial infection acquired later, thus being important a clinical and laboratorial follow-up of children exposed previously to filarial antigens during early periods of human development [24]. Malhotra *et al* performed another interesting study to determine whether maternal filariasis influences the risk of infection by and immunity to *Wuchereria bancrofti* in children [25]. According to this study, they indicated that maternal filarial infection increased childhood susceptibility to *Wuchereria bancrofti* and skewed filaria-specific immunity toward a Th2-type cytokine response [25]. They proposed that results supported the notion that in utero exposure to filarial antigens affected the natural history of filariasis during childhood [25]. Concerning the transmission via blood and blood products, Hira and Husein said that microfilariae of *Wuchereria bancrofti* were also found in donor populations [26]. They noted that while no disease may be induced, allergic reactions due to the breakdown products of dead microfilariae might manifest themselves [26].

1.4. Genetic and Molecular Biology of Bancroftian Filariasis

Genetic is mentioned as an important intrinsic affecting the ability of vectors to transmit pathogens. In addition to the genetic pattern in vector, the effect of genetic polymorphism in human is also mentioned. Hise *et al* examined 906 residents of an area of Papua New Guinea where bancroftian filariasis was endemic for genetic polymorphisms in three innate immunity genes suspected of contributing to susceptibility to infection and lymphatic pathology [27]. They found that there was no association of infection status, lymphedema of an extremity, or hydrocele with chitotriosidase genotype (CHIT1) [27]. In this study, polymorphisms of toll-like receptor-2 and toll-like receptor-4 genes (TLR4 A896G; TLR2 T2178A, G2258A) were not detected except for two individuals heterozygous for a TLR2 mutation (C2029 T) [27].

Based on these results, Hise *et al* indicated that a CHIT1 genotype associated previously with susceptibility to filariasis and TLR2 and TLR4 polymorphisms did not correlate with infection status or disease phenotype in this Melanesian population [27]. Also, there are some applications on using molecular diagnosis for bancroftian filariasis [28].

1.5. Pathophysiology and Clinical Manifestation of Bancroftian Filariasis

Bancroftian filariasis is classified as a lymphatic filariasis. Freedman *et al* noted that despite the common association of filarial infection with elephantiasis, the great majority of those infected were in fact clinically asymptomatic microfilariae carriers [29]. They proposed that infection but not disease exists in these presymptomatic persons [29]. Recently, Freedman *et al* used dynamic radionuclide lymphoscintigraphy to compare 30 limbs from asymptomatic microfilaremic subjects with 16 control limbs [29]. They found increased lymph flow in asymptomatic microfilaremic subjects and they noted that abnormal lymphatic function in these subjects indicated that current passive intervention strategies might need to change if the debilitating sequelae of this parasitic infection were to be avoided [29]. Simonsen and Meyrowitsch suggested that specific anti-sheath-antibodies were associated with an immunologic resistance mechanism that in the endemic community is expressed with highest prevalence in young individuals before development of patent microfilaremia [30]. In addition, several investigators have suggested that females have increased resistance to infection and this is supported by serological studies showing high antibody positivity to adult worm antigens in females [31]. Brabin concluded that the association with the reproductive years suggested a pregnancy-associated mechanism and this had important implications for maternal-fetal interactions and maternal filarial infection might influence the development of immunity in children [31]. Recently, King *et al* compared T cell and cytokine responses in 97 residents of two villages in Papua New Guinea [32]. They concluded that demonstrate that the intensity of exposure to L3 affects lymphocyte responsiveness and cytokine bias possibly by a mechanism that alters antigen presenting cell function [32]. Concerning the development of elephantiasis, the chronic lymphatic obstruction is the main pathogenesis [33].

Concerning the clinical manifestation of bancroftian filariasis, the wide spectrum of manifestations is reported. As previously mentioned, some cases are also asymptomatic. Simonsen *et al* performed an interesting study on the clinical manifestation of bancroftian filariasis in Tanzania [34]. They said that hydrocele was the most common chronic clinical manifestation, with prevalences ranging from 14.5 to 21.3% for all males, and from 52.9 to 62.1% for males [34]. According to this study, microfilaraemia was common in males with hydrocele, and in males of 45 years and above there was no significant difference in microfilariae prevalence between males with (42.5%) and without (55.2%) hydrocele [34]. They also noted that from 0.6 to 3.3% of the inhabitants had elephantiasis, which most often affected the legs [34]. They noted that microfilariae were only detected in the blood from one of 18 individuals with elephantiasis [34]. Similar to the report of Simonsen *et al*, Meyrowitsch *et al* performed another study in Tanzania and reported that hydrocele was the most common clinical manifestation followed by leg elephantiasis [35].

Although testicular hydrocele is the most common clinical manifestation of bancroftian filariasis, its pathogenesis is poorly understood, as is its relationship to inflammatory scrotal nodules following death of adult *Wuchereria bancrofti*. Noroes *et al* said that acute hydrocele occurred frequently following death of adult *Wuchereria bancrofti* and single episodes of scrotal nodule formation [36]. They also noted that chronic hydrocele might develop following 5.1% of these episodes [36]. With respect to hydrocele, Simonsen *et al* recently mentioned against the hypotheses assuming a general negative relationship between microfilaraemia and chronic clinical manifestations in bancroftian filariasis [34].

1.6. Diagnosis of Bancroftian Filariasis

The basic diagnostic method for bancroftian filariasis is based on microscopic examination. Microilariae detection is still a difficult blood smear interpretation [37 - 38]. Apart from simple smear, other preparations such as thick film and lymphatic (buffy coat) smear are available. Interpretation of blood film is an important tool in diagnosis of filariasis [37 - 38]. Recommendation of pre-analytical drug intake to cope the periodicity is set in the endemic area [39 - 40]. The microfilariae of *Wuchereria bancrofti* can be identified in blood smears by their sheath, size (approximate size = 230 - 300 μm in length), and the anterior V spot near the head and posterior V spot near the tail. However, it is still difficult to detect the microfilariae in the slide. Southgate said that sensitive, specific, practical and acceptable screening technique for the field surveillance must be set [41].

Antigen testing is now recognized as the method of choice for detection of *Wuchereria bancrofti* infections [42]. Unlike tests that detect microfilariae, antigen tests can be performed with blood collected during the day or night. However, existing enzyme-linked immunosorbent assay (ELISA) tests for filarial antigenemia are difficult to perform in the field, and this has limited their use in endemic countries [42]. Other more-powerful diagnostic tools than the unique detection of microfilariae by blood smear examination are also mentioned. These include the detection of adult worm circulating antigens in humans, the visualization by ultrasound of living *Wuchereria bancrofti* adult worm on its natural host as well as the human being. and the detection of Wuchereria bancrofti larvae in mosquitoes, using DNA probes [43].

1.7. Treatment

Dreyer *et al* said that the goals of treatment for lymphatic filariasis were: to prevent, reverse, or halt progression of disease; and to interrupt transmission of the parasite [44]. In the past, treatment of lymphatic filariasis has focused primarily on antiparasitic chemotherapy; however, for many of the acute and chronic manifestations of lymphatic filariasis, it is now clear that supportive or other forms of clinical care are even more important than antiparasitic medication in order to prevent worsening of the disease [44]. Dreyer *et al* said that regardless of the clinical manifestations of filarial disease in a particular patient, the following three components of treatment should be considered: supportive or disease specific clinical care (including hygiene and diet), patient education and counseling and finally, antiparasitic chemotherapy with diethylcarbamazine (DEC) and/or the combination of DEC with ivermectin [44]. Dreyer and Noroes said that because of the lack of ideal drug with micro and macrofilaricidal properties, together with the new understand about the disease and the new parameters for monitoring the efficacy of the drug, diethylcarbamazine had back its importance conquered at the begin of its discovery [45].

The prevention is the good method to control this disease. Since this disease is vector-borne transmission, the control of vector is important in primary prevention. In order to control the mosquito, use of bed nest and pesticide should be considered.

Further more details will be presented in the final chapter.

2. Malayan Filariasis

2.1. Introduction and Worldwide Epidemiology of Malayan Filariasis

Malayan or brugian filariasis is the term used for the filariasis that is caused by *Brygia malayi*. This filariasis is another common lymphatic filariasis. Malayan filariasis is endemic in Asia, especially Southeast Asia. There are many reports from Asia concerning the epidemiology of this disease. In Southeast Asia, recent filariasis surveys at Lubuk Mumpo and Datar Lebar, Bengkulu, Sumatera, showed microfilarial rates of 23.9% and 30% respectively [46]. In addition, *Brugia malayi* infections were seen in 7.1% of domestic cats. Triteeraprapab *et al* said that lymphatic filariasis caused by *Brugia malayi* is highly prevalent in Narathiwat province of Thailand. They performed a survey in this area in 2001 [47]. By using the conventional microscopic method, the microfilarial rate of *Brugia malayi* in an endemic area of Narathiwat province in the southern part of Thailand was 1.38 % [47]. They also noted that the lowest microfilarial rate was in the age group less than 15 years (0.37%) [47]. Wiwanitkit also reported the increase prevalence of malayan filariasis due to the immigration of Mynmar into the southern part of Thailand as well [38]. In East Asia, there are also some reports from the southern part of China. However, Duan *et al* noted that since the basic elimination of filariasis in Hunan Province in 1986, the number of residual microfilariemia cases decreased year after year, suggesting that the transmission of filariasis had been interrupted [48].

2.2. Vector and transmission

Malayan filariasis is an important nematode infection. The causative worm is *Brugia malayi*. As previously mentioned, malayan filariasis is a mosquito-borne infection. Mansonia mosquitoes are the main vectors of the *Brugia malayi*. Suzuki *et al* recently performed a study on the vector of malayan filariasis in Indonesia [49]. In the study area, the most prevalent man-biting Mansonia mosquitoes were *Mansonia bonneae* (41%), followed by *Mansonia annulata* (27%), *Mansonia uniformis* (25%) and *Mansonia dives* (7%) [49]. They concluded that the principal vectors of periodic Brugiamalayi in the study area in Bengkulu are four Mansonia species (*Mansonia annulata, Mansonia bonneae, Mansonia uniformis and Mansonia dives*), and that the potential vectors include two Anopheles species (*Anopheles nigerrimus* and *Anopheles peditaeniatus*) [49]. Concerning the life cycle, similar pattern to that of is *Wuchereria bancrofti* mentioned.

In addition to vector transmission, other modes of transmission for malayan filariasis are also documented. Similar to bancroftian filariasis, the transplacental transmission in malayan filariasis is of concern. In 1989, Sanjeevi and Narayanan studied the presence of anti-filarial antibody in the mother and cord blood at the time of delivery was identified by ELISA. They found that 6 out of 29 cases showed IgM against *Brugia malayi* antigen in the cord blood. They concluded that there was a fetal response to maternal filariasis [50].

2.3. Genetic and Molecular Biology of Malayan Filariasis

In 1994, Severson *et al* identified two quantitative trait loci (QTL) affecting susceptibility of the mosquito *Aedes aegypti* to the filarial worm parasite *Brugia malayi* using restriction fragment length polymorphism (RFLP) markers [51]. The first locus, fsb[1,LF178], resides within a 10 cM interval on chromosome 1 and exhibits a recessive effect with respect to susceptibility and the second locus, fsb[2,LF98], resides within a 9 cM interval on chromosome 2 and exhibits an additive effect on susceptibility [51]. In 2002, Gomez-Escobar *et al* defined genomic organisation of two abundant larval transcript (alt) genes from the filarial nematode *Brugia malayi*. They showed relatively strong expression in the gut cells of *Caenorhabditis elegans* for both alt-1 and -2 constructs, commencing in larval worms and continuing into adulthood [52]. Moreover, they also noted that expression was enhanced when constructs contained segments of alt-1 coding and intronic sequence in addition to the 5' UTR [52]. Gomez-Escobar *et al* concluded that the high level of alt transcription in filarial L3s was not due to expression from a multi-copy gene family but to a set of strong promoter elements shared between the two alt genes [52].

2.4. Pathophysiology and Clinical Manifestation of Malayan Filariasis

Malayan filariasis is classified as a lymphatic filariasis. In 1985, Sakamoto *et al* described changes in lymphatic endothelial cells of Brugia-infected cats [53]. According to their study, transmission electron microscopy revealed a decrease in the number of cytoplasmic vesicles in endothelial cells from lymphatic vessels harboring filarial nematodes when compared with similar cells from the contralateral uninfected control vessels, however, the size of the vesicles and their location within the cytoplasm was not changed [53]. They noted that irregular large vacuoles, often containing degenerating organelles, were common in endothelial cells lining Brugia-infected lymphatic vessels [53]. Sakamoto *et al* suggested that damage of cells by living or dead worms or worm products might have a direct effect on the endothelial lining of lymphatic vessels and this might compromise the efficiency of vessels that collect and transport edematous fluid in affected limbs [53].

Several immunopathological processes in Brugia malayi infection are proposed. Sartono *et al* noted that in an area in which brugian filariasis is endemic, when cytokine levels were analyzed as a function of clinical status comparing those who were asymptomatic and amicrofilaremic with those who were microfilaremic, it was found that both interferon (IFN)-gamma and interleukin (IL)-5 were suppressed in microfilariae carriers ($P < .01$ and $P < .001$, respectively), but IL-4 was unabated [54]. In asymptomatic amicrofilaremic subjects, IL-4 production was high in young persons and decreased with age, whereas in microfilaremic subjects, IL-4 increased significantly with age and conversely, IFN-gamma showed a tendency to increase with age in asymptomatic amicrofilaremic subjects but not in microfilaremic subjects [54]. In addition, IL-5 decreased significantly with increasing age in both asymptomatic amicrofilaremic and microfilaremic groups [54]. Sartono *et al* concluded that the length of exposure to and infection with filarial parasites could each exert a substantial effect on the cytokine response profiles of host T cell populations [54].

Concerning the clinical manifestation, similar manifestations to those of *Wuchereria bancrofti* infection are noted. Soh *et al* noted that the main clinical manifestation was cuticular hypertrophy (elephantiasis) [55]. They noted that the elephantiasis appeared more often in the lower extremities than in the upper part of the body, and in the right side than in the left [55]. Some interesting manifestations such as tropical pulmonary eosinophilia can also be seen. Bm2325, a major IgE-inducing antigen of the filarial parasite *Brugia malayi* has been implicated in the pathology of tropical pulmonary eosinophilia, a pulmonary syndrome thought to result from hypersensitivity to microfilariae [56]. Lobos *et al* said that molecular mimicry between the parasite gamma-GT homolog and the host membrane-bound gamma-GT presented in lung epithelial cells likely contributed to the pathogenesis observed in tropical pulmonary eosinophilia [56].

2.5. Diagnosis of Malayan Filariasis

The basic diagnostic method for malayan filariasis is also based on microscopic examination. The microfilariae of *Brugia malayi* can be identified in blood smears by their sheath, size (approximate size = 175 - 260 μm in length), and the terminal and subterminal swelling of the tail. However, it is still difficult to detect the microfilariae in the slide. In addition, in the endemic area, there is a need to differentiate between common micorfilariae from different species.

Table 1. Differentiation between sheathed microfilariae of *Wuchereria bancrofti* and *Brugia malayi*

Species	Length (μm)	Diameter (μm)	Cephalic space	Caudal space	Terminal nucleus
Wuchereria bancrofti	230 -300	7 -10	yes	yes	elongated
Brugia malayi	175 - 260	4 -6	yes	no	round

In addition to the classical microscopic examination, there are also new advanced tests for diagnosis of *Brugia malayi* infection. Several immunological diagnostic tests are developed. An alternative approach for identification of infected individuals is to detect specific parasite antigens in circulation [57]. A WHO initiative to use either an antigen or antibody assay to replace night blood is presently underway [57]. In addition, new molecular biology-based tests are also launched. Recently, species-specific DNA probes have also been developed for *Brugia malayi* [57].

2.6. Treatment and Prevention

The goals of treatment for lymphatic filariasis: prevention, reversation and cutting the transmission of the parasite are applicable for *Brugia malayi* infection [44]. Similar treatments to bancroftian filariasis can be applied for malayan filariasis. Of interest, there are some interesting trials for the alternative medicine to treat malayan filariasis. Recently, Lakshmi *et al* said that the chloroform methanol extract of an unidentified green zoanthus (Phylum Coelenterata, Class Anthozoa) showed promising in vitro adulticidal activity with a lethal concentration of 125 microg/ml on *Brugia malayi* [58].

However, the prevention is also the good method to control this disease.

Partono said that the filarial parasites reproduce slowly, whereas their mosquito vectors were quickly-reproducing opportunists, thus, although vector control could reduce the risk of transmission, the parasite itself would seem a more vulnerable target for prolonged attack [59]. Further more details on vector control will be presented in the final chapter. Concerning the vaccination for malayan filariasis, there some interesting recent reports on this topic. In 2004, Gnanasekar *et al* described a novel phage display method based on an iterative subtraction strategy to identify candidate vaccine antigens of *Brugia malayi*. In this study, a cDNA library of the infective larval stage of B. malayi expressed on the surface of T7 phage was sequentially screened with sera samples from human subjects showing different manifestations of the disease [60]. Gnanasekar *et al* identified five antigens, four of which were previously reported (ALT-2, TPX-2, VAH and COX-2) and the other one was a novel cuticular collagen (Col-4) [60]. They found that ALT-2 appeared to be the most predominantly recognized antigen by the immune sera, therefore, it was decided to evaluate the vaccine potential of recombinant ALT-2 (rALT-2) in a mouse and jird model [60]. The results presented show that immunization with rALT-2 conferred over 73% protection against a challenge infection in the jird model and over 64% protection in the mouse model [60].

3. Brugia Timori and Brugia Pahangi Infections

In additional to *Brugia malayi* infection, the other two common brugian pathogens for humans are *Brugia timori* and *Brugia Pahangi*. Filariasis due to *Brugia timori* is unevenly distributed in Southeast Asia [61]. *Brugia timori* is a pathogenic filarial nematode of humans, replacing the closely related species *Brugia malayi* on some islands in eastern Indonesia and Timor [62]. Similar to *Brugia malayi*, *Brugia timori* infections are seen in the rural areas [61]. Similar vectors for *Brugia malayi* and *Brugia timori* are also mentioned [61]. Recent studies on Alor island show that, locally, *Brugia timori* is still of great public health importance, causing mainly acute filarial fever and chronic lymphedema [62].

As previously mentioned, *Brugia timori* is very similar to *Brugia malayi* in morphology, therefore, the diagnosis usually required confirmation test. Several immunological diagnostic tests are produced to this purpose. Recently, a rapid immunochromatographic dipstick test (Brugia Rapid, BR), based on the detection of anti-filarial IgG4 antibodies that react with a recombinant *Brugia malayi* antigen (BmR1), was evaluated on microfilaraemic and amicrofilaraemic individuals [63]. According to that study, the BR test showed great promise to be employed as a monitoring tool for B. timori in the framework of the Global Program to Eliminate Lymphatic Filariasis (GPELF) [63]. PCR-based assays to detect parasite DNA, in addition to assays for detecting specific antibodies that have been originally developed for *Brugia malayi*, can be used efficiently as diagnostic tools for *Brugia timori* [62]. Fischer *et al* proposed that *Brugia timori* could be effectively detected using the PCR-based assay developed for *Brugia malayi* and could then be differentiated from *Brugia malayi* by other molecular markers [64]. Concerning treatment, Fischer *et al* said that in the framework of the GPELF, a single annual dose of diethylcarbamazine, in combination with albendazole, was found to reduce the prevalence and density of microfilaraemia persistently, therefore, elimination of *Brugia timori* appears to be achievable [62].

Concerning *Brugia pahangi* infection, human infection is considered accidental. However, infection patterns in the cat closely parallel those of Brugia and Wuchereria in humans, therefore, it is used as the animal model for study of human filariasis [65]. Considering human infection, there are some reports on Brugia pahangi infection. In 1989, Hitch *et al* performed a study in Haiti and noted that the levels in children were significantly elevated in humoral immunoreactivity to Brugia pahangi extracts compared to adults [66].

4. Loiasis

Loiasis or eyeworm infection is a human filariasis caused by *Loa Loa* infection. The endemic area for this filariasis is Africa. Filarial loiasis differs from other filariases in that most infected subjects are amicrofilaremic and this difference raises the notion of occult infection [67]. In 1999, Toure *et al* performed a study to evaluate the relationship between the intensity of transmission and incidence of infection [67]. For this purpose, they determined the incidence of loiasis both microscopically and by PCR in 201 subjects from three villages in the province of Haut Ogooue in Gabon [67]. According to this study, they found no significant difference between the three villages with regard to the incidence of microfilaremia [67]. They concluded that the incidence of loiasis is correlated with the intensity of transmission especially in children [67]. Wanji *et al* performed another interesting study in Cameroon [68]. They noted that the occurrence of the infection was largely related to environmental factors favouring the breeding of Chrysops vectors [68]. Since this disease is a fly-borne disease, therefore, more details are not mentioned in this book.

5. Onchocerciasis

Onchocerciasis or river blindness is a human filariasis caused by *Onchocerca volvulus*. Similar to loiasis, this disease is endemic in Africa. It is the world's second leading infectious cause of blindness [69]. It is transmitted to humans through the bite of a blackfly (Simulium species) [69]. These flies breed in fast-flowing streams and rivers, increasing the risk of blindness to individuals living nearby, hence the commonly known name of "river blindness" [69]. Within the human body, the adult female worm (macrofilaria) produces thousands of baby or larval worms (microfilariae) which migrate in the skin and the eye [69 - 70]. Since this disease is not a mosquito-borne disease, therefore, more details are not mentioned in this book.

6. Guinea Worm Infection

Guinea worm infection or *Dracunculus medinensis* infection is another human filariasis. This is an ancient disease and the beginner of the classical sign of medicine. Unlike other human filariasis, this disease is not an arthropod-borne disease. Humans are infected when they ingest water containing copepods [71 - 72]. Then juvenile worms exist intestinal tract and migrate to subcutaneous tissue [71 - 72]. Finally, female worms migrate to skin and produce blisters [71 - 72]. Within the blisters, the juvenile worms are formed [71 - 72]. If these blisters break, the infective juvenile worm can be liberated into the water and then ingested by copepods [71 – 72]. Since this disease is not a mosquito-borne disease, therefore, more details are not mentioned in this book.

Wolbachia Infection

A. Introduction to Wolbachia Infection

Filariasis is a major tropical disease. Inflammatory responses are also a feature of the adverse reaction to filarial chemotherapy that is thought to occur after the release of large amounts of parasite material following treatment. Several factors are believed to contribute to the inflammatory pathogenesis of filariasis, including the parasite, the immune response, and infection of the parasite, *Wolbachia*, a Rickettsia-like endosymbiont found in insects.

Numerous species of various insect orders carry obligatory symbionts such as flagellates, yeasts and bacteria. When these microorganisms are removed by using antibiotics, the insects often show growth reduction or do not survive at all. There are many well-documented cases of insects that carry obligatory intracellular bacteria that alter their host's mode of reproduction [73]. *Wolbachia*, a Rickettsia-like bacteria and an insect endosymbiont is a good example of such a microorganism.

Hertig and Wolbach first observed *Wolbachia* in the ovaries of the mosquito *Culex pipiens*, hence the resulting genus name [74]. It has created much interest in entomology because it is responsible for numerous insect host reproductive modifications. It has also been recovered in reproductive tissues and some somatic tissues of hundreds of diverse arthropod species. The traditional taxonomy of these bacteria has largely been based upon which host they occupy; for example, the current nomenclature for three species in the *Wolbachia* genus are: *Wolbachia pipientis, Wolbachia persica* and *Wolbachia melophagi* (*Culex pipiens* harbours *Wolbachia pipientis,* and so on). However, the new systematic study using the 16S *rRNA* gene, these species that were thought to be closely related are shown to belong to entirely different subdivisions of the *Proteobacteria*; *Wolbachia persica* belongs to the g - *Proteobacteria*, whilst *Wolbachia pipientis* inhabits the a -*Proteobacteria* along with the rest of the *Rickettsia*-like bacteria [75]. *W. melophagi* also is more distantly related than first thought; suprisingly it is more closely related to *Agrobacterium* and other Rhizobacteria [76].

Because of their obligatory intracellular nature, *Wolbachia* has not yet been cultured outside of cells. It is only possible to culture them by inoculation into yolk sacs of chicken eggs or by infecting and maintaining them in host cells in tissue culture lines. However, *Wolbachia* can be observed by using an electron microscope and have been observed as coccoid (~1.0μm in diameter) and bacilliform (0.25 x 1.5μm) gram-negative bacteria. The bacteria are seen to have a third membrane surrounding them, seemingly of host origin. Polymerase chain reaction (PCR) technology has enabled workers to rapidly and easily screen insect populations for the presence of *Wolbachia*. PCR has also enabled the cloning of *Wolbachia*-specific genes, such as *ftsZ* and *wsp*, to elucidate finer *Wolbachia* phylogenies [77].

B. Distribution

Wolbachia spp are extremely abundant; previous studies have estimated that between 16% [78] and 22% [79] of all insect species harbour Wolbachia infections. Extrapolating from the percentage of infected species observed so far to the number of arthropod species in existence globally (which is between 10-30 million) yields a figure of between 1.6 to 6.6 million Wolbachia-infected insect species worldwide. This makes Wolbachia amongst the most abundant and successful endosymbiotic bacteria known [80].

Since Wolbachia's discovery by Hertig and Wolbach, they have been observed in a wide array of parasitoid taxa, from the Aphelinidae, Pteromalidae and Trichogrammatidae of the Hymenoptera to the Tachinidae of the Diptera [81]. Indeed, they have been described in hundreds of arthropod species as diverse as the isopods, crustaceans, and mites, and in all of the major insect orders [78].

C. Transmission

A) Vertical Transfer

Vertical transmission involves the transfer of the *Wolbachia* endosymbionts from the maternal oocyte cytoplasm to the offspring and through the generations of that specific taxon. This is also known as "cytoplasmic inheritance".

B) Horizontal (Intertaxon) Transfer

Evidence for horizontal transfer was provided by Werren [78], who found that *Wolbachia* in a fly (*Protocalliphora*) and its parasitoid (*Nasonia giraulti*) have been nearly identical *ftsZ* gene sequences, and therefore are phylogenetical extremely close. This suggests that multiple horizontal transfers have taken place, but only relatively recently, and only between the *Trichogramma* species in that monophyletic group [81]. Therefore, vertical transmission was the main form of *Wolbachia* transfer in *Trichogramma* until horizontal transmission occurred a short time ago between members of a group of closely related species, perhaps before the speciation of a common ancestor occurred. This suggests that both types of transmission do indeed occur.

D. Relation of *Wolbachia* and Filarial Nematodes, What Is the Clinical Application?

These intracellular bacteria have been observed in various species of filarial nematodes. The endosymbiont is widespread in filarial nematodes, including all of the major pathogenic filariae of humans [82]; *Wuchereria bancrofti*, *Brugia malayi* and *Onchocerca volvulus*. Of the filarial species investigated so far, using PCR, only two, the rodent filaria *Acanthocheilonema viteae*, and the deer filaria *Onchocerca flexuosa*, appear to be free of symbionts.

In filarial species positive for *Wolbachia*, all isolates examined have been found to harbour this bacteria, with bacteria showing identical or nearly identical gene sequences throughout the geographical distribution of the worm [83]. In addition, the phylogeny of *Wolbachia* endosymbionts is congruent with the phylogeny of their host nematodes. The distribution and phylogenetic patterns of *Wolbachia* in filarial nematodes indicate that the association is stable and specific, and suggest a long coevolutionary history [83]. Thus, co-adaptation and reciprocal dependence between filarial nematodes and their *Wolbachia* can be expected.

To cure filarial diseases, it is necessary to destroy the adult worms in a patient. Drugs which destroy immature worms are available, but as yet there are no safe drugs which kill adult worms (macrofilaricides). Novel targets on which studies are being supported include glutathione-S-transferase, lipid modification enzymes, tubulin, and the endosymbiont *Wolbachia* [84 – 85]. Due to a recent study, the effective effect of tetracycline on the embryogenesis of the canine filaria Dirofilaria immitis was reported [86]. Also, similar effect of tetracycline on three different species of filarial nematodes, *Brugia malayi*, *Brugia pahangi*, and *Dirofilaria immitis* was also mentioned in another study. Due to this study, tetracycline was capable of inhibiting L3 to L4 molting within a dosage range similar to that reported for susceptible rickettsial organisms. However, Wolbachia DNA could still be detected in nematodes from tetracycline-treated cultures [87]. In conclusion, a number of studies suggest that killing the symbiotic bacteria that live inside the worm with antibiotics could be an effective therapy especially if combined with existing drugs (e.g. Ivermectin) [88]. Finally, Wiwanitkit proposed that the worms are weakened by killing the bacteria, and the adult worms produce fewer larvae [88].

DIROFILARIASIS

The infection caused by filarial parasites is an important problem for the tropical countries including to Thailand. Apart from human filarial parasites, there are also other filarial parasites such as *Dirofilaria* species. Human dirofilariasis is another group of filarial parasite infestation that can be occasionally found [89]. Cases of dirofilariasis infection occur widely throughout European, African, Middle Eastern, and Asian countries [89].

1. Dirofilaria Repens Infection

1.1. Introduction to Dirofilaria Repens

Here, *Dirofilaria repens*, a not uncommon human dirofilariasis [90], infestation is reviewed. It is usually misunderstood as a tumor; diagnosis is usually made by accidental finding in the histology section of the nodule. Because this parasite is not uncommon in human beings, therefore, the physicians should know the important pathophysiology of this dirofilariasis. *Dirofilaria repens*, or the other name *Nochtiella repens*, is classified into the Phylum Netamoda of Animal Kingdom. It is one of the filarial worms, which is the parasite relatively common in animals. Dogs, foxes and cats are the definitive hosts and principal reservoirs of the parasite. In these animals, this worm acts as the lymphohematopoietic parasites. This canids and felids' parasite, usually nonpathogenic to humans, but can be transmitted to man by mosquito (many species of Culicidae) bites [91]. There is a report of presence of *Dirofilaria repens* and an insect immunocyte (plasmatocyte) in a human subcutaneous nodule, induced by a mosquito bite [92 - 93]. Therefore, this nematode is confirmed for mode of transmission to humans by the vector mosquito bite. More than one worm can be demonstrated from a single inoculum

In humans the parasite dies before reaching sexual maturity and the result is an inconspicuous granulomatous reaction in the subcutaneous tissue [94]. Therefore, the human organism is an accidental host while the dog is the reservoir [95].

The diagnosis of this parasite in human is usually histological - derived by identification of the parasite. The excision biopsy shows the presence of a dead or alive, usually, female worm that measures 220-660 microns across; the central intestine and the genital organs (two uteri) are located in the pseudocoelom; the thick, multilayered cuticle is provided with 95-105 sharp, longitudinal ridges, the latter being separated from each other by a distance of 12 microns; the circumferential muscle cell layer, covering the inner side of the cuticle, is bilaterally interrupted by the large chord cells, two to five nuclei of which are discernible in each cross section [90].

The diagnostic difficulties that can be detected arise when regressive phenomena render the parasite's morphologic characteristics largely or completely unrecognizable. These phenomena are due to the death of the filaria inside the inflammatory nodule weeks or months prior to surgical removal, and to the consequent invasion of inflammatory cells. They start at the nematode's natural orifices (mouth, vulva, anus, and cloaca) and gradually spread throughout its body. In cases of difficult diagnosis, therefore, it is recommended that the nodule be sectioned at different points comprising caudal, cephalic and middle body aspects, so as to reveal the few morphologic features that are still recognizable and which may afford a correct diagnosis [96].

Another difficulties can be found is the differential diagnosis of *Dirofilaria repens* and *Dirofilaria immitis* due to the lack of a diagnostic method which would make possible the routine identification of these parasites as developing larvae either in the vector or in unsuitable hosts, including man. This is very important point, especially for the area where the two nematodes are symmetric. Therefore the PCR-based and immunohistochemistry method are also developed for the case of ambiguous identification of mature and immature adult worms [97 – 98].

Serological diagnosis of this parasite in human is not mentioned as definitive diagnosis tool. Cross-reaction of serological response among the filarial worms is observed. Sometimes mixed infection of this dirofilaria and other types can be detected [99]. In the present day, there are a number of reported cases of this human dirofilariasis. As of today, over 410 cases of *Dirofilaria repens* infections in man are recorded in world literature [100]. Cases of this zoonotic dirofilariasis infection, caused by *Dirofilaria repens*, occur widely throughout European, African, Middle Eastern, and Asian countries [101]. In Thailand, although this parasite can be found in dogs and cats but there is no specific report of human dirofilariasis. Infection of dogs with all of filarial worm ranges from 12% to 37%. The high incidence of dirofilariasis in dogs is of great interest compared to the low incidence in humans. The prevalence of endemic subcutaneous dirofilariosis is probably underestimated as the clinical expression is non-specific and spontaneous cure is common. The occurrence of common host animals and insect vectors makes dirofilarias is a potential danger for public health [102].

1.2. Clinical Manifestation of Human Dirofilaria Repens Infestation

As already mentioned, the manifestation of this human dirofilariasis is not mainly involvement of hematolymphopoietic tissue. Blood hypereosinophilia was exceptionally observed. To best of our knowledge, microfilariae have been found in the blood of only one patient [103]. More than 100 cases of this human dirofilariasis are reported. From literature review, the clinical manifestation of this human dirofilariasis can be categorized as:

Subcutaneous Nodule

Subcutaneous containing a helminth is the main clinical manifestation of this human dirofilariasis. Except in rare cases, the parasite was located subcutaneously, and nested in a nodule [104]. The common chief complaint of the patients is having a painful subcutaneous swelling [105]. The subcutaneous locations described are: skull, cheek, breast [106], inguinal area [107], buttocks, arms and legs [99]. Diagnosis is usually derived after histological examination of the nodule or by accidental extraction and morphological study of the worm. In the majority of the cases the diagnosis has been misinterpreted, the lesions being first seen as malignant or benign tumours or foreign-body granuloma [107 – 108]. The diagnosis of epidermoid cyst is frequently suggested. History taking does not always reveal traveling or animal contact history. The helminth is discovered when the nodule is opened, also providing successful cure.

Eye Manifestation

Ocular manifestation of this human dirofilariasis is another common manifestation of this disease [109]. The patient usually presented with suddenly appeared conjunctival swelling [105]. Inflammatory reaction (episcleritis, chemosis, orbital cellulitis) associated with the passage of the nematode under the Tenon's capsule can be found. Intraorbital cavity [100] and inside vitreous body lesion [110] are also mentioned.

In clinical practice, the infections have mostly been misdiagnosed as a neoplasia, usually benign but sometimes malignant. Under the assumption of an intraorbital lesion, the endoscopic transnasal revision of the orbital cavity was suggested, as this approach promised to be least traumatic and best suited for the lesion, resulting in complete removal of the worm. In unclear lesions in the head and neck, and infection with *Dirofilaria repens* should be considered as a differential diagnosis [100]. In ocular manifestation, the simple extraction of the worm cures the patient.

Uncommon Manifestation

In general, this parasite is able to migrate from the inoculation site to other districts (such as lung and eye) [94]. But sometimes such a localization in a human can be observed [111]. The findings of a worm during a pancreatectomy and in a perirectal nodule have also been reported [111]. Furthermore, cases of testicular location with painful symptoms have been observed [111]. Histological examination of the nodule and morphological study of the worm diagnosed these cases [89].

2. Dirofilaria Immitis Infection

Dirofilaria immitis infection is widely known as heartworm infection. Canine heartworm disease is a mosquito vectored illness resulting from parasitization by the filariid worm *Dirofilaria immitis* [112]. While presenting some danger to humans, the filariid has its greatest impact on the canine population [112]. Haddock said that while its distribution was known in general terms, much research remained to be done to assess the pattern of distribution as well as the impact of *Dirofilaria immitis* on canine populations and their human owners for many locales [112]. Humans are considered as an accidental host for *Dirofilaria immitis*.

Although benign, this zoonosis, of which *Dirofilaria immitis* is the major etiological agent, represents a medical problem since it produces symptoms which may be confused with neoplasia and thus may subject patients to unnecessary thoracic surgery [113]. Muro *et al* said that infection with immature worms has been found in humans, who develop nodules, mainly in subcutaneous tissue or in lung parenchyma arising from branches of the pulmonary artery [114]. In humans, the parasites do not usually reach the adult stage and microfilaremia is absent, as has been shown by diagnosis using invasive methods for removing the nodules [114]. Rodrigues-Silva *et al* said that this parasitic infection remains underdiagnosed [113]. They also said that the importance of a differential diagnosis between dirofilariasis and pulmonary neoplasia was emphasized in cases where there is a solitary subpleural nodule ("coin lesion") present [113]. They proposed that the development and improvement of modern immunological diagnostic techniques were essential to distinguish this benign disease from other pathological conditions and thus avoid unnecessary surgery [113].

REFERENCES

[1] Filariasis. Available at http://www.chclibrary.org/micromed/00048410.html

[2] Dirofilariasis Information. Available at http://www.diseasesdatabase.com/ddb31226.htm

[3] Dhanda V, Das PK, Lal R, Srinivasan R, Ramaiah KD. Spread of lymphatic filariasis, re-emergence of leishmaniasis and threat of babesiosis in India. *Indian J. Med Res.* 1996; 103: 46-54.

[4] Raccurt CP. Dirofilariasis, an emerging and underestimated zoonoses in France. *Med. Trop. (Mars).* 1999; 59: 389-400.

[5] Ault SK. Environmental management: a re-emerging vector control strategy. *Am. J. Trop. Med. Hyg.* 1994; 50(6 Suppl): 35-49.

[6] Hoerauf A. Control of filarial infections: not the beginning of the end, but more research is needed. *Curr. Opin. Infect. Dis.* 2003; 16: 403-10.

[7] Brown KR, Phillips SM. Tropical diseases of importance to the traveler. *Adv. Intern. Med.* 1984;29: 59-84.

[8] Hochberg N, Ryan ET. Medical problems in the returning expatriate. *Clin. Occup. Environ. Med.* 2004; 4: 205-19.

[9] Muro A, Genchi C, Cordero M, Simon F. Human dirofilariasis in the European Union. *Parasitol. Today.* 1999; 15: 386-9.

[10] Schlotthauer JC, Harrison EG Jr, Thompson JH Jr. Dirofilariasis-- an emerging zoonosis? *Arch. Environ. Health.* 1969; 19:897-900.

[11] Ottesen EA, Ramachandran CP. Lymphatic filariasis infection and disease: control strategies. *Parasitology Today.* 1995; 11: 129 –31.

[12] Hassan AN. Bancroftian filariasis: spatial patterns, environmental correlates and landscape predictors of disease risk. *J. Egypt Soc. Parasitol.* 2004; 34: 501-13.

[13] Melrose WD. Lymphatic filariasis: new insights into an old disease. *Int. J. Parasitol.* 2002; 32: 947-60.

[14] de Almeida AB, Freedman DO. Epidemiology and immunopathology of bancroftian filariasis. *Microbes Infect.* 1999; 1: 1015-22.

[15] Kron M, Walker E, Hernandez L, Torres E, Libranda-Ramirez B. Lymphatic filariasis in the Philippines. *Parasitol. Today.* 2000; 16: 329-33.

[16] Kazura JW, Bockarie MJ. Lymphatic filariasis in Papua New Guinea: interdisciplinary research on a national health problem. *Trends Parasitol.* 2003; 19: 260-3.

[17] Rocha EM, Fontes G. Bancroftian filariasis in Brazil. *Rev. Saude Publica.* 1998; 32: 98-105.

[18] Njenga SM, Muita M, Kirigi G, Mbugua J, Mitsui Y, Fujimaki Y, Aoki Y. Bancroftian filariasis in Kwale district, Kenya. *East Afr. Med. J.* 2000; 77: 245-9.

[19] Gyapong JO, Kyelem D, Kleinschmidt I, Agbo K, Ahouandogbo F, Gaba J, Owusu-Banahene G, Sanou S, Sodahlon YK, Biswas G, Kale OO, Molyneux DH, Roungou JB, Thomson MC, Remme J. The use of spatial analysis in mapping the distribution of bancroftian filariasis in four West African countries. *Ann. Trop. Med. Parasitol.* 2002; 96: 695-705.

[20] The Filarial Genome Network. Available at http://www.math.smith.edu/~sawlab/fgn/pnb/wuchban.html

[21] Triteeraprapab S, Kanjanopas K, Suwannadabba S, Sangprakarn S, Poovorawan Y, Scott AL. Transmission of the nocturnal periodic strain of Wuchereria bancrofti by Culex quinquefasciatus: establishing the potential for urban filariasis in Thailand. *Epidemiol. Infect.* 2000; 125: 207-12.

[22] Calheiros CM, Fontes G, Williams P, Rocha EM. Experimental infection of Culex (Culex) quinquefasciatus and Aedes (Stegomyia) aegypti with Wuchereria bancrofti. *Mem. Inst. Oswaldo Cruz.* 1998; 93: 855-60.

[23] Rao KR, Venkatanaryana M, Naidu YD, Narasimham MV, Viswanatham R, Rao CK. Transplacental transmission in bancroftian filariasis. *Indian J. Med. Res.* 1984; 79: 495-6.

[24] Pires ML, Ferreira RS, Araujo S, Albuquerque R, Remigio Neto J, Da Silva AS, Dreyer G. Transplacental passage of Wuchereria bancrofti microfilariae in newborns of microfilaremic mothers. *Rev. Inst. Med. Trop. Sao Paulo.* 1991; 33: 91- 5 25.

[25] Malhotra I, Ouma JH, Wamachi A, Kioko J, Mungai P, Njzovu M, Kazura JW, King CL. Influence of maternal filariasis on childhood infection and immunity to Wuchereria bancrofti in Kenya. *Infect. Immun.* 2003; 71: 5231-7.

[26] Hira PR, Husein SF. Some transfusion-induced parasitic infections in Zambia. *J. Hyg. Epidemiol. Microbiol. Immunol.* 1979; 23: 436-44.

[27] Hise AG, Hazlett FE, Bockarie MJ, Zimmerman PA, Tisch DJ, Kazura JW. Polymorphisms of innate immunity genes and susceptibility to lymphatic filariasis. *Genes Immun.* 2003; 4: 524-7.

[28] Thanomsub BW, Chansiri K, Sarataphan N, Phantana S. Differential diagnosis of human lymphatic filariasis using PCR-RFLP. *Mol. Cell Probes.* 2000; 14: 41-6.

[29] Freedman DO, de Almeido Filho PJ, Besh S, Maia e Silva MC, Braga C, Maciel A, Furtado AF. Abnormal lymphatic function in presymptomatic bancroftian filariasis. *J. Infect. Dis.* 1995; 171: 997-1001.

[30] Simonsen PE, Meyrowitsch DW. Bancroftian filariasis in Tanzania: specific antibody responses in relation to long-term observations on microfilaremia. *Am. J. Trop. Med. Hyg.* 1998; 59: 667-72.
[31] Brabin L. Sex differentials in susceptibility to lymphatic filariasis and implications for maternal child immunity. *Epidemiol. Infect.* 1990; 105: 335-53.
[32] King CL, Connelly M, Alpers MP, Bockarie M, Kazura JW. Transmission intensity determines lymphocyte responsiveness and cytokine bias in human lymphatic filariasis. *J. Immunol.* 2001; 166: 7427-36.
[33] Aben-Athar J. Mechanism producing elephantiasis in filariasis (F. wucheria and F. bancrofti). *Rev. Bras. Med.* 1951; 8: 89-94.
[34] Simonsen PE, Meyrowitsch DW, Makunde WH, Magnussen P. Bancroftian filariasis: the pattern of microfilaraemia and clinical manifestations in three endemic communities of Northeastern Tanzania. *Acta Trop.* 1995; 60: 179-87.
[35] Meyrowitsch DW, Simonsen PE, Makunde WH. Bancroftian filariasis: analysis of infection and disease in five endemic communities of north-eastern Tanzania. *Ann. Trop. Med. Parasitol.* 1995; 89: 653-63.
[36] Noroes J, Addiss D, Cedenho A, Figueredo-Silva J, Lima G, Dreyer G. Pathogenesis of filarial hydrocele: risk associated with intrascrotal nodules caused by death of adult Wuchereria bancrofti. *Trans. R. Soc. Trop. Med. Hyg.* 2003; 97: 561-6.
[37] 37. Triteeraprapab S. Update in lymphatic filariasis: A re-emerging disease of Thailand. *Chula. Med. J.* 1996; 41: 611 – 22.
[38] Wiwanitkit V. Prevaelnce of filariasis in Myanmar migrant workers in Bangsaparn district, Prachuab Kiri Khan province Thailand. Presented at the Joint international Tropical Medicine Meeting 2001. Bangkok: Thailand, 2001
[39] Shutidamrong C, Phantana S. The periodicity of microfilaria in Thailand. *Commun. Dis. J.* 1986; 12: 227 – 39.
[40] Wongcharoenyong S, Thammapalo S, Veerawathanaporn P. Filarial control in Myanmar worker by single dose diethylcarbamzine citrate (DEC). *W. Epidemiol. Surveil. Rep.* 1997; 28: 89-92.
[41] Southgate BA. Recent advances in the epidemiology and control aspects of transmission. *Tran. R. Soc. Trop. Med. Hyg.* 1984; 18(Suppl): 19 – 25.
[42] Weil GJ, Lammie PJ, Weiss N. The ICT Filariasis Test: A rapid-format antigen test for diagnosis of bancroftian filariasis. *Parasitol. Today.* 1997; 13: 401- 4.
[43] Nicolas L. New tools for diagnosis and monitoring of bancroftian filariasis parasitism: The polynesian experience. *Parasitol. Today.* 1997; 13: 370-5.
[44] Dreyer G, Dreyer P, Noroes J. Recommendations for the treatment of bancroftian filariasis in symptomless and diseased patients. *Rev. Soc. Bras. Med. Trop.* 2002; 35: 43-50.
[45] Dreyer G, Noroes J. Diethylcarbamazine in the treatment of Bancroft's filariasis. *Rev. Soc. Bras. Med. Trop.* 1997; 30: 229-40.
[46] Sudomo M, Hanifah A, Mak JW, Lim BL. A study of malayan filariasis in Lubuk Mumpo and Datar Lebar villages in Lais Regency, North Bengkulu, Sumatera, Indonesia. Southeast. *Asian J. Trop. Med. Public Health.* 1982; 13: 584-89.
[47] Triteeraprapab S, Karnjanopas K, Porksakorn C, Sai-Ngam A, Yentakam S, Loymak S. Lymphatic filariasis caused by Brugia malayi in an endemic area of Narathiwat Province, southern of Thailand. *J. Med. Assoc. Thai.* 2001; 84 Suppl 1, S182-8.

[48] Duan J, Li Q, Li Z, Tang L, Zou Y. SurveilLance on filariasis after its basic elimination in Hunan Province. *Zhongguo Ji Sheng Chong Xue Yu Ji Sheng Chong Bing Za Zhi.* 1998; 16: 291-5.

[49] Suzuki T, Sudomo M, Bang YH, Lim BL. Studies on Malayan filariasis in Bengkulu (Sumatera), Indonesia with special reference to vector confirmation. *Southeast Asian J. Trop. Med. Public Health.* 1981; 12: 47-54.

[50] Sanjeevi CB, Narayanan PR. Antifilarial and anti PPD IgM antibodies in cord blood. *Indian J. Pediatr.* 1989; 56: 207-11.

[51] Severson DW, Mori A, Zhang Y, Christensen BM. Chromosomal mapping of two loci affecting filarial worm susceptibility in Aedes aegypti. *Insect. Mol. Biol.* 1994; 3: 67-72.

[52] Gomez-Escobar N, Gregory WF, Britton C, Murray L, Corton C, Hall N, Daub J, Blaxter ML, Maizels RM. Abundant larval transcript-1 and -2 genes from Brugia malayi: diversity of genomic environments but conservation of 5' promoter sequences functional in Caenorhabditis elegans. *Mol. Biochem. Parasitol.* 2002; 125: 59-71.

[53] Sakamoto M, Meier JL, Folse DS, Ewert A. Perturbation of lymphatic endothelial cells in experimental Brugia malayi infections. *Microcirc. Endothelium. Lymphatics.* 1985; 2: 487-98:

[54] Sartono E, Kruize YC, Kurniawan A, Maizels RM, Yazdanbakhsh M. Depression of antigen-specific interleukin-5 and interferon-gamma responses in human lymphatic filariasis as a function of clinical status and age. *J. Infect. Dis.* 1997; 175: 1276-80.

[55] Soh CT, Lee KT, Im SW, Lee JH. Clinical manifestation of Brugia malayi infection in Korea. Kisaengchunghak. *Chapchi.* 1996; 4: 1-6.

[56] Lobos E, Zahn R, Weiss N, Nutman TB. A major allergen of lymphatic filarial nematodes is a parasite homolog of the gamma-glutamyl transpeptidase. *Mol. Med.* 1996; 2: 712-24.

[57] McReynolds LA, Poole C, Hong Y, Williams SA, Partono F, Bradley J. Recent advances in the application of molecular biology in filariasis. *Southeast Asian J. Trop. Med. Public Health.* 1993; 24 Suppl 2: 55-63.

[58] Lakshmi V, Saxena A, Pandey K, Bajpai P, Misra-Bhattacharya S. Antifilarial activity of Zoanthus species (Phylum Coelenterata, Class Anthzoa) against human lymphatic filaria, Brugia malayi. *Parasitol. Res.* 2004; 93: 268-73.

[59] Partono F. Diagnosis and treatment of lymphatic filariasis. *Parasitol. Today.* 1985; 1: 52-7.

[60] Gnanasekar M, Rao KV, He YX, Mishra PK, Nutman TB, Kaliraj P, Ramaswamy K. Novel phage display-based subtractive screening to identify vaccine candidates of Brugia malayi. *Infect. Immun.* 2004; 72: 4707-15.

[61] Mak JW. Filariasis in Southeast Asia. *Ann. Acad. Med. Singapore.* 1981; 10: 112-9.

[62] Fischer P, Supali T, Maizels RM. Lymphatic filariasis and Brugia timori: prospects for elimination. *Trends Parasitol.* 2004; 20: 351-5.

[63] Supali T, Rahmah N, Djuardi Y, Sartono E, Ruckert P, Fischer P. Detection of filaria-specific IgG4 antibodies using Brugia Rapid test in individuals from an area highly endemic for Brugia timori. *Acta Trop.* 2004; 90: 255-61.

[64] Fischer P, Wibowo H, Pischke S, Ruckert P, Liebau E, Ismid IS, Supali T. PCR-based detection and identification of the filarial parasite Brugia timori from Alor Island, Indonesia. *Ann. Trop. Med. Parasitol.* 2002; 96: 809-21.

[65] Grenfell BT, Michael E, Denham DA. A model for the dynamics of human lymphatic filariasis. *Parasitol. Today.* 1991; 7: 318-23.

[66] Hitch WL, Lammie PJ, Eberhard ML. Heightened anti-filarial immune responsiveness in a Haitian pediatric population. *Am. J. Trop. Med. Hyg.* 1989; 41: 657-63.

[67] Toure FS, Deloron P, Egwang TG, Wahl G. Relationship between the intensity of Loa loa filariasis transmission and prevalence of infections. *Med. Trop. (Mars).* 1999; 59: 249-52.

[68] Wanji S, Tendongfor N, Esum M, Atanga SN, Enyong P. Heterogeneity in the prevalence and intensity of loiasis in five contrasting bioecological zones in Cameroon. *Trans. R. Soc. Trop. Med. Hyg.* 2003; 97: 183-7.

[69] Onchocerciasis. Available at http://www.who.int/pbd/blindness/onchocerciasis/en/

[70] Stingl P. Onchocerciasis. *MMW Fortschr. Med.* 2004; 146: 44-5.

[71] Greenaway C. Dracunculiasis (guinea worm disease). *CMAJ.* 170, 495-500 (2004)

[72] Cairncross S, Muller R, Zagaria N. Dracunculiasis (Guinea worm disease) and the eradication initiative. *Clin. Microbiol. Rev.* 2002; 15: 223-46.

[73] Van Meer MMM, Stouthamer R. Cross-order transfer of Wolbachia from Muscidifurax uniraptor (Hymenoptera pp.Pteromalidae) to Drosophila simulans (Diptera pp. Drosophilidae). *Heredity.* 1999; 82: 163-169.

[74] Vavre F, Girin C, Bouletreau M. Phylogenetic status of a fecundity-enhancing Wolbachia that does not induce thelytoky in Trichogramma. *Insect. Mol. Biol.* 1999; 67-72.

[75] HertigM. The rickettsia, Wolbachia pipentis (gen. et sp.n.) and associated inclusions of the mosquito Culex pipens. *Parasitology.* 1936; 28: 453 – 86.

[76] O'Meill SL, Giordano R, Colbert AME, Karr TL, Robertson HM. 16 S rRNA phylogenetic analysis of the bacterial ensymbionts assocaited with cytoplasmic incompatability in insects. *Proc. Natl. Acad. Sci. USA.* 1992; 89: 2699 - 702.

[77] Braig H, Zhou W, Dobson SL, ONeill SL. Cloning and Characterisation of a gene encoding the major surface protein of the bacterial endosymbiont Wolbachia pipientis. *J. Bacteriol.* 1998; 180: 2373-2378.

[78] Werren JH. Biology of Wolbachia. *Ann. Rev. Entomol.* 1997; 42: 587-609.

[79] West SA, Cook JM, Werren JH, Godfray HCJ. Wolbachia in two insect host-parasitoid communities. *Mol. Ecol.* 1998; 7: 1457-1465.

[80] Wilkinson T. Wolbachia come of age. *Trend. Ecol. Evol.* 1998; 13: 213-214.

[81] Cook JM, Butcher RDJ. The transmission and effects of Wolbachia bacteria in parasitoids. *Res. Pop. Ecol.* 1999; 41:15-28.

[82] Taylor MJ, Hoerauf A. Wolbachia bacteria of filarial nematodes. *Parasitol Today.* 1999; 15: 437-442.

[83] Taylor MJ, Bilo K, Cross HF, Archer JP, Underwood AP. 16S rDNA phylogeny and ultrastructural characterization of Wolbachia intracellular bacteria of the filarial nematodes Brugia malayi, B. pahangi and Wuchereria bancrofti. *Exp. Parasitol.* 1999; 91 356-361.

[84] Smith HL, Rajan TV. Tetracycline inhibits development of the infective-stage larvae of filarial nematodes in vitro. *Exp. Parasitol.* 20001; 95: 265-70.

[85] aylor MJ, Bandi C, Hoerauf AM, Lazdins J. Wolbachia bacteria of filarial nematodes: a target for control? *Parasitol. Today.* 2000; 16: 179-80.

[86] Genchi C, Sacchi L, Bandi C, Venco L. Preliminary results on the effect of tetracycline on the embryogenesis and symbiotic bacteria (Wolbachia) of Dirofilaria immitis. An update and discussion. *Parassitologia.* 1998; 40: 247-9.

[87] Smith HL, Rajan TV. Tetracycline inhibits development of the infective-stage larvae of filarial nematodes in vitro. *Exp. Parasitol.* 2000; 95: 265-70.

[88] Wiwanitkit V. Wolbachia infection in filarial nematodes, new trend in the study on macrofilaricides. *Songklanagarind. Med. J.* 2001; 19: 235 – 9.

[89] Wiwanitkit V, Chongboonprasert C. Dirofilaria repens : a minor human filarial parasite. *Chula Med. J.* 2002; 46: 463 – 8.

[90] Jelinek T, Schulte-Hillen J, Loscher T. Human dirofilariasis. *Int. J. Dermatol.* 1996; 35: 872-5.

[91] Pampiglione S, Bortoletti G, Fossarello M, Maccioni A. Human dirofilariasis in Sardinia: 4 new cases. Review of published cases. *Pathologica.* 1996; 88: 472-7.

[92] Pampiglione S, Gupta AP. Presence of Dirofilaria repens and an insect immunocyte (plasmatocyte) in a human subcutaneous nodule, induced by a mosquito bite. *Parassitologia.* 1998; 40: 343-6.

[93] Orihel TC, Helentjaris D, Alger J. Subcutaneous dirofilariasis: single inoculum, multiple worms. *Am. J. Trop. Med. Hyg.* 1997; 56: 452-5.

[94] Fini M, Perrone A, Vagliani G, Andreini C, Salvi G, Misuriello G, Di Silverio A. A case of human dirofilariasis (D. repens) of the spermatic cord. Minerva. *Urol. Nefrol.* 1992; 44: 129-31.

[95] Desruelles F, Marty P, Perrin C, De Saint Florent JD, Lacour JP, Le Fichoux Y, Ortonne JP. Endemic subcutaneous Dirofilaria repens filariasis in Southern France. *Ann. Dermatol. Venereol.* 1989; 125: 423-4.

[96] Pampiglione S, Rivasi F, Canestri-Trotti G. Pitfalls and difficulties in histological diagnosis of human dirofilariasis due to Dirofilaria (Nochtiella) repens. *Diagn. Microbiol. Infect. Dis.* 1999; 34: 57-64.

[97] Favia G, Lanfrancotti A, della Torre A, Cancrini G, Coluzzi M. Advances in the identification of Dirofilaria repens and Dirofilaria immitis by a PCR-based approach. *Parassitologia.* 1997; 39: 401-2.

[98] Cancrini G, Favia G, Giannetto S, Merulla R, Russo R, Ubaldino V, Tringali R, Pietrobelli M, Del Nero L. Nine more cases of human infections by Dirofilaria repens diagnosed in Italy by morphology and recombinant DNA technology. *Parassitologia.* 1999;40:461-6.

[99] Giannetto S, Pampiglione S, Santoro V, Virga A. Research of canine filariasis in Trapani province (western Sicily). Morphology on SEM of male Dirofilaria repens. *Parassitologia.* 1997; 39: 403-5.

[100] .Braun H, Koele W, Stammberger H, Ranner G, Groll R. Endoscopic removal of an intraorbital "tumor": a vital surprise. *Am. J. Rhinol.* 1999; 13, 469- 72.

[101] Ruiz-Moreno JM, Bornay-Llinares FJ, Prieto Maza G, Medrano M, Simon F, Eberhard ML. Subconjunctival infection with Dirofilaria repens: serological confirmation of cure following surgery. *Arch. Ophthalmol.* 1998; 116: 1370-2

[102] Vakalis NC, Himonas CA. Human and canine dirofilariasis in Greece. *Parassitologia.* 1997; 39: 389-91.

[103] Marty P. Human dirofilariasis due to Dirofilaria repens in France. A review of reported cases. *Parassitologia.* 1997; 39: 383-6.

[104] Guillot P, Dachary D, Dallot M, Cadiergues MC, Bain O. Cutaneous dirofilariasis from Dirofilaria repens. A case contracted in Gironde. *Ann. Dermatol. Venereol.* 1998; 125: 105-7.

[105] Gutierrez Y, Misselevich I, Fradis M, Podoshin L, Boss JH. Dirofilaria repens infection in northern Israel. *Am. J. Surg. Pathol.* 1995; 19:1088-91.

[106] Pampiglione S, Di Palma S, Bono A, Bartoli C, Pilotti S. Breast infection due to Dirofilaria repens: report of two new Italian cases and revision of the literature. *Parassitologia.* 1998; 40: 269-73.

[107] Pampiglione S, Elek G, Palfi P, Vetesi F, Varga I. Human Dirofilaria repens infection in Hungary: a case in the spermatic cord and a review of the literature. *Acta Vet. Hung.* 1999; 47: 77-83.

[108] Pampiglione S, Canestri Trotti G, Rivasi F. Human dirofilariasis in Italy. *Ann. Parasitol. Hum .Comp.* 1991; 66: 195-203.

[109] Rouhette H, Marty P, Zur C, Bain O, Fenollar S, Gastaud P. Ocular filariasis: not strictly tropical. Ophthalmologica. 1999; 213: 206-8.

[110] Vasilkova D, Klisenbauer D, Juhas T, Moravec F, Uhlikova M, Hubner J, Konakova G .Isolation of Dirofilaria repens in vitreoretinal findings. *Cesk. Oftalmol.* 1992; 48: 274-7.

[111] Pampiglione S, Arlotta MR, Carla TG, D'Ambrosio E, Filotico R, Primiceri O, Vetrugno M. Human dirofilariasis in southern Italy. *I. The Puglia Region.* Pathologica. 1994; 86: 528-32.

[112] Haddock KC. Canine heartworm disease: a review and pilot study. *Soc. Sci. Med.* 1987; 24: 225-46.

[113] Rodrigues-Silva R, Moura H, Dreyer G, Rey L. Human pulmonary dirofilariasis: a review. *Rev. Inst. Med. Trop. Sao Paulo.* 1995; 37: 523-30.

[114] Muro A, Genchi C, Cordero M, Simon F. Human dirofilariasis in the European Union. *Parasitol. Today.* 1999; 15: 386-9.

Chapter XIV

Borreliosis

Introduction to Borreliosis

Borreliosis is a group of diseases caused by *Borrelia* spp. The most well known infection is Lyme disease. Lyme borreliosis is a zoonotic disease transmitted by ticks and caused by the spirochete *Borrelia burgdorferi* [1]. There are cases of the infection reported at least since the beginning of last century, although a complete description of the disease is available only since 1982 [1]. Clinical presentation consists generally of a characteristic skin rash, known as erythema migrans, and a variety of systemic manifestations, which evolve in stages, along months to years [1].

Another important infection is relapsing fever caused by *Borrelia recurrentis*. This disease is characterized by a febrile stage lasting for 3 to 10 days, ending by crisis and recurring at intervals about a week [2 -3]. Relapsing fever Borrelia infections have attracted little attention in recent years; however, where endemic, these infections still result in considerable illness and death [2 - 3].

Pathogenic Organism

Borrelia is a spirochete. *Borrelia burgdorferi* is a spirochete which is the causative agent of Lyme disease, the most common tick-borne disease in the USA. *B. burgdorferi* is the cause of a mysterious outbreak of arthritis near the community of Lyme in the late 1970s [4 - 6]. The effort was a long one, as the microbe that causes Lyme disease turned out to be difficult to culture [6]. It was finally isolated by Willy Burgdorfer and colleagues from an infected deer tick, and since then has been cultured hundreds of times from both ticks and ill patients. The strain was named *B. burgdorferi* in honor of Dr. Burgdorfer [6]. The reservoirs for the spirochete are the white-footed mouse and the white-tailed deer. Transmission is accomplished by the bite of infected deer ticks [4 – 5]. Contact with the tick usually occurs in areas of brush and tall grass [4 – 5]. Borrelia may have a length of 20-30um but a width of only .2-.3um. When *B. burgdorferi* is Gram-stained, the cells stain a weak Gram-negative by default, as safranin is the last dye used [4]. Borrelia, like most spirochetes, does have an outer membrane that contains an LPS-like substance, an inner membrane, and a periplasmic space which contains a layer of peptidoglycan [4]. Their cell wall is gram negative in construction containing an outer membrane with LPS, but they stain only weakly in the Gram stain [6]. Therefore, it has a Gram-negative bacterial type cell wall, despite its staining characteristics. Unlike *Treponema pallidum*, *B. burgdorferi* can be cultivated in vitro. However, the bacterium is fastidious and requires a very complex growth medium [4]. The medium used to grow *B. burgdorferi* is called Barbour-Stoenner-Kelly (BSK) medium [4]. It contains over thirteen ingredients in a rabbit serum base. *B.burgdorferi* has an optimal temperature for growth of 32 C, in a microaerobic environment. Even under optimal conditions, the generation time is slow, about 12-24 hours [4]. This spirochete have 7-11 endoflagella that form a structure that is called an axial filament similar to that seen for *T. pallidum* [6]. *B. burgdorferi* cells are long and thin: 10-30 m in length and 0.2-0.5m in width. Similar to *T. pallidum,* they are nearly invisible in the light microscope and are viewed using a dark field microscope or by fluorescent antibody stain [6]. Interestingly, molecular analysis has shown isolates to be phenotypically and genotypically divergent [6]. The microbe contains a linear chromosome of ~900 kB and 21 plasmids, of which 9 are also linear [6]. In additional to an unusual genome comprised of a linear chromosome, it has the largest plasmid complement of any characterized bacterium [7]. Certain plasmid-encoded elements are required for virulence and viability, both in vitro and in vivo [7]. Cell division in this organism must involve an interesting mechanism to keep track of that many separate DNA molecules and replicate the linear ones [6]. The mechanism for the unusual genome plasticity in the linear replicons has remained elusive. The enzymatic machinery (the telomere resolvase ResT) responsible for generating the hairpin ends from replicative intermediates has recently been shown to also perform a reverse reaction that fuses telomeres on unrelated replicons [8]. Infrequent stabilization of such fusion events over evolutionary time provides the first proposed biochemical mechanism for the DNA rearrangements that are so prominent in the linear replicons of *B. burgdorferi* [8]. Certain features of *B. burgdorferi* have hampered the development of an effective system of genetic analysis, but basic tools are now available and their application has begun to provide information about the identities and roles of key bacterial components in both the tick vector and the mammalian host [9]. Increased genetic analysis of *B. burgdorferi* should advance our understanding of the infectious cycle and the pathogenesis of Lyme disease [9].

Considering *B. recurrentis*, it has a similar microbiological property to *B. burgdorferi.* Its outer sheath encloses axial fibrils wrapped around protoplasmic cylinder[10]. Axial fibrils originate at both poles and may overlap at center of cell [10]. It is usually associated with poverty, crowding, and warfare [10]. There are many strains of *B. recurrentis*. There are at least 18 strains, A1 to A18 of this spirochete. Isolates can be cultured in BSK II medium. Relapsingfever strains should be maintained by thrice weekly subculturing, the dissimilarity between *B. recurrentis* and American tickborne relapsing-fever strains, Lyme-associated strains, and other borreliae was highlighted by the whole DNA-DNA hybridization studies.

Comparison of the DNA sequence of *B. recurrentis* with the sequence of a strain of an African tick-borne relapsing-fever borrelia (*B. duttonii*) revealed that these organisms are closely related, but differ in 4 bp in the 16S rRNA gene (26) and in 1 bp in the flagellin gene [11]. e differences in the 16S RNA gene and the flagellin gene sequences of *B. recurrentis* and *B. duttonii* suggest that there is selective pressure to maintain the flagellin gene without mutation [11]. Phylogenetic trees based on either the 16S RNA gene sequence or the flagellin gene sequence gave similar cluster patterns, confirming the relationship of *B. recurrentis*, *B.*

duttonii, and *B. crocidurae*, which are more distantly related to relapsing-fever strains of Spanish origin [11]. According to the study of Ras et al, *B. crocidurae, B. duttonii, B. recurrentis*, and *B. hispanica*. Another cluster comprised tow main branches with *B. coriaceae, B. lonestari*, and *B. miyamotoi* on one side and *B. parkeri, B. turicatae*, and *B. hermsii* on the other side [12].

LYME DISEASE

Lyme disease is due to infection with *B. burgdorferi* and the body's immune response to the infection. In Europe, the rash (then called erythema chronicum migrans or ECM) was first described at the beginning of the 20th century [13]. The neurologic manifestations and the association with *Ixodes* ticks were recognized by the mid 1930s and were known as tick-borne meningoencephalitis [13]. In the United States, Lyme disease was not recognized until the early 1970s, when an outbreak of childhood arthritis occurred in the Lyme [13].

A. Pathogenesis

B burgdorferi is transmitted from host to host by the Ixodes, or deer tick. The life cycle of the Ixodes tick and B burgdorferi is important, as it relates to the epidemiology of this infection. The Ixodes tick is born as a larval tick in the summer and feeds only once [14]. Sawari et al proposed that the risk for Lyme disease in campers and staff was much higher than that of the general population despite the use of tick-exposure precautions [14]. Focused interventions need to be put in place in summer camps to prevent transmission of Lyme disease [14]. Ticks exposed to a temperature cycle exhibited a unimodal pattern of activity, similar to that exhibited by ticks exposed to both light and temperature cycles at the same time of year, whereas those exposed to a light cycle exhibited a bimodal pattern of activity [15]. Although the difference did not quite reach statistical significance, there is a possibility that temperature is a stronger entraining agent for tick diurnal activity than is light, an unusual situation [15]. Its preferred host is the common field mouse, but other animals apparently suffice [13]. Mice do not appear to develop Lyme disease, but they do carry the bacteria [13]. The following spring, it becomes a nymph and again feeds only once, with its preferred host again being the field mouse [13]. Even if a tick feeds on an infected animal, it may not pick up the infection [13]. In the fall, the nymph becomes an adult and feeds a single time. Its preferred host is the white-tailed deer [13]. The change in diurnal activity pattern from fall to spring suggests that ticks are adjusting their strategy for host finding, possibly in relation to remaining stored food supplies or host activity, and may have practical implications for sampling carried out to track tick populations [15]. Thus, unless the tick feeds on an infected host before feeding on a person, an individual cannot be infected from that tick bite [13]. Dissemination of B. burgdorferi from the site of a tick bite likely occurs, in part, via attachment to host plasmin and subsequent degradation of glycoproteins. Previous immunological studies indicated that the Lyme disease spirochete, B. burgdorferi, expresses Erp outer surface proteins during mammalian infection [16]. As naive tick larvae acquired B. burgdorferi by feeding on infected mice, essentially all transmitted bacteria produced Erp proteins, also suggestive of continual Erp expression during mammalian infection [16]. Shortly after the larvae acquired bacteria, Erp production was drastically downregulated [16]. The expression of Erp proteins on B. burgdorferi throughout mammalian infection is consistent with their hypothesized function as factor H-binding proteins that protect the bacteria from host innate immune responses [16]. Although the strong proinflammatory B. burgdorferi lipoproteins have been implicated in the induction of inflammation, they do not seem to act exclusively through Toll-like receptor (TLR) engagement. In fact, mice that are deficient for MyD88, a component of the TLR signaling pathway, manifest similar or increased recruitment of cells into B. burgdorferi -infected tissues [17]. By contrast, the absence of the chemokine receptor CXCR2 results in reduced inflammation [17]. Overall, these findings highlight the complexity of Lyme disease pathogenesis and identify chemokine pathways as novel therapeutic targets for the control of B. burgdorferi -induced inflammation [17].

The pathogenesis of the disease in its early stages is associated largely with the presence of viable bacteria at the site of inflammation. The capacity of a pathogen to use a secreted arthropod protein to help it colonize the mammalian host is shown [18]. According to an animal model study [18], the binding of Salp15 protected B. burgdorferi from antibody-mediated killing in vitro and provided spirochetes with a marked advantage when they were inoculated into naive mice or animals previously infected with *B. burgdorferi* [18]. Moreover, RNA interference-mediated repression of salp15 in I. scapularis drastically reduced the capacity of tick-borne spirochaetes to infect mice [18]. Whereas in the later stages of disease, autoimmune features seem to contribute significantly [19].In addition, it has been suggested that chronic persistence of B. burgdorferi in affected tissues is of pathogenic relevance [19]. Much speculation has surrounded the possibility that autoimmune mechanisms are involved in chronic symptoms [20]. It is clear that T cells and macrophages are intimately associated with the pathogenesis of arthritis and that immune mechanisms are involved in other aspects of disease. Inflammation directed at persistence of Borrelial antigens is a plausible explanation for persisting arthritis [21]. Humoral immunity plays a protective role, prompting interest in vaccine development [1]. Significant variation in certain of the outer surface proteins suggests that multiple proteins, peptides, or chimeric vaccines may be needed to provide a sufficiently broad humoral protective response [21]. Long-term exposure of the host immune system to spirochaetes and/or borrelial compounds may induce chronic autoimmune disease [19]. However, in most cases, involvement of autoimmunity in Lyme disease has not received experimental support [20]. The exception is in a small group of patients with chronic arthritis whose abnormal joint symptoms persist after apparent elimination of the bacteria [20]. Autoimmunity based on molecular mimicry may play a role in the pathogenesis of Lyme disease [21].There is an interesting animal model study by Cadavid et al [22]. In this work, the predominant cells in the inflammatory infiltrate were T cells and plasma cells and the deposition of antibody and complement in inflamed muscles [22]. The spirochetal load was very high while the animals were immunosuppressed but decreased to minimal levels when immunocompetence was restored [22].

B. Clinical Manifestation

Lyme borreliosis in humans is an inflammatory disease affecting multiple organ systems, including the nervous system, cardiovascular system, joints and muscles. Infection and immunity are believed to be the two main factors indicating the severity of this disease. Clinical manifestations of this disease can be divided into 3 stages: localized, disseminated, and persistent [13]. The first 2 stages are part of the early infection, while persistent disease is considered late infection while stage 3 of disease usually occurs within 1 year of infection [13]. Important clinical manifestations of Lyme disease include the followings:

Cutaneous Manifestation

About 80% of all Lyme borreliosis cases represent skin manifestations (dermatoborrelioses) [23]. The three characteristic dermatoborrelioses are erythema migrans, borrelial lymphocytoma, and acrodermatitis chronica atrophicans, which occur in different stages of the disease [23]. Erythema migrans is the hallmark of early Lyme borreliosis, whereas acrodermatitis chronica atrophicans is the characteristic manifestation of late Lyme borreliosis [23]. Erythema migrans is an erythematous lesion that increases in size over several days [13]. Multiple lesions can be observed in half of the patients and are usually not the result of multiple tick bites. It may be asymptomatic or it may itch or burn. It often occurs at or near the site of the tick bite, which may be an area not normally visualized by individuals, such as the axilla, groin, or popliteal areas [13]. The rash may not be observed until it is already full size [13]. Antibiotic treatment is necessary for all stages and manifestations of Lyme borreliosis [23]. Doxycycline is the antibiotic of choice for most patients with dermatoborrelioses [23]. Untreated, the rash will persist for 2-3 weeks. Approximately 30 % of all patients with erythema migrans develop no further manifestations of Lyme disease, while the other patients develop further symptoms [13]. These may be associated with lymphadenopathy and symptoms such as fever and myalgias, which may be described by the patient as flu-like in nature [13]. It should be notd that hematogenous dissemination of Borrelia causes flu like symptoms up to meningitis and multiple erythemata migrantia on the skin [24].

Lyme Arthritis

Lyme arthritis is one of the most common clinical manifestations of Lyme borreliosis. It is caused by an intraarticular infection with *B. burgdorferi*. The arthritis usually presented as a migratory polyarticular process involving bursae, tendons, and joints, which evolves over 1-2 days into a monoarticular process involving the knee, ankle, and wrist in decreasing frequency. In two thirds of patients, the first episode occurs within 6 months of the erythema migrans lesion. Untreated, the episodes last approximately a week [13]. With time, these episodes become less frequent and severe and involve fewer joints. Even without treatment, the recurrent episodes usually resolve over a decade. The DRB1*0101 allele and the DRB1*0101-DQB1*0501 haplotype may be relevant to the development of infection with strains from the least invasive genotypes of B. burgdorferi and have a strong association with arthritis [25]. A small number of bacteria are liable to provoke severe arthritis by inducing mechanisms (including the induction of cytokines and chemokines) that amplify the inflammatory response. The cellular immune response against *B. burgdorferi* is characterised by a predominant T helper cell type 1 (Th1) pattern that appears to be inadequate to overcome the infection [26]. Because of good public education, the incidence of Lyme arthritis and other late-stage symptoms has not increased in tandem with the increases in early infection [27]. In most cases, Lyme arthritis may be cured by antibiotic therapy [26]. However, about 10% of Lyme arthritis patients do not respond sufficiently to antibiotic treatment. Two not mutually exclusive pathogenetic concepts of these treatment-resistant cases will be discussed in the present study: persistent infection and infection-induced immunopathology [26]. There have been major advances in the understanding of the pathogenesis of Lyme arthritis. The understanding of mechanisms of arthritis in Lyme borreliosis may also shed light on the mechanisms of disease in other infectious and noninfectious arthritides [27].

Neurological Manifestation

Neurological manifestations consist of chronic lymphocytic meningitis, cranial neuritis and radiculoneuritis associated to varying degrees [28].Lesions of the central nervous system, which occur long after the *B. burgdorferi* infection, are thought to represent a tertiary stage of Lyme disease [28]. Cranial nerve palsies is the most common neurologic manifestation, particularly in children. More than half of children with neurologic symptoms have a facial palsy, usually a bilateral type. The palsy lasts less than 8 weeks and can spontaneously resolve. Meningitis is also another important neurological manifestation. There seemed to be clinical benefit as well as a decrease of spinal fluid pleocytosis and spinal proteins [29]. Nervous system infection with Borrelia burgdorferi frequently causes meningitis and rarely causes encephalomyelitis. Altered cognitive function also can occur in the absence of central nervous system infection [30]. Recently developed serodiagnostic tools, such as the C6 assay, and appropriate use of Western blotting promise to improve diagnostic accuracy [30]. Intravenous high-dose antibiotic is the treatment of choice [29]. According to the observation of Skoldenberg, almost half of the patients were treated more than 4 weeks after the onset of symptoms and 15% of the patients had persisting or progressive symptoms between 4 and 11 months [29]. No significant symptoms of Herxheimer reaction were demonstrated [29]. There is an interesting neuroloigical manifestation namely Meningoradiculoneuritis (Bannwarth syndrome). This syndrome is characterized by severe radicular pain (due to neuritis), with a prominent nocturnal component [13]. Luckily, the meningitis may be relatively mild [13].

Cardiac Borreliosis

Lyme carditis is typically characterized by varying degrees of intermittent atrioventricular block occurring within weeks of infection with *B. burgdorferi* [31 - 32]. Myocarditis and/or pericarditis may occur [31]. This usually presents with fever and syncope due to AV block. Tachyarrhythmias, myopericarditis, mild cardiac muscle dysfunction are other common cardiac manifestations [33]. The level of AV block varies and fluctuates so that the symptoms may be intermittent. The block rarely lasts longer than a week; a temporary pacemaker rarely is required. Patients with atrioventricular block have good prognosis. Most cases resolve within 1 to 2 weeks [33]. Temporary, but almost never permanent, cardiac pacing may be required for some patients [33]. The diagnosis of Lyme carditis should be supported by the presence of concurrent erythema migrans, or by positive results of 2-step laboratory testing for antibodies to *B. burgdorferi* [31]. False positive results may occur, emphasizing the importance of clinical judgment in attributing specific manifestations to *B. burgdorferi* infection [31]. Carditis generally resolves spontaneously, but antimicrobial therapy can shorten symptom duration and prevent potential cardiac and non-cardiac sequelae

[31]. Cardiac manifestations generally resolve spontaneously, but antimicrobial therapy can shorten symptom duration and prevent potential cardiac and non-cardiac sequelae [31]. Cardiac manifestations of Lyme disease are treatable with antibiotics [33]. The prognosis for Lyme carditis is excellent [31].

Malaise and Fatigue

These are the most common findings after the skin lesion in early infection. Symptoms consistent with fibromyalgia/chronic fatigue syndrome develop even after adequate treatment. Treib et al said that it was worth examining whether an antibiotic therapy should be considered in patients with chronic fatigue syndrome and positive Borrelia serology [34]. Fatigued patients did show a surprisingly high rate of unexplained minor CSF abnormalities suggestive of CNS or meningeal dysfunction [35].

Ocular Borreliosis

Conjunctivitis and episcleritis are the most frequent manifestations of the early stage [36]. Neuro-ophthalmic disorders and uveitis occur in the second stage whereas keratitis, chronic intraocular inflammation and orbital myositis have been reported in the third stage of borreliosis [36]. Topical corticosteroids can be used for anterior segment inflammation [37]. An antibiotic therapeutic trial can be used for posterior segment or neuroophthalmic disease [37]. Systemic corticosteroids without concomitant antibiotics should not be used in the treatment of ocular Lyme disease [37]. If ocular Lyme disease is discovered and treated early, response to therapy usually is satisfactory [37].

C. Diagnosis of Lyme Disease

Serological test is the widely used method for diagnosis of Lyme disease. ELISA technique is the most widely used test [38]. Most laboratories use an assay based on purified flagella antigen [38]. The two-tier approach with Western Blot as confirmatory testing is not recommended since the contribution to the diagnostic specificity is only marginal [38]. If a tick bite is followed within three weeks by flue-like or neurological symptoms, or joint swelling in the vicinity of the bite, a serological investigation work-up should be carried out [39]. In the early stage, however, borrelia-specific antibodies can be detected in only 30-80% of the patients. However, during the further course of the illness, the specific IgM and IgG antibody titers almost always increase [39]. Considerable improvement has been achieved in detection of *B. burgdorferi* by culture, particularly of blood specimens during early stages of disease. A screening assay is recommended as the first step. When the ELISA is reactive, it is followed by immunoblot (IgM, IgG) [40]. The reactive diagnostic bands should be clearly identified; this is easy if recombinant antigens are used. Identification of diagnostic bands is difficult in the conventional blot and should be done by monoclonal antibodies [40]. Progress has been made in the sensitivity of the recombinant blot using additional antigens as p58 and homologues of Osp17 [40]. In neuroborreliosis the determination of the CSF/serum index is indicated (investigation of paired serum and CSF from the same day) [40]. Culturing plasma and increasing the volume of material cultured have accomplished this [41]. Further improvements might be obtained if molecular methods are used for detection of growth in culture and if culture methods are automated [41]. Unfortunately, culture is insensitive in extracutaneous manifestations of Lyme disease [41]. New developments in the diagnosis of Lyme disease are the development of PCR tests [42]. PCR and culture have high sensitivity on skin samples of patients with erythema migrans whose diagnosis is based mostly on clinical recognition of the lesion [41]. PCR on material obtained from extracutaneous sites is in general of low sensitivity, with the exception of synovial fluid [41]. PCR on synovial fluid usually shows a high in patients with untreated or partially treated Lyme arthritis, therefore, PCR might be a helpful confirmatory test in these patients [41]. Currently, the best use of PCR is for confirmation of the clinical diagnosis of suspected Lyme arthritis in patients who are IgG immunoblot positive [41].

D. Treatment of Lyme Disease

Prompt antimicrobial therapy using oral agents such as doxycycline or amoxicillin is successful among more than 90% of patients [43]. Treatment with antibiotics is reasonable in all stages of Lyme borreliosis and for all clinical manifestations; however, it has been most effective early in the course of the illness [44]. The choice of antibiotic depends upon many factors including the efficacy, pharmacokinetic profile, side effects, expected compliance and price. For the majority of manifestations the most effective antibiotic, the optimal dosage, and the most appropriate duration of treatment have not been exactly determined [44]. Inadequate penetration of oral agents into the CNS may result in the development of overt neuroborreliosis [43]. Therapy with penicillin or tetracycline hastens the resolution of stage I symptoms [45]. Treatment duration normally ranges between 10 days and three weeks [45]. Tetracycline or doxycycline appears to be more effective than penicillin in preventing the development of late Lyme disease [45]. Although intravenous penicillin G and ceftriaxone are both effective for the treatment of late Lyme disease, many clinicians consider ceftriaxone to be the agent of choice [45]. The parenteral agent ceftriaxone is the drug of choice for severe acute and chronic infections, due to good penetration into CSF, convenient single daily dosage regimen and proven high efficacy in clinical trials involving a wide variety of disseminated infections [43]. Regardless of therapeutic agent, there appears to a small minority of patients who do not respond; such cases may be due to long-term persistence of borrelial cysts and to misdiagnoses based solely on seropositivity [43]. Several adjunct therapies are available, including hyperbaric oxygen therapy and immune system supplements, but clinical trials have yet to be conducted [43]. Whether exposed patients from endemic areas should receive antimicrobial prophylaxis is controversial [45]. Further clinical studies are needed to determine optimal therapy for the various stages of Lyme disease, particularly Lyme arthritis [45].

Relapsing Fever

Relapsing fever is a rapidly progressive and severe septic disease caused by certain *Borrelia* spirochetes. The disease is divided into two forms, i.e., epidemic relapsing fever, caused by *B. recurrentis* and transmitted by lice, and the endemic form, caused by several *Borrelia* species, such as *B. duttonii*, and transmitted by soft-bodied ticks [46]. The spirochetes enter the bloodstream by the vector bite and live persistently in plasma even after the development of specific antibodies [46]. This leads to fever relapses and high mortality and clearly indicates that the *Borrelia* organisms utilize effective immune evasion strategies [46].

A. Pathogenesis

The vector of this disease is the infected human body louse (*Pediculus humanus humanus*). Lice become infected by feeding on a spirochetemic patient. The ingested spirochetes enter the gut and cross the epithelium into the hemolymph. Transmission to humans occurs by contamination of abraded skin with hemolymph from a crushed infected louse. This tick borne disease is an old disease with a long history [2]. Relapsing fever Borrelia infections have attracted little attention in recent years; however, where endemic, these infections still result in considerable illness and death [2]. Despite the marked antimicrobial drug susceptibility of these organisms, therapy is often delayed through lack of clinical suspicion. With increasing travel, infections may be imported, through exotic relapsing fever infection or through resurgence of infected disease vectors [2]. Although louseborne relapsing fever is now geographically limited, it was once of global importance [2]. Relapsing fever is transmitted to humans by 2 vectors, ticks and lice. The human body louse, *Pediculus humanus*, is the specific vector (*Pediculus pubis* is not a vector) [47]. Louse-borne relapsing fever is more severe than the tick-borne variety. Soft ticks of the genus *Ornithodoros* spread the tick-borne variety [47]. The responsible *Borrelia* species are identified closely with its tick vector. *Borrelia parkeri* infects *Ornithodoros parkeri*; *Borrelia hermsii* is the agent transmitted by tick bite by *Ornithodoros hermsii* [47]. Soft ticks feed for short periods of time, and the *Borrelia* organisms are inoculated within minutes [47]. This is an important distinction from other tick-borne diseases such as Lyme disease [47]. The pathogenic organisms usually invade the endothelium and this can produce a low-grade disseminated intravascular coagulation and thrombocytopenia [47]. Giyard et al said that bhpA encodes a unique and functional serine protease in relapsing fever spirochaetes [48]. This periplasmic enzyme may prevent the accumulation of proteins damaged by the innate immune response and contribute to the ability of the relapsing fever spirochaetes to achieve high cell densities in blood [48]. Production of a serine protease provides resistance to oxidative stress and killing by neutrophils [48].

The direct, complement-independent, bactericidal activity of antibodies is a critical mechanism of host defense against infection [49]. Alugupalli et al said that B1b cells generated the T-independent IgM required for the control and resolution of relapsing fever borreliosis [50]. Connolly et al said that IgM is bactericidal in the absence of complement and is part of the polyclonal Ab response that mediates the clearance of this bacterium from the blood [51]. They found that purified monoclonal IgM caused direct structural damage to the outer membrane of the spirochete, in the absence of complement [51]. They concluded that the direct, complement-independent, bactericidal activity of antibodies was a critical mechanism of host defense against infection [51]. The relapse phenomenon occurs because of genetically programmed shifting of outer surface proteins of the *Borrelia* that allows a new clone to avoid destruction by antibodies directed against the majority of the original infecting organisms [47]. Thus, the person clinically improves until the new clone multiplies sufficiently to cause another relapse [47].

B. Clinical Manifestation

The disease usually develops within 3-18 days after exposure to the spirochete. As with all the tick-borne diseases, the season of onset and epidemiologic history suggesting possible tick exposure are important clues [47]. *Ornithodoros* ticks often frequent caves and decaying woodpiles [47]. A classical flu-like symptom is the most common presentation of relapsing fever. Fever, headache, myalgia, arthralgia, weakness and anorexia can be seen in acute infection. Basically, the first acute febrile infection lasts for 3 – 7 days. Sometimes, fatal shock can be seen. The relapse usually occurs within 1 – 2 weeks after the first febrile infection. However, subsequent relapses tend to be less severe.

Tick-Borne Relapsing Fever

Tick-borne relapsing fever is characterized by recurring fevers separated by afebrile periods and is accompanied by nonspecific constitutional symptoms [52]. It occurs after a patient has been bitten by a tick infected with a Borrelia spirochete. The diagnosis of tick-borne relapsing fever requires an accurate characterization of the fever and a thorough medical, social, and travel history of the patient [52]. Most cases have been acquired from exposure to rustic tick-infested cabins and caves [53]. Findings on physical examination are variable; abdominal pain, vomiting, and altered sensorium are the most common symptoms [52]. Initial symptoms include sudden onset of fever, chills, headache, arthralgias, and myalgias [54]. Patients may suffer several febrile episodes or relapses unless they are diagnosed and treated promptly because the pathogenic spirochetes are able to alter their outer surface proteins and, thus, escape the infected host's immune response [54]. Laboratory confirmation of tick-borne relapsing fever is made by detection of spirochetes in thin or thick blood smears obtained during a febrile episode [52]. The diagnosis of this condition early in its course can save clinicians and patients the anxiety and cost of the work-up of a fever of unknown origin [55]. Le said that since vacationing in the national parks and forests has become increasingly popular among many American families, tick-borne relapsing fever should be considered in any patient with an acute or recurrent fever of unknown origin who exhibits nonspecific symptoms of an undifferentiated viral illness [55].

Louse-Borne Relapsing Fever

Louse-borne relapsing fever is characterized by recurring fevers, similar to tick-borne relapsing fever. However, the number of relapses of louse-borne is different from tick-borne fever. The number of relapses for louse-borne fever is usually fewer. According to a recent observation by Ramos et al [56], most the cases were children under 15 years of age. In this report [56], the adult cases were far more likely to present with headache, musculo-skeletal pains, dizziness and bleeding than the children. The overall level of case fatality was 6.4% and death appeared to be significantly associated with adulthood, delay in consultation and the presence of vomiting [56]. According to another study by Bognolo et al, the common clinical features of the disease were fever, headache, chills, abdominal pain, epistaxis, hepatomegaly, splenomegaly, petechial rash and jaundice [57]. Observed complications were pneumonia in 14% and central nervous system involvement in 10% [57].

C. Diagnosis of Relapsing Fever

The easiest method for diagnosis of relapsing fever is the detection of organism in the blood smear. Of interest, the spirochete can be determined in the peripheral blood smear during peak of fever. Visualizing spirochetes in smears of peripheral blood during a febrile episode is the clue for making a definitive diagnosis. Multiple smears (both thick and thin, using Wright and Giemsa stains) may need to be examined. Quantitative buffy coat (QBC) analysis can improve the diagnosis [58]. In vitro experiments showed that QBC analysis may be as much as 100-fold more sensitive than thick smear [58]. Diagnosis can be confirmed by intraperitoneal inoculation of blood specimens from patients into laboratory mice [58]. Presently, advanced molecular biology technique can be applied for diagnosis of relapsing fever. PCR test targeting the glycerophosphodiester phosphodiesterase (GlpQ) gene can be used to detect infection in the blood of suspected relapsing fever patients [59]. According to a recent study by Halperin et al, this method is highly effective [59].

D. Treatment of Relapsing Fever

Medical therapy is recommended for relapsing fever. Symptomatic treatment for fever such as antipyretic drug should be prescribed. To get rid of the pathogen, antimicrobial pathogen is required. A clinical trial was conducted in order to evaluate the efficacy of procaine penicillin and tetracycline, respectively, in the treatment of louse-borne relapsing fever. According to this work, relapses occurred most often in the group receiving the lowest dose of penicillin, and decreased with increasing dosage of penicillin; none of the patients treated with oral tetracycline had a relapse [60]. The duration of spirochetemia after treatment was much longer after antibiotic treatment [61]. However, following the antimicrobial treatment, patients may develop a Jarisch-Herxheimer reaction, which can be severe, especially in louse-borne relapsing fever when patients' host defenses may be otherwise compromised [47]. This reaction has been reported to occur in 50% of patients with relapsing fever [47]. The reaction produces apprehension, diaphoresis, fever, tachycardia, and tachypnea with an initial pressor response followed rapidly by hypotension. It should be noted that this reaction can be fatal [47]. As mortality is linked to severe Jarisch-Herxheimer-like reactions, and most relapses are clinically mild and easily treated, using low-dose penicillin to initiate the treatment of relapsing fever is more favorable [60].

References

[1] Roca B. Lyme borreliosis *Med. Clin. (Barc).* 2006;127:265-8.

[2] Cutler SJ. Possibilities for relapsing fever reemergence. *Emerg. Infect. Dis.* 2006;12:369-74.

[3] Gangaidzo IT. Forgotten diseases: relapsing fever. Cent Afr J Med. 2004;50:73-5.

[4] Borrelia burgdorferi. Available online at http://www.bacteriamuseum.org/species/borrelia.shtml

[5] Lyme disease. Available online at textbookofbacteriology.net/Lyme.html

[6] Borrelia burgdorferi. Available online at http://www.bact.wisc.edu/Microtextbook

[7] Stewart PE, Byram R, Grimm D, Tilly K, Rosa PA. The plasmids of Borrelia burgdorferi: essential genetic elements of a pathogen. *Plasmid.* 2005;53:1-13.

[8] Chaconas G. Hairpin telomeres and genome plasticity in Borrelia: all mixed up in the end. *Mol. Microbiol.* 2005;58:625-35.

[9] Rosa PA, Tilly K, Stewart PE. The burgeoning molecular genetics of the Lyme disease spirochaete. *Nat. Rev. Microbiol.* 2005;3:129-43.

[10] Borrelia. Available online at www.life.umd.edu/classroom/bsci424/PathogenDescriptions/Borrelia.htm

[11] Cutler SJ, Moss J, Fukunaga M, Wright DJ, Fekade D, Warrell D. Borrelia recurrentis characterization and comparison with relapsing-fever, Lyme-associated, and other Borrelia spp. *Int. J. Syst. Bacteriol.* 1997;47:958-68.

[12] Ras NM, Lascola B, Postic D, Cutler SJ, Rodhain F, Baranton G, Raoult D. Phylogenesis of relapsing fever Borrelia spp. *Int. J. Syst. Bacteriol.* 1996;46:859-65.

[13] Lyme disease. Available online at http://www.emedicine.com/med/topic1346.htm

[14] Sarwari AR, Strickland T, Pena C, Burkot TR. Tick exposure and Lyme disease at a summer camp in Maryland. *W. V. Med. J.* 2005;101:126-30.

[15] Madden SC, Madden RC. Seasonality in diurnal locomotory patterns of adult blacklegged ticks (Acari: Ixodidae). *J. Med. Entomol.* 2005;42:582-8.

[16] Miller JC, von Lackum K, Babb K, McAlister JD, Stevenson B. Temporal analysis of Borrelia burgdorferi Erp protein expression throughout the mammal-tick infectious cycle. *Infect. Immun.* 2003;71:6943-52.

[17] Guerau-de-Arellano M, Huber BT. Chemokines and Toll-like receptors in Lyme disease pathogenesis. *Trends Mol. Med.* 2005;11:114-20.

[18] Ramamoorthi N, Narasimhan S, Pal U, Bao F, Yang XF, Fish D, Anguita J, Norgard MV, Kantor FS, Anderson JF, Koski RA, Fikrig E. The Lyme disease agent exploits a tick protein to infect the mammalian host. *Nature.* 2005;436:573-7.

[19] Singh SK, Girschick HJ. Lyme borreliosis: from infection to autoimmunity. *Clin. Microbiol. Infect.* 2004 ;10:598-614.

[20] Bolz DD, Weis JJ. Molecular mimicry to Borrelia burgdorferi: pathway to autoimmunity? *Autoimmunity.* 2004;37:387-92.

[21] Sigal LH. Lyme disease: a review of aspects of its immunology and immunopathogenesis. *Annu. Rev. Immunol.* 1997;15:63-92.

[22] Cadavid D, Bai Y, Dail D, Hurd M, Narayan K, Hodzic E, Barthold SW, Pachner AR. Infection and inflammation in skeletal muscle from nonhuman primates infected with different genospecies of the Lyme disease spirochete Borrelia burgdorferi. *Infect. Immun.* 2003 ;71:7087-98.

[23] Mullegger RR. Dermatological manifestations of Lyme borreliosis. *Eur. J. Dermatol.* 2004;14:296-309.

[24] Hofmann H. Lyme borreliosis. Cutaneous manifestation. *Hautarzt.* 2005;56:783-95

[25] Wormser GP, Kaslow R, Tang J, Wade K, Liveris D, Schwartz I, Klempner M. Association between human leukocyte antigen class II alleles and genotype of Borrelia burgdorferi in patients with early lyme disease. *J. Infect. Dis.* 2005;192:2020-6.
[26] Franz JK, Priem S, Rittig MG, Burmester GR, Krause A. Studies on the pathogenesis and treatment of Lyme arthritis. *Wien. Klin. Wochenschr.* 1999;111:981-4.
[27] Hu L. Lyme arthritis. *Infect. Dis. Clin. North Am.* 2005;19:947-61.
[28] Masson C. Neurologic aspects of Lyme disease. *Presse Med.* 1987;16:72-5.
[29] Skoldenberg B, Stiernstedt G, Karlsson M, Wretlind B, Svenungsson B. Treatment of Lyme borreliosis with emphasis on neurological disease. *Ann. N. Y. Acad. Sci.* 1988;539:317-23.
[30] Halperin JJ. Central nervous system Lyme disease. *Curr. Neurol. Neurosci. Rep.* 2005;5:446-52.
[31] Haddad FA, Nadelman RB. Lyme disease and the heart. *Front Biosci.* 2003;8:s769-82.
[32] Bartunek P, Gorican K, Mrazek V, Nemec J, Zapletalova J, Varejka P, Sklenar T, Bina R, Rozmarova P, Veiser T. Cardiac abnormalities of lyme borreliosis. *Cas. Lek. Cesk.* 2005;144 Suppl 1:30-6.
[33] Gresik P, Oczko-Grzesik B, Kepa L. Cardiac manifestations of Lyme borreliosis. *Przegl. Epidemiol.* 2004;58:589-96.
[34] Treib J, Grauer MT, Haass A, Langenbach J, Holzer G, Woessner R. Chronic fatigue syndrome in patients with Lyme borreliosis. *Eur. Neurol.* 2000;43:107-9.
[35] Coyle PK, Krupp LB, Doscher C, Amin K. Borrelia burgdorferi reactivity in patients with severe persistent fatigue who are from a region in which Lyme disease is endemic. *Clin. Infect. Dis.* 1994;18 Suppl 1:S24-7.
[36] Zagorski Z, Biziorek B, Haszcz D. Ophthalmic manifestations in Lyme borreliosis. *Przegl. Epidemiol.* 2002;56 Suppl 1:85-90.
[37] Zaidman GW. The ocular manifestations of Lyme disease. *Int. Ophthalmol. Clin.* 1997;37:13-28.
[38] Dessau RB, Bangsborg JM, Jensen TP, Hansen K, Lebech AM, Andersen CO. Laboratory diagnosis of infection caused by Borrelia burgdorferi. *Ugeskr. Laeger.* 2006;168:2805-7.
[39] Hofmann H. Early diagnosis of Lyme borreliosis. *MMW Fortschr. Med.* 2006;148:32, 34, 36.
[40] Aguero-Rosenfeld ME, Wang G, Schwartz I, Wormser GP. Diagnosis of lyme borreliosis. *Clin. Microbiol. Rev.* 2005;18:484-509.
[41] Wilske B. Microbiological diagnosis in Lyme borreliosis. *Int. J. Med. Microbiol.* 2002;291 Suppl 33:114-9.
[42] van Dam AP. Recent advances in the diagnosis of Lyme disease. *Expert Rev. Mol. Diagn.* 2001;1:413-27.
[43] Taylor RS, Simpson IN. Review of treatment options for lyme borreliosis. *J. Chemother.* 2005;17 Suppl 2:3-16
[44] Strle F. Principles of the diagnosis and antibiotic treatment of Lyme borreliosis. *Wien Klin. Wochenschr.* 1999;111:911-5.
[45] Goodwin SD, Sproat TT, Russell WL. Management of Lyme disease. *Clin. Pharm.* 1990;9:192-205.

[46] Meri T,Cutler SJ, Blom AM, Meri S, Jokiranta T S. Relapsing fever spirochetes *Borrelia recurrentis* and *B. duttonii* acquire complement regulators C4b-binding protein and factor H. *Infect. Immun.* 2006; 74: 4157–4163.
[47] Relapsing fever. Available online at http://www.emedicine.com/emerg/topic590.htm
[48] Guyard C, Battisti JM, Raffel SJ, Schrumpf ME, Whitney AR, Krum JG, Porcella SF, Rosa PA, DeLeo FR, Schwan TG. Relapsing fever spirochaetes produce a serine protease that provides resistance to oxidative stress and killing by neutrophils. *Mol. Microbiol.* 2006;60:710-22.
[49] Connolly SE, Thanassi DG, Benach JL. Generation of a complement-independent bactericidal IgM against a relapsing fever Borrelia. *J. Immunol.* 2004;172:1191-7.
[50] Alugupalli KR, Gerstein RM, Chen J, Szomolanyi-Tsuda E, Woodland RT, Leong JM. The resolution of relapsing fever borreliosis requires IgM and is concurrent with expansion of B1b lymphocytes. *J. Immunol.* 2003;170:3819-27.
[51] Connolly SE, Thanassi DG, Benach JL. Generation of a complement-independent bactericidal IgM against a relapsing fever Borrelia. *J. Immunol.* 2004;172:1191-7.
[52] Roscoe C, Epperly T. Tick-borne relapsing fever. *Am. Fam. Physician.* 2005;72:2039-44
[53] Dworkin MS, Schwan TG, Anderson DE Jr. Tick-borne relapsing fever in North America. *Med. Clin. North Am.* 2002;86:417-33, viii-ix.
[54] Rawlings JA. An overview of tick-borne relapsing fever with emphasis on outbreaks in Texas. *Tex. Med.* 1995;91:56-9.
[55] Le CT. Tick-borne relapsing fever in children. *Pediatrics.* 1980;66:963-6.
[56] Ramos JM, Malmierca E, Reyes F, Wolde W, Galata A, Tesfamariam A, Gorgolas M. Characteristics of louse-borne relapsing fever in Ethiopian children and adults. *Ann. Trop. Med. Parasitol.* 2004;98:191-6.
[57] Borgnolo G, Denku B, Chiabrera F, Hailu B. Louse-borne relapsing fever in Ethiopian children: a clinical study. *Ann. Trop. Paediatr.* 1993;13:165-71.
[58] van Dam AP, van Gool T, Wetsteyn JC, Dankert J. Tick-borne relapsing fever imported from West Africa: diagnosis by quantitative buffy coat analysis and in vitro culture of Borrelia crocidurae. *J. Clin. Microbiol.* 1999;37:2027-30.
[59] Halperin T, Orr N, Cohen R, Hasin T, Davidovitch N, Klement E, Kayouf R, Baneth G, Cohen D, Yavzori M. Detection of relapsing fever in human blood samples from Israel using PCR targeting the glycerophosphodiester phosphodiesterase (GlpQ) gene. *Acta Trop.* 2006;98:189-95.
[60] Seboxa T, Rahlenbeck SI. Treatment of louse-borne relapsing fever with low dose penicillin or tetracycline: a clinical trial. *Scand. J. Infect. Dis.* 1995;27:29-31.
[61] Perine PL, Teklu B. Antibiotic treatment of louse-borne relapsing fever in Ethiopia: a report of 377 cases. *Am. J. Trop. Med. Hyg.* 1983;32:1096-100.

Chapter XV

Schistosomiasis

Introduction

Schistosomiasis, also known as bilharzia, is a parasitic disease that leads to chronic ill health. It is the major health risk in the rural areas of Central China and Egypt and continues to rank high in other developing countries [1]. Schistosomiasis has been recognized since the time of the Egyptian pharaohs. The worms responsible for the disease were eventually discovered in 1851 by Theodor Bilharz, a young German pathologist, from whom the disease took its original name, Bilharziasis [1]. The disease is indicated either by the presence of blood in the urine or, in the case of intestinal schistosomiasis, by initially atypical symptoms which can lead to serious complications involving the liver and spleen [1].

The main forms of human schistosomiasis are caused by five species of the flatworm, or blood flukes, known as schistosomes: *Schistosoma mansoni, Schistosoma japonicum, Schistosoma mekongi, Schistosoma intercalatum* and *Schistosoma haematobium*. The last species, *Schistosoma haematobium*, causes urinary schistosomiasis and affects millions of people in the developing countries, especially in the Africa Continent [1 – 2]. Schistosomiasis of the urinary bladder and the large intestine may cause severe diseases of the urinary tract or the liver. However, all species cannot be seen in peripheral blood smear examination. Precise data on epidemiology, morbidity, post-treatment resolution, reinfection, and resurgence of schistosomiasis could be helpful in establishing purposeful treatment plans for the disease in endemic populations [2]. Here, the author performed a literature review to summarize the clinical reports on urinary schistosomiasis from tropical Asian countries in Southeast and South Asia.

Urinary Schistosomiasis

1. Epidemiology

1.1. Southeast Asia

In Thailand, *S. japonicum* and *S. mekongi*, which cause intestinal schistosomiasis can be seen especially in the northeastern region. Concerning the urinary schistosomiasis, its prevalence is low. In this work, the author reviews all case reports of the urinary schistosomiasis in Thailand and only two literatures [3 – 4] can be detected. The first case is the worker who went back from working as miner in Africa and presented to the physician with the complaint of hematuria. He was treated as urinary tract infection but not improve. The confirmed diagnosis of this case was from both urine sediment and histological finding. The second case is the foreigner who went to the physician at the private hospital with the complaint of prolonged intermittent hematuria and abnormal calcification was presented in the radiography. The confirmed diagnosis of this case was from histological finding. Conclusively, the common characteristics of the two cases are a) past history of living in the endemic area, Africa, b) male subject, c) presentation as hematuria, d) middle aged (30 - 40 years old) and e) confirmed diagnosis by histological finding. Pantongrag-Brown *et al* [4] proposed that although urinary schistosomiasis never occurs in local Thai population, knowledge of the disease is still important in the present day when international traveling is quite common. Concerning the other Indochina countries, Laos, Cambodia, Vietnam and Myanmar, these countries are limited for resource and clinical reports from these countries are usually unavailable. Although there are some reports on the survey on *S. japonicum*-like [5 – 6]. In this area, there is no report on urinary schistosomiasis.

Table 1. Case reports of urinary schistosomiasis among the Thais

Author	year	Sex	Age (year)	nationality	presentation	diagnosis
Ariyaprakai and Chalermsanyakorn [3]	1986	Male	37	Thai	Hematuria for 4 month, Eosinophilia	Histological study from transurethral endoscopy, 24 hour urine examination
Pantongrag-Brown et al [4]	1997	Male	31	Mali	Hematuria on and off for 3 years, nocturia	Radiological findings, Histological study from transurethral endoscopy

In Malaysia, there is only one previous case report of urinary schistosomiasis. In 1992, Hung and Shekar reported an imported case of S. haematobium infection presenting with hematuria and proteinuria [7]. The patient failed to respond to multiple antibiotic treatment and was successfully treated with praziquantel [7]. Indeed, Greer *et al* proposed that that even among a stable population at risk of Malaysian schistosomiasis the prevalence was low [8]. They also mentioned that *S. malayensis* , a zoonotic infection in man, was unlikely to become a significant public health problem [8]. In Singapore, there is no report of urinary schistosomiasis. There was only one case report of an 83 year-old female with Schistosoma japonicum infection presenting with bloody diarrhoea [9]. Concerning Indonesia, Izhar *et al* said that schistosomiasis in Indonesia was limited to two very isolated areas, the Napu and Lindu valleys, in the province of Central Sulawesi [10]. The disease was initially found in 1937 in the village of Tomado [10]. However, to present, there is no case report of urinary schistosomiasis in Indonesia. Similarly, there was no report of urinary schistosomiasis from Brunei. In the Phillipines, the *S. japonicum* infection can be seen and documented as an important problem [11]. But there is no case report of urinary schistosomiasis.

Conclusively, Schistosomiasis in Southeast Asia, caused by *S. japonicum*, *S. mekongi* and *S. japonicum*-like, have been reported from different countries [12], however, the clinical report on urinary schistosomiasis is very rare. The control measures of schistosomiasis had been implemented in the Philippines and Indonesia [12]. Concerning the parasite, although some Schistostoma species can be detected in Southeast Asia with considerable infective rate, the specific species, which causes urinary schistosomiasis has never been detected. However, since the *Schistostoma* spp might share the common snail intermediate host, therefore, there is a possibility in transferring of *S. haematobium* parasite. Nevertheless, the Southeast Asia has the same climate, tropical, as the known endemic area of this parasite therefore the possibility can be strengthened. In addition, at present there are a lot of Southeast Asian workers who migrate to the endemic area for work and the workers who go aboard and return might get infected [13].

1.2. South Asia

Concerning the tropical South Asia, urinary schistosomiasis is sporadically reported. Amonkar *et al* said that this disease was a much less common occurrence though not unknown in India [14]. They also reported a case of schistosoma induced squamous carcinoma of the bladder which was not a common association in India [14]. There are some surveys on the intermediate host of the pathogen [15] and there are also some reports on the development of diagnostic tool for urinary schistosomiasis [16]. Recently Brown reported a test on Enzyme-linked immunosorbent assay (ELISA) in Gimvi village, India, using antigens derived from S. haematobium and S. mansoni adult worms [16]. Brown noted that the patients excreting schistosome ova in urine elicited positive ELISA titres, whereas patients who were previously positive but are no longer passing viable eggs were negative for ELISA [16]. In Pakistan, the urinary schistosomiasis is also sporadic. Recently, Khalid and Mahmood noted that schistosomiasis should be included as a viable differential for hematuria in travelers in Pakistan [17]. In Sri Lanka, the prevalence of urinary schistosomiasis is lower than the previously mentioned countries. The imported case is also reported [18].

Conclusively, there are sporadic case reports of urianry schistosomiasis in South Asia. The prevalence on this disease in South area is actually higher than Southeast Asia. One explanation is due to the geography. The South Asia is nearer to the Middle East, the endemic area in non- tropical Asia, than the Southeast Asia. It can be seen that the prevalence of urinary schistosomiasis in decreased in the eastern part of the South Asia, next to Southeast Asia, especially in Bangaladesh.

1.3. Africa

As previously mentioned, Africa is the highly endemic area for urinary schistosomiasis. For example, Egypt is the country with highly endemicity of this infection. Several surveillance and program for this disease have been continuously launched within this country [19]. Assessing prevalence of hematuria by interview is commonly used as a rapid method to identify communities for mass treatment of *S. haematobium* infection [20]. van der Werf said that there was a strong positive association between prevalence of hematuria and infection, but no effect of recall period length [20]. This suggests that the choice of recall period is of minor importance in control programs or studies based on reported hematuria [20].

2. Life Cycle of Pathogen [21]

The adult *S. haematobium* lives in the venous plexus within the pelvic area and passes the eggs, penetrating into bladder cavity via urinary bladder wall. The urinated eggs contain miracidia which can hatch outside when pass into the water. The hatching miracidia will penetrate the snail intermediate host and further develop into mother sporocyst, daughter sporocyst and cercaria, chronologically (about 4 – 8 weeks). *Biomphalaria pfeifferi* is the most common the most prevalent first intermediate host species [22]. Cercaria is an infective stage and will go out of the snail into the water. The cercaria will penetrate into the skin of animals or humans during swimming or bathing. The cercaria will further penetrate into the venous vessel within 1 – 2 days then pass to the circulation and finally reach the pelvic venous plexus. Activities that require behaviour and attitude modification have been identified and encouraged as components in the control of schistosome-attributable morbidity (in the absence of pipe-borne water) [23].

3. Pathophysiology

It has been suggested that immunologic factors, rather than transmission factors, may play a particularly important role in the regulation of schistosome populations [24]. Support for this view comes from several studies of the epidemiology of *S. haematobium* infection, although evidence is accumulating from both field and laboratory studies that immunity in schistosomiasis need not be a concomitant immunity [24]. Correlations between immunologic parameters such as peripheral blood eosinophil counts and specific anti-worm immunoglobulin E (IgE) antibody levels, and apparent resistance to reinfection following chemotherapy have been reported and used as evidence in favor of the existence of an acquired immunity [24]. However, Hagan et al noted that antibody-dependent, complement-independent killing of schistosomula of *S. haematobium* by eosinophils was barely detectable and did not differ between reinfected and non reinfected groups [25]. These observations suggest that subjects with elevated counts are less susceptible to reinfection but the mechanisms involved are not apparent [25].

The infection does not cause as problem as its chronic complication, carcinoma of urinary bladder. *S. haematobium* infection is strongly associated with urinary bladder cancer. Although numerous explanations have been proposed for this association, the nature of this relationship remains unresolved [26]. A dysregulation of cell proliferation is occurring during cystitis in these patients, however, the extent to which this alteration affects the level of chromosomal breakage is yet to be determined [26 - 27].

4. Clinical Manifestation and Laboratory Diagnosis

Significant symptoms for this infection are visible hematuria, dysuria, suprapubic pain and strangury [28]. The sensitivity and specificity of these symptoms were too low for them to be recommended as distinct clinical diagnostic criteria [28]. Okoli et al found that about 50 % of the patients infected with *S. haematobium* had visible hematuria, followed by suprapubic pains (24.3%) and painful micturition (11.0%) [29]. They also found that although 10. 5% of the sampled subjects with eggs of *S. haematobium* showed no visible hematuria, 14.6% clearly demonstrated hematuria [29]. In their study, prevalence was higher in males than in females and in subjects 11-20 years of age, while prevalence varied among different occupational groups, with farmers ranking the highest [29]. Correlation between the degree of hematuria and the intensity of infection and between intensity of infection with age and/or gender could partly explain these variations [30]. Severe infection can cause obstruction of urinary tract. Obstructed urine flow results in hydroureter and hydronephrosis [21, 31].

For laboratory diagnosis, urinalysis becomes the simplest tool. The presence of characteristic eggs in the urinary sediment is the usual means of diagnosing a *S. haematobium* infection [32]. *S. haematobium* egg is an elongated oval shape egg with a thinner shell and a prominent long spine. Hassan et al performed another interesting comparative study to evaluate urinalysis reagent strips versus microscopical examination [33]. According to their report, the specificity of strips and microscopical examination in detection of hematuria was 100%, while that for proteinuria was 97% as detected by strips [33]. These results show that urinalysis strips cannot be used as an alternative to microscopic examination of urine for the presence of *S. haematobium* eggs [33]. Additionally, the small and less commonly encountered miracidium stage of S. haematobium may also be present in the urine, which is another means of diagnosing urinary tract schistosomiasis [32]. For diagnosis, the best fitted model was able to provide estimates of sensitivity for each age/gender stratum as a function of the intensity of infection, which could not be done by using the two-by-two table approach [30]. A decrease in sensitivity adjusted for intensity of infection above 10 years of age among males is discussed [30]. For pathology examination, among the general histopathological changes, an active chronic infection with a chiefly granulomatous reaction is noted [34]. Calcification, pseudotumorous polypoid formations, ulcerations, obliterating fibrous lesions, epithelial transformations such as hyperplasia, metaplasia and dysplasia follow later [34]. These changes are followed at the various sites by diverse clinical and morphological complications-posthaemorrhagic anaemia, adhesions, serious obstructions of urogenital openings and its consequences and, finally, an increased risk of pavement-cell carcinoma of the bladder [34].

5. Treatment and Prevention

The standard treatment of acute schistosomiasis with praziquantel is ineffective and can aggravate clinical outcome during this phase [35]. Randomized trials have shown, however, that older, cheaper agents may be more cost-effective in controlling *S. haematobium* in some endemic areas [36]. Since schistosomiasis continues to rank, following malaria, at the second position of the world's parasitic diseases in terms of the extent of endemic areas and the number of infected people, therefore, prevention and control for this infection is necessary

[37]. For disease control, the elimination of snail vectors by applications of chemicals succeeds when the entire infested foci are isolated [38]. The development of a vaccine against schistosomiasis is necessary in order to reduce the risk of reinfection after drug treatment [39]. Recent reports converge on a message strongly supporting the existence of naturally acquired human immunity to this infection and reinforcing the hypothesis that at least partial protection can be achieved by artificial means [39]. Interestingly, although all of the vaccine molecules characterized are situated in the tegument, their exposure on the parasite surface, in most instances, is transient and/or non-essential [40]. The properties of four of these immunogens, glutathione-S-transferase (P26,28), paramyosin (Sm97), GP38, and GP18 are widely discussed [40]. Despite the identification and recombinant synthesis of several promising protective antigens, vaccination of humans against schistosomiasis remains in the realm of fantasy [40].

Intestinal Schistosomiasis

1. Epidemiology

The intestinal schistosomiasis can be seen worldwide. *S. japonicum* is more common in Far East and Southeast Asia while *S. Mansoni* and S. *intercalatum* are more common in Africa. For *S. mekongi*, it is a new discovered species with high endemicity in the area called "emerald triangle" of Indochina between Thai, Laos and Cambodia. Globally, schistosomes infect 1 in 30 people. A few countries have eradicated the disease, and many more are working towards it [41]. The human measurements most widely used in schistosomiasis epidemiology are based on the prevalence of active infections in the community [42]. Prevalence classifies subjects as positive or negative for the presence of eggs, and is recorded as the proportion or percentage positive [42]. In practice, the easiest measurements to obtain and the most widely used are the qualitative indicators (prevalence, cure rate and annual incidence) but they are relatively insensitive and reveal only gross changes [42]. The most informative is annual incidence although it may be hard to obtain in high prevalence areas where uninfected subjects may confined to atypical age groups such as very young children [42]. The WHO is promoting efforts working towards this goal. In some cases, urbanization, pollution, and/or consequent destruction of snail habitat has reduced exposure, with a subsequent decrease in new infections [41]. Physicians around the world need to remain aware of this common parasitic infection.

2. Life Cycle of Pathogen

Similar life cycle to that of *S. haematobium* can be seen. However, the main different are the site of infection. For *S. mansoni*, the infection site is at the inferior mesenteric venous system. For *S. japonicum*, the infection site is at the superior mesenteric, inferior mesenteric and rectal venous systems. Since the sites of infection for Schistosoma species causing intestinal schistosomiasis is near the intestine, penetrating into the intestinal lumen via intestinal wall can be seen in the life cycle. Another difference among the species causing intestinal schistosomiasis is the difference of intermediate hosts.

Table 2. Intermediate hosts for different species of Schistosoma

Species	Intermediate hosts
S. mansoni	*Biomphalaria glabrata*
S. japonicum	*Oncomelania nosophora*
S. mekongi	*Neotricula aperta*
S. intercalatum	*Biomphalaria crystallinus*

3. Pathophysiology

For *S. mansoni*, there are several animal models on its pathogenesis. In a study, electroblotted sera from *S. mansoni*-infected and control uninfected mice displayed different antigenic profiles when probed with the cross-reactive anti-human fibrinogen antibodies, suggesting an alteration in mouse host fibrinogen metabolism as a result of the parasitic infection [43]. Doenhoff et al said that modulation of fibrinogen metabolism might be a factor in a recently discovered anti-atherogenic effect exerted by schistosomes [43]. De Jonge et al performed another study on the presence and effects on intestinal contractility of somatostatin (SOM) and its receptor, SSTR2A relating to motility-related dysfunctions [44]. They found that schistosomiasis influenced the distribution and expression levels of SOM and SSTR2A in the murine ileum, which might explain the changed motility pattern [44]. In addition, Silva et al proposed that increasing the E (max) of two vasoconstrictors, possibly by increasing membrane depolarisation through a more effective opening of Cl (Ca) channels, with calcium entering through L-type Ca (2+) channels corresponded for *S. mansoni* altered portal vein physiology [45].

For *S. japonicum*, there are also many animal model researches for its pathogenesis. Balemba et al found that neuronal nitric oxide synthase activity was increased during granulomatous inflammation in the colon and caecum of pigs infected with *S. japonicum*. The apparent alterations in the activities of enzymes responsible for the generation of nitric oxide showed possible alterations in the NO mediated non-adrenergic non-cholinergic reflexes in the enteric nervous tissue [46]. These alterations might contribute to impaired intestinal motility and absorption, and other pathophysiological conditions seen during *S. japonicum* infections [46].

4. Clinical Manifestation and Laboratory Diagnosis

The signs and symptoms of infection usually occur during three phases: penetrating of skin, egg formation within venous plexus and penetrating of the intestinal wall, and healing. For penetrating of skin, the skin signs and symptoms can be observed. Cercarial dermatitis is caused by the infestation of the skin by cercariae of nonhuman schistosomes whose commonest hosts are aquatic birds [47]. Human contamination can occur during swimming in fresh water infested with cercariae [47]. Its geographic distribution is worldwide and is increasingly described in France during the summer months [47]. Gui et al found that *S. japonicum* might escape from local tissue reactions in the skin, due to its rapid migration, might induce only poor lymphocyte proliferation [48]. As a possible consequence, *S. japonicum* may establish more efficiently than *S. mansoni* [48]. Concerning the clinical manifestation, a diffuse eruption composed of prurigenous maculopapules appears within the 24 hours following exposure. Regression is spontaneous within one day to three weeks [47, 49].

For egg formation within venous plexus and penetrating of the intestinal wall, several clinical manifestations are noted. Pathology usually results from parasite eggs that lodge in the intestines and liver [50]. Intestinal schistosomiasis is most often asymptomatic and presents with occult gastrointestinal bleeding [50]. Generally, the patient present with fever, rigor, watery diarrhoea and notes intermittent generalised giant urticarial wheals, which is known as acute schistosomiasis or Katayama fever. *Schistosoma* spp living in the portal vein and/or mesenteric vein of patients, producing numerous eggs can eventually induce multiple granulomas in the liver and the intestine [51]. Cuison et al proposed that the presence of *Schistosoma* spp in the portal vein is beneficial to the parasites, not only for receiving enriched nutrition from the blood of the portal vein, but also for inducing immunological tolerance in the hosts [51]. Sometimes, the eggs within the venous system could be blown and entrapped in other organs causing complications. Such complications are liver and neurological complications. The presence of eggs in the central nervous system (CNS) induces a cell-mediated periovular granulomatous reaction [52]. When eggs reach the CNS during the early stages of the infection or during evolution of the disease to its chronic forms, large necrotic-exudative granulomas are found [52].

For healing, fibrosis can be seen and can induce clinical symptoms. Hepatosplenic schistosomiasis develops insidiously because of cumulative fibrotic injury[53]. Stigmata of liver failure are absent unless comorbid viral or alcoholic hepatitis is present. Patients with end-stage hepatosplenic schistosomiasis die from variceal hemorrhage [53].

For laboratory diagnosis, intestinal schistosomiasis can be detected by microscopic examination. Microscopic identification of eggs in stool is the most practical method for diagnosis. The examination can be performed on a simple smear (1 to 2 mg of fecal material). Since eggs may be passed intermittently or in small amounts, their detection will be enhanced by repeated examinations and/or concentration procedures (such as the formalin-ethyl acetate technique) [50]. In addition, for field surveys and investigational purposes, the egg output can be quantified by using the Kato-Katz technique (20 to 50 mg of fecal material) or the Ritchie technique [50]. For the measurement of eggs in the feces of presenting patients the scientific unit used is epg or eggs per gram. Stool examination should be performed when infection with *S. mansoni* or *S. japonicum* is suspected [50, 53].

Table 3. Ova characteristics for different species of Schistosoma

Species	Ova characters
S. haematobium	Yellowish brown, 112 – 170 microns by 40 – 70 microns in diameter, with a colorless terminal spine
S. mansoni	Size and color are similar to that of *S. haematobium*, with lateral spine pointing toward the narrow pole
S. japonicum	More spheroidal, 70 – 100 microns by 50 – 60 microns in diameter, with a rudimendary spine as a small notch

Diagnosis of schistosomiasis is also confirmed by finding eggs in biopsy specimens [53]. Antischistosome antibodies may identify infected tourists returning from endemic areas [53]. However, the reliability of this test is still questionable [54]. Circulating schistosome antigens distinguish current from past infections [53]. Antigen levels are often significantly lower than those of antibodies, but, theoretically, are directly related to the number of worms present [42]. Continuously improving techniques now allow detection of very low antigen levels [42]. Levels tend to be more stable than egg counts but the relationship between egg counts and antigen levels is not always perfect [42]. Although antigen tests often confirm suspected light infections with sparse eggs, negative antigen tests still occur in subjects passing eggs [42]. However, the most accurate method for diagnosis at present is PCR base method, however, it is expensive and is not recommended for routine usage.

5. Treatment and Control

For cercarial dermatitis, treatment is symptomatic in the majority of patients. The optimal prevention, for bathers, is to swim in sufficiently deep water [47]. Concerning the other forms of clinical manifestation, specific chemotherapy is needed. Two safe, effective drugs, praziquantel and metrifonate, are now available for schistosomiasis and are included in the WHO Model List of Essential Drugs [53]. Praziquantel is the first schistosomicidal drug of choice. An initial single dose (40 mg/kg) of praziquantel [55]. Adding with prednisolone 40 mg once daily for 5 days is also recommended [55]. It is therefore safe and beneficial to give corticosteroid with chemotherapy in acute schistosomiasis (Katayama fever) [55]. It is effective against all forms of infection with few, and only transient, side effects. Tawfik et al found that the duration of infection prior to treatment is a determining factor in subsequent expression of immune reactivity [56]. In addition, Xiao et al found that the concentrations of praziquantel and periods of drug exposure causing gross tegumental damage to *Schistosoma* spp in vitro correlated with the peak serum levels and time course of unchanged praziquantel associated with reduction of worm burden in vivo [57]. Thus, stage-specific resistance of S. mansoni to praziquantel does occur in vitro and correlates better with the tegumental than the muscular action of the drug [57]. Most cases of hepatosplenic schistosomiasis resolve after effective treatment [50, 53]. Oxamniquine is used exclusively in Africa and South America. Even though re-infection may occur after treatment, the risk of developing severely diseased organs is diminished and even reversed in young children [53]. In most areas, a reduction in the overall number of cases is maintained for 18-24 months and in other areas for up to five years without further intervention [53]. Prophylactic propranolol may prevent hemorrhage in praziquantel-treated patients with high-grade varices. Sclerotherapy is also efficacious [50, 53]. When necessary, patients with hepatosplenic schistosomiasis tolerate decompressive surgery well [50, 53].

For prevention, Schistosomiasis control is a long-term commitment. While short-term objectives to reduce prevalence can be achieved (up to 75% within two years in many endemic areas), surveillance and maintenance must continue for 10-20 years [53]. Treatment and re-treatment strategies for schistosomiasis is recommended [58]. The simplest approach is mass chemotherapy with a curative dose of praziquantel. However, this is sometimes impossible in most endemic areas, if only because of the high cost of praziquantel, therefore, alternatives included targeted chemotherapy, treating only infected subjects after examining everyone in the community to diagnose those infected; selective, targeted chemotherapy, treating only those subjects with heavy infections; and selective, targeted chemotherapy, treating subjects in defined, high-risk groups, with mass treatment, can be used [42]. Approaches differ for controlling the various forms of schistosomiasis and must be adapted according to the epidemiology resources and culture of each country [53]. New techniques should also be applied for adding the success to the control program. Bayesian geostatistical analysis is a powerful and statistically robust tool for identifying high prevalence areas in a heterogeneous and imperfectly known environment [59].

REFERENCES

[1] Schistosomiasis. Available on *http://www-micro.msb.le.ac.uk/224/Schisto.html.*

[2] Bichler KH, Feil G, Zumbragel A, Eipper E, Dyballa S. Schistosomiasis: a critical review. *Curr. Opin. Urol.* 2001;11:97-101

[3] Ariyaprakai W, Chalermsanyakorn P. Urinary schistosomiasis in a Thai: a case report. *J. Med. Assoc. Thai.* 1986;69:33-6

[4] Pantongrag-Brown L, Prasopsanti K, Kojalern S. Radiographic findings in urinary tract schistosomiasis : a case report. *Chula. Med. J.* 1997; 41 : 745-751

[5] Duong TH, Barrabes A, Bacq Y, Fournon M, Combescot C. Schistosoma mekongi bilharziasis along the Mekong River and its affluents, the Mun and Tonle Sap Rivers. General review. *Med. Trop.* (Mars) 1987;47:321-8

[6] Allen AM, Taplin D, Legters LJ, Ferguson JA. Letter: Schistosomes in Vietnam. *Lancet.* 1974;1:1175-6

[7] Hung LC, Shekar KC. Schistosoma haematobium infection in Malaysia--a case report. *Med. J. Malaysia.* 1992;47:328-30

[8] Greer GJ, Dennis DT, Lai PF, Anuar H. Malaysian schistosomiasis: description of a population at risk. *J. Trop. Med. Hyg.* 1989 Jun;92:203-8

[9] Lam KN, Chew SK, Lim KH, Swaminathan I, Chew LS. Schistosomiasis in Singapore--a case report. *Ann. Acad. Med. Singapore.* 1991;20:394-5

[10] Izhar A, Sinaga RM, Sudomo M, Wardiyo ND. Recent situation of schistosomiasis in Indonesia. *Acta Trop.* 2002;82:283-8

[11] Blas BL, Rosales MI, Lipayon IL, Yasuraoka K, Matsuda H, Hayashi M. The schistosomiasis problem in the Philippines: a review. *Parasitol. Int.* 2004;53:127-34

[12] Harinasuta C. Epidemiology and control of schistosomiasis in Southeast Asia. *Southeast Asian J. Trop. Med. Public Health.* 1984;15:431-8

[13] Bergquist NR. Schistosomiasis: from risk assessment to control. *Trends Parasitol.* 2002l;18:309-14

[14] Amonkar P, Murali G, Krishnamurthy S. Schistosoma induced squamous cell carcinoma of the bladder. *Indian J. Pathol. Microbiol.* 2001;44:363-4

[15] Sathe BD, Pandit CH, Chanderkar NG, Badade DC, Sengupta SR, Renapurkar DM. Sero-diagnosis of schistosomiasis by ELISA test in an endemic area of Gimvi village, India. *J. Trop. Med. Hyg.* 1991;94:76-8

[16] Brown DS. A mistaken report of the occurrence in India of the freshwater snail Bulinus and its relation to transmission of Schistosoma. *Ann. Trop. Med. Parasitol.* 1997;91:225-7

[17] Khalid SE, Mahmood SM. Schistosomiasis--a viable differential for hematuria in travelers in Pakistan. *J. Pak. Med. Assoc.* 2001;51:325-7

[18] Wijesundera MS, Beligaswatte AM, Prematilleke MN, Seneviratne MP. Urinary schistosomiasis acquired in Mali, West Africa. I. Case report of Schistosoma haematobium infection in a Sri Lankan with a note on the parasitic life cycle and the risk of local transmission. *Ceylon Med. J.* 1986;31:181-7

[19] Abdel-Wahab MF, Esmat G, El-Boraey Y, Ramzy I, Medhat E, Strickland GT.The epidemiology of schistosomiasis in Egypt: methods, training, and quality control of clinical and ultrasound examinations. *Am. J. Trop. Med. Hyg.* 2000;62:17-20.

[20] van der Werf MJ, Borsboom GJ, de Vlas SJ. No effect of recall period length on prevalence of self-reported hematuria in Schistosoma haematobium-endemic areas. *Trans. R. Soc. Trop. Med. Hyg.* 2003;97:373-4.

[21] Paul JF, Verma S, Berry K. Urinary schistosomiasis. *Emerg. Med. J.* 2002;19:483-4.

[22] Bagalwa M, Baluku B. The distribution of freshwater molluscs the intermediate hosts of human schistosomas in Katan, south-Kivu. *Med. Trop. (Mars).* 1997;57:369-72.

[23] Useh MF, Ejezie GC. Modification of behaviour and attitude in the control of schistosomiasis. 1. Observations on water-contact patterns and perception of infection. *Ann. Trop. Med. Parasitol.* 1999;93:711-20.

[24] Hagan P. Immunity and morbidity in infection due to Schistosoma haematobium. *Am. J. Trop. Med. Hyg.* 1996;55:116-20.

[25] Hagan P, Wilkins HA, Blumenthal UJ, Hayes RJ, Greenwood BM. Eosinophilia and resistance to Schistosoma haematobium in man. *Parasite Immunol.* 1985;7:625-32.

[26] Rosin MP, Saad el Din Zaki S, Ward AJ, Anwar WA. Involvement of inflammatory reactions and elevated cell proliferation in the development of bladder cancer in schistosomiasis patients. *Mutat. Res.* 1994;305:283-92.

[27] Rosin MP, Anwar WA, Ward AJ. Inflammation, chromosomal instability, and cancer: the schistosomiasis model. *Cancer Res.* 1994;54(7 Suppl):1929s-1933s.

[28] Ekanem EE, Ejezie GC, Asindi AA, Antia-Obong OE. Urinary symptoms and blood pressure of children with Schistosoma haematobium infection in south-eastern Nigeria. *East Afr. Med. J.* 1995;72:486-9.

[29] Okoli CG, Iwuala MO. The prevalence, intensity and clinical signs of urinary schistosomiasis in Imo state, Nigeria. *J. Helminthol.* 2004;78:337-42.

[30] Etard JE. Modelling sensitivity, specificity and predictive values of hematuria testing using reagent sticks in the diagnosis of Schistosoma haematobium infection. *Bull. Soc. Pathol. Exot.* 2004;97:24-8.

[31] Neal PM. Schistosomiasis--an unusual cause of ureteral obstruction: a case history and perspective. *Clin. Med. Res.* 2004;2:216-27.

[32] Procop GW, Mendez JC, Schneider SK, Rosenblatt JE. Diagnostic value of a miracidium in urinary sediment. *Diagn. Cytopathol.* 1999;20:34-7.

[33] Hassan SI, Talaat M, el Attar GM. Evaluation of urinalysis reagent strips versus microscopical examination of urine for Schistosoma haematobium. *J. Egypt. Soc. Parasitol.* 1994;24:603-9.

[34] Zampachova V. Pathology of urogenital schistosomiasis. *Klin. Mikrobiol. Infekc. Lek.* 2006;12:138-42.

[35] Jaureguiberry S, Perez L, Paris L, Bricaire F, Danis M, Caumes E. Invasive schistosomiases. *Presse Med.* 2005;34:1641-5.

[36] King CH, Mahmoud AA. Drugs five years later: praziquantel. *Ann. Intern. Med.* 1989;110:290-6.

[37] Utzinger J, Xiao S, N'Goran EK, Bergquist R, Tanner M. The potential of artemether for the control of schistosomiasis. *Int. J. Parasitol.* 2001;31:1549-62.

[38] Saliternik Z. The specific methods of control and eradication of schistosomiasis in Israel. *Trop. Geogr. Med.* 1979;31:175-84.

[39] Bergquist R. Prospects of vaccination against schistosomiasis. *Scand. J. Infect. Dis. Suppl.* 1990;76:60-71.

[40] Sher A, James SL, Correa-Oliveira R, Hieny S, Pearce E. Schistosome vaccines: current progress and future prospects. *Parasitology.* 1989;98 Suppl:S61-8.

[41] Schistosomiasis. Available online at http://en.wikipedia.org/wiki/Schistosomiasis

[42] Sturrock RF. Harmonization of research and control in schistosomiasis. *Mem. Inst. Oswaldo Cruz.* 1992;87 Suppl 4:45-53.

[43] Doenhoff MJ, Stanley RG, Pryce D, Curtis RC, Parry H, Griffiths K, Jackson CL. Identification of a fibrinolytic enzyme in Schistosoma mansoni eggs and modulated blood fibrinogen metabolism in S. mansoni-infected mice. *Parasitology.* 2003;126:231-4.

[44] De Jonge F, Van Nassauw L, De Man JG, De Winter BY, Van Meir F, Depoortere I, Peeters TL, Pelckmans PA, Van Marck E, Timmermans JP. Effects of Schistosoma mansoni infection on somatostatin and somatostatin receptor 2A expression in mouse ileum. *Neurogastroenterol. Motil.* 200315:149-59.

[45] Silva CL, Lenzi HL, Silva VF, Paulo FO, Noel F. Cellular mechanisms involved in the increased contraction of portal veins from Schistosoma mansoni-infected mice. *Parasitol. Res.* 2003;89:16-22.

[46] Balemba OB, Mortensen K, Semuguruka WD, Hay-Schmidt A, Johansen MV, Dantzer V. Neuronal nitric oxide synthase activity is increased during granulomatous inflammation in the colon and caecum of pigs infected with Schistosoma japonicum. *Auton. Neurosci.* 2002;99:1-12.

[47] Bouree P, Caumes E. Cercarial dermatitis. *Presse Med.* 2004;33:490-3

[48] Gui M, Kusel JR, Shi YE, Ruppel A Schistosoma japonicum and S. mansoni: comparison of larval migration patterns in mice. *J. Helminthol.* 1995;69:19-25.

[49] Al-Karawi KS, Al-Amro Al-Akloby OM, Mugharbel RM. Ectopic cutaneous schistosomiasis. *Int. J. Dermatol.* 2004;43:550-1.

[50] Elliott DE. Schistosomiasis. Pathophysiology, diagnosis, and treatment. *Gastroenterol. Clin. North Am.* 1996;25:599-625.

[51] Cuison A, Tasaka K, Chuang CK, Minai M, Yoshikawa H, Nakajima Y. Schistosome eggs in the portal vein can induce tolerance. *Int. J. Parasitol.* 1995;25:993-8.

[52] Pittella JE. Neuroschistosomiasis. *Brain Pathol.* 1997;7:649-62.

[53] Schistosomiasis. Available online at http://www.who.int/mediacentre/factsheets/fs115/en/index.html

[54] Thors C, Holmblad P, Maleki M, Carlson J, Linder E. Schistosomiasis in Swedish travellers to sub-Saharan Africa: Can we rely on serology? *Scand. J. Infect. Dis.* 2006;38:794-9.

[55] Ong EL, Ellis ME. Acute schistosomiasis (Katayama fever): corticosteroid as adjunct therapy. *Scand. J. Infect. Dis.* 1989;21:473-4.

[56] Tawfik AF, Carter CE, Colley DG. Effects of anti-schistosomal chemotherapy on immune responses, protection and immunity. I. Changes in cellular and humoral responses. *Am. J. Trop. Med. Hyg.* 1986 ;35:100-9.

[57] Xiao SH, Catto BA, Webster LT Jr. Effects of praziquantel on different developmental stages of Schistosoma mansoni in vitro and in vivo. *J. Infect. Dis.* 1985;151:1130-7.

[58] Magnussen P. Treatment and re-treatment strategies for schistosomiasis control in different epidemiological settings: a review of 10 years' experiences. *Acta Trop.* 2003;86:243-54.

[59] Clements AC, Lwambo NJ, Blair L, Nyandindi U, Kaatano G, Kinung'hi S, Webster JP, Fenwick A, Brooker S. Bayesian spatial analysis and disease mapping: tools to enhance planning and implementation of a schistosomiasis control programme in Tanzania. *Trop. Med. Int. Health.* 2006;11:490-503.

INDEX

A

B

C

F

G

M

O

P

Q

R

S

T

U

V

W

Y

Z